W9-BSH-134

Routine Screenings

The key to maintaining health is heading off problems before they occur by going to your doctor for regular checkups and keeping to a schedule of health screenings. Keep in mind, though, that these recommendations aren't set in stone; your doctor should tailor a screening schedule to meet your needs.

For men and women:

- **Basic physical:** Every 3 years for healthy adults under age 40, every 2 years from 40 to 50, and every year after 50.
- **Electrocardiogram (ECG or EKG):** Every 3 years after age 30 if your doctor thinks that you're at risk for heart disease, or every 3 to 4 years after 50 if you're not at risk.
- **Colorectal cancer screening:** Experts generally recommend annual testing after age 50. Adults at risk of colon and rectal cancer, including people with a strong family or personal history of colon and rectal disease, should be screened earlier and more often.

For men:

- **Digital rectal examination (DRE):** Every year after age 40.
- **Prostate-specific antigen test:** Every year after age 50.
- **Testicular examination:** Annually by a professional, along with monthly self-examinations, starting in adulthood.

For women:

- **Gynecological exam:** Annually after age 18 and for women who are sexually active.
- **Mammogram:** Annually for women over age 50 and for women at risk of breast cancer. Women ages 40 to 49 should decide with their practitioners whether to have annual mammograms.

For children:

- **Metabolic screening:** Immediately after birth.
- **Routine visits:** Well-baby visits every 2 to 3 months in the first 2 years of life, with annual examinations each year after age 2.
- **Hemoglobin test:** At 9 months of age.
- **Lead test:** At 9 months of age.
- **Vision and hearing test:** At 3 years of age.

For seniors:

- **Polypharmacy:** *Polypharmacy* is what experts call the problem of the complicated mix of over-the-counter and prescription drugs that many older people take. As a preventive measure, sit down with your doctor regularly and go over the medications that you're taking.
- **Hearing and vision testing:** Unfortunately, hearing and sight often deteriorate with aging. Regular testing can help catch problems early.
- **Nutrition testing:** Because some older adults have trouble getting enough vitamins and minerals, your physician should monitor your nutrition.
- **Flu and pneumonia vaccination:** Older adults are more vulnerable to the flu and the complications it can cause. To prevent problems, the Centers for Disease Control and Prevention recommends an annual flu vaccine and an annual pneumonia vaccine for everyone over the age of 65.

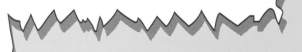

Using Common Home Remedies

You probably have the following common household products on hand, and they can be used to relieve everyday ailments.

- **Acetaminophen:** A painkiller and fever reducer for children and for people who are allergic to aspirin
- **Alcohol (rubbing):** A mild topical antiseptic or germ killer that cools and soothes certain cases of irritated skin
- **Ammonia:** Used as "smelling salts" for fainting and to neutralize insect bites
- **Baking soda:** When scantily applied, a soothing treatment for sunburn to reduce pain, itching, and inflammation
- **Benzalkonium chloride:** A detergent-type cleanser and disinfectant for treating wounds
- **Boric acid:** A weak germ and fungus killer used as a dusting powder
- **Calamine lotion:** Used to treat rashes, sunburns, and other minor heat burns that don't result in blisters
- **Egg white:** Used to soothe the stomach and retard the absorption of some poisons
- **Epsom salts:** A soothing treatment for wounds when dissolved in water; also used to make wet dressings for wounds
- **Flour:** When made into a thin paste, used to soothe the stomach and retard the absorption of some poisons
- **Hydrogen peroxide:** A germ killer when it comes into direct contact with bacteria
- **Milk:** Used to soothe the stomach and retard the absorption of some poisons
- **Milk of magnesia:** Used as a universal antidote for poisoning, in small doses as an antacid for stomach upset, and as a laxative
- **Petroleum jelly:** A skin softener and protective ointment used on wound dressings
- **Powdered (dry) mustard:** Used to induce vomiting in certain cases of poisoning
- **Salt (table salt):** Used to induce vomiting in certain cases of poisoning
- **Soap suds (not detergent):** Used as an antidote for poisoning by certain metal compounds
- **Starch:** When cooked and made into a thin paste, soothes the stomach and retards the absorption of some poisons
- **Vinegar:** Treats a number of problems, including jellyfish stings, sunburns, yeast infections, alkali burns, and swimmer's ear

Putting Together a Medical Record

You may assume that your doctor or hospital has all your pertinent medical information, but this is unfortunately not always the case. For each family member, make sure to record the following information:

- Conditions or diseases that run in the family
- Vital statistics: blood types, heights, weights, cholesterol levels, blood pressures, and immunization records
- Personal medical histories: medical problems and treatments
- Preventive screenings and results
- Known allergies, allergy symptoms, and treatments
- Hospital and laboratory records
- Gynecological and prenatal records for women
- Over-the-counter and prescription medications used
- Vision and hearing test results

Praise For Family Health For Dummies

"Once or twice in a century, the paths of medical science, common sense, and clarity intersect. *Family Health For Dummies* has captured all three. A lightning strike of useful and healthy information."
— Dr. Philip P. Gerbino, President, University of the Sciences in Philadelphia

"In my lectures as president of the UCLA Center on Aging, I often say, 'You can't turn the clock back — but you *can* rewind it!' That's what my friend Charles Inlander is all about in this practical guide to living *better,* longer."
— Art Linkletter, Author, Entertainer, TV Star, and President of the UCLA Center on Aging

"This book is priceless! It covers the ABCs of almost every family health question. Next to living in perfect health yourself comes the wonderful knowledge of what to do and *not* to do in any emergency. Read it before you need it!"
— Bonnie Prudden, Bonnie Prudden School and Pain Erasure Clinic

"Consumer power at its best! *Family Health For Dummies* opens the door to authentic, practical, and up-to-date health and medical information. This is an essential resource for family health."
— Dr. Lowell S. Levin, Professor Emeritus, Yale School of Public Health

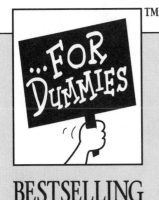

References for the Rest of Us! ™

BESTSELLING BOOK SERIES FROM IDG

Do you find that traditional reference books are overloaded with technical details and advice you'll never use? Do you postpone important life decisions because you just don't want to deal with them? Then our *...For Dummies®* business and general reference book series is for you.

...For Dummies business and general reference books are written for those frustrated and hard-working souls who know they aren't dumb, but find that the myriad of personal and business issues and the accompanying horror stories make them feel helpless. *...For Dummies* books use a lighthearted approach, a down-to-earth style, and even cartoons and humorous icons to diffuse fears and build confidence. Lighthearted but not lightweight, these books are perfect survival guides to solve your everyday personal and business problems.

> *"More than a publishing phenomenon, 'Dummies' is a sign of the times."*
>
> — The New York Times

> *"A world of detailed and authoritative information is packed into them..."*
>
> — U.S. News and World Report

> *"...you won't go wrong buying them."*
>
> — Walter Mossberg, Wall Street Journal, on IDG Books' *...For Dummies* books

Already, millions of satisfied readers agree. They have made *...For Dummies* the #1 introductory level computer book series and a best-selling business book series. They have written asking for more. So, if you're looking for the best and easiest way to learn about business and other general reference topics, look to *...For Dummies* to give you a helping hand.

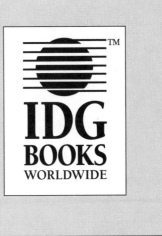

IDG BOOKS WORLDWIDE ™

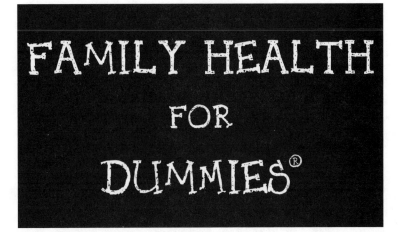

FAMILY HEALTH FOR DUMMIES®

by Charles B. Inlander, Karla Morales, & the People's Medical Society

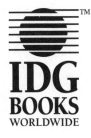

IDG Books Worldwide, Inc.
An International Data Group Company

Foster City, CA ♦ Chicago, IL ♦ Indianapolis, IN ♦ New York, NY

Family Health For Dummies®

Published by
IDG Books Worldwide, Inc.
An International Data Group Company
919 E. Hillsdale Blvd.
Suite 400
Foster City, CA 94404
www.idgbooks.com (IDG Books Worldwide Web site)
www.dummies.com (Dummies Press Web site)

Library of Congress Catalog Card No.: 98-89041

ISBN: 0-7645-5121-3

Printed in the United States of America

10 9 8 7 6 5 4 3 2 1

1O/RV/RS/ZY/IN

Distributed in the United States by IDG Books Worldwide, Inc.

Distributed by Macmillan Canada for Canada; by Transworld Publishers Limited in the United Kingdom; by IDG Norge Books for Norway; by IDG Sweden Books for Sweden; by Woodslane Pty. Ltd. for Australia; by Woodslane (NZ) Ltd. for New Zealand; by Addison Wesley Longman Singapore Pte Ltd. for Singapore, Malaysia, Thailand, and Indonesia; by Norma Comunicaciones S.A. for Colombia; by Intersoft for South Africa; by International Thomson Publishing for Germany, Austria and Switzerland; by Distribuidora Cuspide for Argentina; by Livraria Cultura for Brazil; by Ediciencia S.A. for Ecuador; by Ediciones ZETA S.C.R. Ltda. for Peru; by WS Computer Publishing Corporation, Inc., for the Philippines; by Contemporanea de Ediciones for Venezuela; by Express Computer Distributors for the Caribbean and West Indies; by Micronesia Media Distributor, Inc. for Micronesia; by Grupo Editorial Norma S.A. for Guatemala; by Chips Computadoras S.A. de C.V. for Mexico; by Editorial Norma de Panama S.A. for Panama; by Wouters Import for Belgium; by American Bookshops for Finland. Authorized Sales Agent: Anthony Rudkin Associates for the Middle East and North Africa.

For general information on IDG Books Worldwide's books in the U.S., please call our Consumer Customer Service department at 800-762-2974. For reseller information, including discounts and premium sales, please call our Reseller Customer Service department at 800-434-3422.

For information on where to purchase IDG Books Worldwide's books outside the U.S., please contact our International Sales department at 317-596-5530 or fax 317-596-5692.

For information on foreign language translations, please contact our Foreign & Subsidiary Rights department at 650-655-3021 or fax 650-655-3281.

For sales inquiries and special prices for bulk quantities, please contact our Sales department at 650-655-3200 or write to the address above.

For information on using IDG Books Worldwide's books in the classroom or for ordering examination copies, please contact our Educational Sales department at 800-434-2086 or fax 317-596-5499.

For press review copies, author interviews, or other publicity information, please contact our Public Relations department at 650-655-3000 or fax 650-655-3299.

For authorization to photocopy items for corporate, personal, or educational use, please contact Copyright Clearance Center, 222 Rosewood Drive, Danvers, MA 01923, or fax 978-750-4470.

is a trademark under exclusive license to IDG Books Worldwide, Inc., from International Data Group, Inc.

About the Authors

Charles B. Inlander, President of the People's Medical Society, is a highly acclaimed health commentator on public radio's *Marketplace.* He is a faculty lecturer at the Yale University School of Medicine and writes regularly for *Nursing Economics, The New York Times, Glamour,* and *Boardroom.*

Karla Morales, Vice President of Editorial Services and Communications for the People's Medical Society, has coauthored several best-selling books, including *Take This Book to the Obstetrician with You* and *Getting the Most for Your Medical Dollar.*

The People's Medical Society is the nation's largest nonprofit consumer health organization. Its mission is to provide consumers with up-to-date health information from health care professionals and the latest medical research. Its health care experts have published more than 70 health titles and are frequently seen on such television programs as *Oprah, Today,* and *Good Morning America.*

ABOUT IDG BOOKS WORLDWIDE

Welcome to the world of IDG Books Worldwide.

IDG Books Worldwide, Inc., is a subsidiary of International Data Group, the world's largest publisher of computer-related information and the leading global provider of information services on information technology. IDG was founded more than 30 years ago by Patrick J. McGovern and now employs more than 9,000 people worldwide. IDG publishes more than 290 computer publications in over 75 countries. More than 90 million people read one or more IDG publications each month.

Launched in 1990, IDG Books Worldwide is today the #1 publisher of best-selling computer books in the United States. We are proud to have received eight awards from the Computer Press Association in recognition of editorial excellence and three from Computer Currents' First Annual Readers' Choice Awards. Our best-selling ...For Dummies® series has more than 50 million copies in print with translations in 31 languages. IDG Books Worldwide, through a joint venture with IDG's Hi-Tech Beijing, became the first U.S. publisher to publish a computer book in the People's Republic of China. In record time, IDG Books Worldwide has become the first choice for millions of readers around the world who want to learn how to better manage their businesses.

Our mission is simple: Every one of our books is designed to bring extra value and skill-building instructions to the reader. Our books are written by experts who understand and care about our readers. The knowledge base of our editorial staff comes from years of experience in publishing, education, and journalism — experience we use to produce books to carry us into the new millennium. In short, we care about books, so we attract the best people. We devote special attention to details such as audience, interior design, use of icons, and illustrations. And because we use an efficient process of authoring, editing, and desktop publishing our books electronically, we can spend more time ensuring superior content and less time on the technicalities of making books.

You can count on our commitment to deliver high-quality books at competitive prices on topics you want to read about. At IDG Books Worldwide, we continue in the IDG tradition of delivering quality for more than 30 years. You'll find no better book on a subject than one from IDG Books Worldwide.

John Kilcullen
Chairman and CEO
IDG Books Worldwide, Inc.

Steven Berkowitz
President and Publisher
IDG Books Worldwide, Inc.

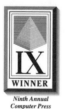

Eighth Annual
Computer Press
Awards ≥1992

Ninth Annual
Computer Press
Awards ≥1993

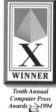

Tenth Annual
Computer Press
Awards ≥1994

Eleventh Annual
Computer Press
Awards ≥1995

IDG is the world's leading IT media, research and exposition company. Founded, in 1964, IDG had 1997 revenues of $2.05 billion and has more than 9,000 employees worldwide. IDG offers the widest range of media options that reach IT buyers in 75 countries representing 95% of worldwide IT spending. IDG's diverse product and services portfolio spans six key areas including print publishing, online publishing, expositions and conferences, market research, education and training, and global marketing services. More than 90 million people read one or more of IDG's 290 magazines and newspapers, including IDG's leading global brands — Computerworld, PC World, Network World, Macworld and the Channel World family of publications. IDG Books Worldwide is one of the fastest-growing computer book publishers in the world, with more than 700 titles in 36 languages. The "...For Dummies®" series alone has more than 50 million copies in print. IDG offers online users the largest network of technology-specific Web sites around the world through IDG.net (http://www.idg.net), which comprises more than 225 targeted Web sites in 55 countries worldwide. International Data Corporation (IDC) is the world's largest provider of information technology data, analysis and consulting, with research centers in over 41 countries and more than 400 research analysts worldwide. IDG World Expo is a leading producer of more than 168 globally branded conferences and expositions in 35 countries including E3 (Electronic Entertainment Expo), Macworld Expo, ComNet, Windows World Expo, ICE (Internet Commerce Expo), Agenda, DEMO, and Spotlight. IDG's training subsidiary, ExecuTrain, is the world's largest computer training company, with more than 230 locations worldwide and 785 training courses. IDG Marketing Services helps industry-leading IT companies build international brand recognition by developing global integrated marketing programs via IDG's print, online and exposition products worldwide. Further information about the company can be found at www.idg.com.   10/8/98

Cartoons at a Glance

By Rich Tennant

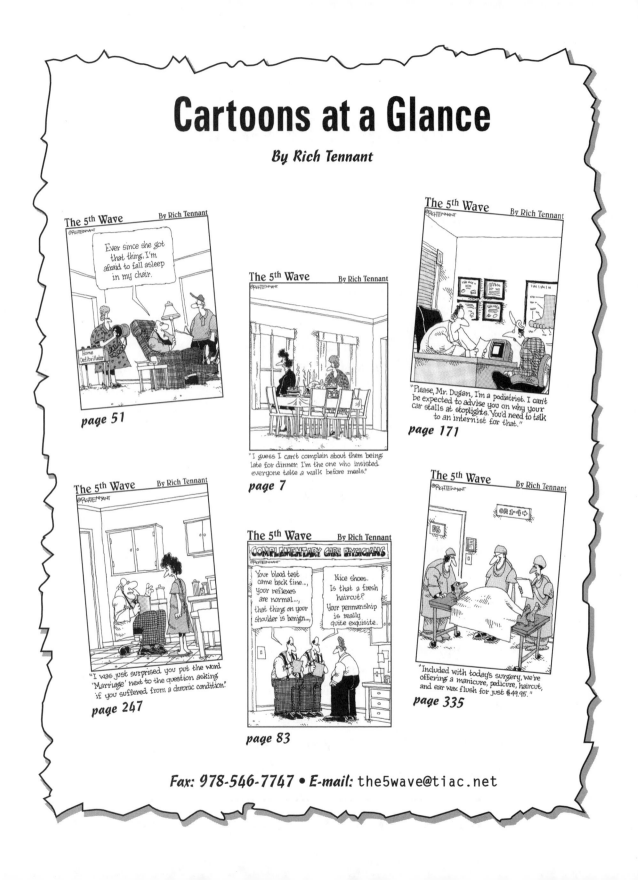

Contents at a Glance

Publisher's Acknowledgments

We're proud of this book; please register your comments through our IDG Books Worldwide Online Registration Form located at http://my2cents.dummies.com.

Some of the people who helped bring this book to market include the following:

Acquisitions and Editorial

Senior Project Editor: Pamela Mourouzis

Executive Editor: Tammerly Booth

Copy Editor: Gwenette Gaddis

Technical Reviewers: Brian Chicoine, M.D.; Edward A. Blumen, M.D.

Editorial Manager: Colleen Rainsberger

Editorial Assistant: Darren Meiss

Editorial Coordinator: Maureen F. Kelly

Special Help

Ted Cains, Johnathan Malysiak, Karen S. Young

Production

Project Coordinator: Karen York

Layout and Graphics: Lou Boudreau, J. Tyler Connor, Maridee V. Ennis, Angela F. Hunckler, Brent Savage, Jacque Schneider, Brian Torwelle

Special Art: Kathryn Born, Certified Medical Illustrator

Proofreaders: Christine Berman, Kelli Botta, Rachel Garvey, Nancy Price, Rebecca Senninger, Ethel M. Winslow, Janet M. Withers

Indexer: Steve Rath

General and Administrative

IDG Books Worldwide, Inc.: John Kilcullen, CEO; Steven Berkowitz, President and Publisher

IDG Books Technology Publishing: Brenda McLaughlin, Senior Vice President and Group Publisher

Dummies Technology Press and Dummies Editorial: Diane Graves Steele, Vice President and Associate Publisher; Mary Bednarek, Director of Acquisitions and Product Development; Kristin A. Cocks, Editorial Director

Dummies Trade Press: Kathleen A. Welton, Vice President and Publisher; Kevin Thornton, Acquisitions Manager

IDG Books Production for Dummies Press: Michael R. Britton, Vice President of Production and Creative Services; Cindy L. Phipps, Manager of Project Coordination, Production Proofreading, and Indexing; Kathie S. Schutte, Supervisor of Page Layout; Shelley Lea, Supervisor of Graphics and Design; Debbie J. Gates, Production Systems Specialist; Robert Springer, Supervisor of Proofreading; Debbie Stailey, Special Projects Coordinator; Tony Augsburger, Supervisor of Reprints and Bluelines

Dummies Packaging and Book Design: Robin Seaman, Creative Director; Kavish + Kavish, Cover Design

♦

The publisher would like to give special thanks to Patrick J. McGovern, without whom this book would not have been possible.

♦

Authors' Acknowledgments

We may be dummies, but we're not dumb enough to try to convince you that this entire book was created, researched, and produced by just the two of us named on the front cover. Many others deserve our grateful acknowledgment for their contributions in making this book a reality.

From the People's Medical Society, we especially thank and acknowledge Janet Worsley Norwood, who served as the editorial project manager for the book. She pushed, shoved, and cajoled everything and everyone with her usual aplomb, skill, and talent. She made this a painless project for all of us. Special kudos to other People's Medical Society staffers: Jennifer Hay, Michael Donio, Annette Doran, and Lehigh University intern Sara Zuckerman. Each made significant contributions through editing, researching, and writing skills.

Special thanks to Professor George Annas for updating his medical rights quiz. Dr. Annas is one of the nation's leading authorities on consumer health rights and is a good friend of the People's Medical Society.

Many talented and dedicated writers contributed to this book. Our special thanks to Kathleen Blease, Mary Erpel, Martha Capwell Fox, Robert C. Goldberg, Thomas Harper, John Hillman, Gerald Irving, Lisa Kane, Luci S. Patalano, Maria G. Richard, John Riddle, and Gail Snyder.

Over the years, Gail Ross has been a major reason books from the People's Medical Society have reached print. As our literary agent, board member, and great friend, she was instrumental in bringing IDG Books and the People's Medical Society together.

And speaking of IDG Books, we have worked with many publishers and editors over the years, but this has been one of the most enjoyable collaborations we have ever encountered. We are sincerely grateful to IDG Books Executive Editor Tammerly Booth, who conceived of this project and wanted us as a partner. Working with her has been a sheer delight. We are equally thankful for the wonderful guidance of Pam Mourouzis, the Senior Project Editor at IDG. Her contribution is on every page, and all of her efforts have made this a better book. And then there are the unsung heroes of this book: Gwenette Gaddis, who copy edited the final manuscript; Kathryn Born, who illustrated the book; and Drs. Brian Chicoine and Edward A. Blumen for their comprehensive technical review.

Table of Contents

. . . .

Bring your own medications and vitamins to the hospital 351
Donate blood 352
Join an ambulance service 352
Borrow medical equipment when possible 352
Make a living will 353
Avoid weekend hospital admissions 353

Appendix A: Glossary of Medical Terms *355*

Appendix B: Common Medical Abbreviations *369*

Index *373*

Book Registration Information .... *Back of Book*

Introduction

● ●

*H*ealth is on everyone's mind these days — as it should be. But with more information at your fingertips than ever before, it's easy to get confused about what's best when it comes to your family's medical care.

Even so, we're convinced that this book is not for everyone. Some people are so bright, so on top of things, that owning a copy of *Family Health For Dummies* would be a total waste of time for them. You may be one of those people.

In an effort to save you about 20 bucks, we've devised a short "Do I Need This Book?" quiz. Take it now, before you plunk down your hard-earned cash (or if you already have, before you break the book's spine enough that the bookstore won't take it back). If you pass the quiz, congratulations: You're a health care genius (and we recommend that you tackle *Gray's Anatomy* in the third Hungarian edition). But if you fail the quiz — and don't be dismayed if you do — this book contains information that can help you improve your family's health and the care that you receive.

Circle T (true) or F (false):

T   F   1. My mother-in-law is a medical expert, and I believe everything she says.

T   F   2. My doctor is so competent that he or she never fails the annual state license test.

T   F   3. No one sees my medical record without my knowledge.

T   F   4. President Clinton's health plan has worked perfectly since it was passed into law.

The correct answers:

1. F. *Our* mothers-in-law are the only medical experts — just ask them.

2. F. Not one state requires a doctor to take another exam after that doctor has been licensed in that state.

3. F. Your medical record is routinely passed around without your knowledge.

4. F. Clinton's health plan might have worked, but it never got passed.

Scoring is quite simple. If you answered T to any one of the four questions, you need this book. But even if you answered every question correctly (and it's hard for us to believe that you think our mothers-in-law know more than yours), you probably need this book. That's because your family's health is too important to leave to guesswork. For yourself, your child, your spouse, and your parent, the more you know about how to stay healthy, what can go wrong, and what to do if something does go wrong, the more likely you and your family will thrive.

About This Book

This is a truly unique health guide. First, it's not just about one gender, one health problem, or one age range. Plenty of books like that are out there, and many of them are quite helpful. But this book has it all — it's for every member of the family. It's a reference book that you'll refer to almost daily because it helps you deal with the health and medical problems that confront your family each day. From medical conditions affecting the kids to those affecting Grandma, it's all here in these pages.

But this book is not just about conditions; it's a total family health strategy. We tell you what to stock in your medicine cabinet, how to check your medical records, and how to choose health care providers. And that's not all. Are you confused about health insurance and all those abbreviations involved — HMO, POS, PPO, and so on? This book answers those questions, too.

What's also unique about *Family Health For Dummies* is where the information comes from. This is not a book of opinions. It's not one doctor's or hospital's views on health care. This information comes directly from the most reliable sources. We don't just get on the telephone looking for a doctor to confirm our viewpoint — and believe us, that's more common than you think! No, we scour medical journals from around the world. We go to the best medical schools, talk to the most renowned scholars, and even go for second opinions to confirm the suggestions we make. In other words, what you read here has been checked and rechecked.

Foolish Assumptions

Remember that a book about health cannot do certain things. For example, an accurate diagnosis can't be made from a book. Nor can the correct dosage of a medication be prescribed. This book is a guide that you should use in conjunction with your medical professionals. Don't make the foolish assumption that you can do it all alone.

How This Book Is Organized

We've made this book easy to use and easy to read by dividing it into six parts. Each part stands alone — meaning that you can open the book to just about any page (without having to read the preceding ten pages) and still get the information you need. Here's an overview of what you can find in each part.

Part I: Taking Charge of Your Family's Health

Being prepared and informed is half the battle when it comes to health care. In this part, we help you find the right attitude about your family's health and your role in it. We also explain how to prepare your family for whatever may arise — both by keeping your body well maintained with good eating and exercise habits and by telling you which screenings should be done when.

Part II: Health Begins at Home

Health isn't just about what happens when you go to the doctor. Lots of medical conditions and "emergencies" are treated at home, so you need to be prepared and know what to do in case something happens to someone in your family. In this part, we tell you what things to keep on hand at home and also describe the various mishaps that can occur and what to do about them.

Part III: You Can Get There from Here: Navigating the Medical Landscape

These days, it's hard to forget that health care is a business. The medical landscape can be a bewildering place for consumers, and that confusion and uncertainty can affect the quality of the care you seek for yourself and your family. That's why we've included a whole part about the business of health. Here you can find information about choosing a doctor or other practitioner, selecting a medical setting, undergoing tests and surgeries, and managing medications. We also walk you through the insurance process and take a look at complementary, or "alternative," therapies.

Part IV: Different Strokes: Kids, Teens, Moms, and Dads

Although many health principles apply to every member of the family, everyone in the family has some unique needs and concerns. The chapters in this part address each category individually: children, adolescents, women, and men.

Part V: Managing Medical Conditions

If you have a medical condition, whether it's chronic or acute, you're sure to want more information about it. We can't tell you everything you need to know about every medical condition there is in a book this size, but we can give you an overview of common conditions to help you recognize when there's a problem, what that problem might be, and what can be done about it. Here you can find details about the symptoms, tests, and treatments for a number of medical problems. This part also contains a chapter on sexual health and related conditions.

Part VI: The Part of Tens

The Part of Tens is a traditional element in ..._For Dummies_ books. These short chapters are packed with great tips and useful information. In our book, we've included a list of ten things you can do to improve your family's health, ten ways to make the most of your doctor's visit, and ten ways to stretch your medical dollar.

Icons Used in This Book

To help you navigate this book a little more efficiently, we've included some icons in the margins to point to various types of information. Following are the icons we've used and what they mean:

This icon indicates a tip that can help you take better care of your family's health.

This icon lets you know that you need to exercise extra caution.

This icon shows you where we have defined one of those troubling health-related terms.

 This icon points to paragraphs that talk specifically about children's health.

 This icon highlights information that's especially pertinent to seniors.

 This icon helps you navigate your way through the maze of the health care business, providing tips to help you become a more savvy consumer and get the best care for your family.

 This icon points to methods that you can use at home on your own to improve your family's health.

 This icon lets you know when it's time to consult a medical professional.

 This icon sits beside information that is important to remember.

Where to Go from Here

Because this book doesn't require you to read it cover to cover, you can start anywhere you like. If you have a specific problem that you'd like information about, go to the pertinent section in Part V. If you're interested in finding out what you can do to improve your family's health in general, start at Chapter 1. Wherever you start, remember that you can play a big role in determining how healthy you and your family can be in the years to come.

Part I
Taking Charge of
Your Family's Health

The 5th Wave   By Rich Tennant

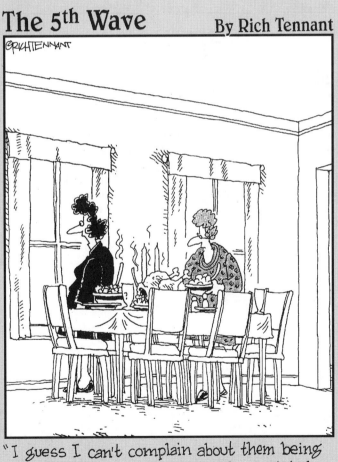

"I guess I can't complain about them being late for dinner. I'm the one who insisted everyone take a walk before meals."

In this part . . .

You always know where to find your house keys and your car keys, right? (Okay, *most* of the time you can find those keys.) You've read books that tell you the keys to success and financial freedom. And somewhere someone knows the key to eternal happiness. But what you want right now are the keys to good health for yourself and your family. Well, you've come to the right place. This part gives you a solid foundation in key areas of health: food, fitness, and prevention. Let this section open the door to your family's good health.

Chapter 1

Getting Healthy, Wealthy, and Wise

So what's the big deal about family health, anyway? When the kids are sick, you take them to the doctor. What could be easier than that?

Technically speaking, of course, you're not referring to health when you're talking like that — you're talking about *illness*. What we want to deal with here is *health,* something that starts long before trips to the doctor and means much more than getting prescriptions filled. In this chapter, you can find out what optimal health really means, how much attitude matters in heading off illness at the pass, and when to realize that a trip to the doctor is the best course of action.

Understanding What "Health" Is

Think of the traditional phrase you use when you swear — solemnly, that is, not profanely — "I, so-and-so, being of sound mind and body . . . ." That, in a nutshell, is what we mean by good health.

By this definition, health encompasses more than just the body and its functions. You can work out on the treadmill every day, eat right, and pass a basic physical with flying colors and still not be healthy if your mind and spirit — that is, your emotional health — are off-kilter.

Rev those engines!

The body is a miracle machine. Like a machine, it has plenty of working parts, uses fuel (food, of course), and works to serve your needs. Like a miracle, it's able to heal on its own, and it can adapt itself to suit its current state. If you're starving in the desert, for example, your body automatically slows its metabolic processes to help conserve fuel. If you start calling on your body to do regular heavy lifting, it builds up your muscle strength to accommodate you.

The body wouldn't be a machine, however, if it didn't break down now and then. A host of adversaries — viruses, genetic triggers, or simply too much wear-and-tear — can cause illness to occur.

That's where regular maintenance comes in. Although you can't protect against everything that might go wrong, you can try to keep your body in good working order — and in good health — by following the same basic rules that you follow with any other sort of machine:

- ✔ Give it the right type of fuel (in other words, eat well).

- ✔ Run it regularly (or, get enough exercise).

- ✔ Have routine inspections to make sure that everything is in order (see your doctor for regular checkups).

Ghost in the machine: The mind-body connection

The mind and the body are hopelessly entangled, so the way you feel physically greatly affects your emotional state, and vice versa. The relationship is complex, with all sorts of brain chemicals and automatic reactions coming into play.

The link between emotional stress and the body is one of the most well understood. The instant stress hits — say you have a near-miss on the freeway — your heart starts pumping faster, your muscles tense, and your adrenaline begins to flow. All this happens to prepare your body for an emergency, to make sure that you have the energy to deal with what may occur. And stress isn't all bad. Oftentimes, a stress reaction can carry you through circumstances that you wouldn't survive otherwise. Think of planning a wedding or pulling an all-nighter the evening before an exam.

The ways in which your physical condition can affect your mental state are also numerous. Most people aren't in the best of moods when they're run-down, and kids tend to get cranky when they've missed a nap. In addition, physical problems and changes can bring on emotional conditions. Brain chemicals afire, Vincent van Gogh, who suffered from a manic-depressive disorder, experienced frenzied periods of artistic inspiration complicated with bouts of depression as part of his illness.

All in the family

So what about *family* health? What's that? Basically, the challenge of keeping your whole family in that state of "sound mind and body" — from the kids to your spouse or significant other to your parents and relatives.

By nature, family health is a little bit of everything. You'll find yourself dealing with a range of ages, maybe dealing one day with the needs of an infant and the next those of an elderly parent. A chronic disease may contrast with a scraped knee that you can kiss and make better. A variety of settings may confront you, too. Although good health begins at home, it ranges far and wide — from the basketball court to the intensive care unit.

Being prepared for every circumstance that may befall you and your loved ones is impossible. Yet you can start to manage your health, and that of your family, after you become familiar with the issues and guidelines that govern their well-being.

Being Proactive

Lose right now the thought that health is a state of being or is something that *happens* to you.

Instead, you need to take control of your family's health. Don't get us wrong — many factors, such as genetic makeup, environmental factors, and just plain chance, can adversely affect your body and your mind. It's all too true that bad things happen to good people. But you can do a great deal to boost your own health and the health of your family. Probably more than you think!

It's time to be proactive when

> ✔ **Everyone is healthy:** No one wants to think about going to the doctor when feeling fine, but scientists have done the research, and it's been scientifically proven that an ounce of prevention equals a pound of cure. Even if you have no ouches, groans, or aches, keeping up with regular checkups is important for everyone in the family. We cover this topic in Chapter 3.

✔ **Illness strikes:** This is the time when you need to put your health know-how to work. When you know what you're dealing with and what options you have, you're better able to make the right decisions regarding your own or your family's care. Find out more about specific conditions in Parts IV and V.

✔ **You're navigating the health care system:** You know that dealing with physicians, hospitals, and insurance agencies can be taxing — but can it really affect health? Without a doubt! How well you communicate with your doctor, how you negotiate with your insurance company, how assertive you are in demanding your rights as a health-care consumer definitely play a role — positive or negative — in the care you receive. Part III is dedicated to this information.

"But," you say, "that means I'll be thinking about health practically all the time!" True enough. Practicing proactive health is an ongoing endeavor, one to which you could probably devote much of your lifetime. Sounds dreary, but think about the consequences. With enough time and effort, you and your family can enjoy even longer, happier, healthier lifetimes. Nice reward, huh? Enough to make up for the time you spend being proactive.

The Doctor Is In

Although books like this one can provide a lot of good information on different conditions and health in general, many times seeking the advice of a professional is important. A host of health care practitioners are available to help you stay healthy, from dietitians and acupuncturists to surgeons and cardiologists — and we talk about their different roles in Chapters 6 and 7.

Remember that this book, and others like it, is no substitute for professional care. We can give you the information you need to make informed decisions concerning your health, but most matters regarding health require medical supervision.

Another reason to be proactive

When someone's down and out, the optimists among us like to offer cheerfully, "At least you've got your health!" But if you're really proactive about your health, you could have even more than a fit mind and body — a few extra dollars in your pocket. Taking control of your health also means being a wise medical consumer: choosing the right doctors, pharmacy, medications, and services for your family (and your family's pocketbook). It also means asking plenty of questions, like "Where did this extra charge come from on my hospital bill?" In the end, you could save a bundle on care and come out ahead in the health department.

Chapter 2

Figuring in Food and Fitness

● ●

In This Chapter

▶ Discovering all you need to know about nutrition

▶ Exercising for health

▶ Combating stress

● ●

*T*ake a look at pretty much any study about health risks, and you'll find the experts recommending two of the best ways to keep yourself and your family healthy: eating right and exercising regularly. Whether it's heart disease, cancer, arthritis, or fatigue, the basic diet and exercise guidelines can help prevent and stave off illness. They can boost emotional health, too. How could you not feel better about yourself when you feel and look pretty good?

Where health is concerned, plenty of factors are out of your control — accidents, genetic tendencies, and germs running rampant during the flu season, to name a few. But you're definitely in charge of what you eat and how you move! Use that control to your — and your family's — advantage.

Becoming a Nutrition Nut

Most Americans eat well, but not wisely. We consume more than enough calories, but not nearly enough of most of the nutrients we need to be truly healthy. And our less-than-wonderful eating habits do more than make us fat; four of the ten leading causes of death — heart disease, stroke, diabetes, and some cancers — are directly related to diet. So finding out how to eat right not only adds life to your years; it can help you live longer and healthier.

 Foods contain more than 40 nutrients, and you need all of them in amounts that vary from large to microscopic. Scientists classify the nutritional components of food as either *macronutrients* and *micronutrients*. We'll start your crash-course in nutrition with explanations of these two classes of nutrients.

Macronutrients

The body is a machine, and machines need fuel. And what fuels your body? Carbohydrates, proteins, and fats. You need these macronutrients in fairly large quantities every day because they supply the body with fuel.

Carbohydrates

Carbohydrates supply the principle source of fuel, *glucose*. All parts of the body — brain, nervous system, organs, and muscles — rely on this fuel. There are two kinds of carbs:

- ✓ **Simple carbohydrates** are sugars, such as table sugar, honey, and the sugars found in fruits.
- ✓ **Complex carbohydrates** are starches, such as those in flour, potatoes, and rice.

Dietary fiber is a carbohydrate, although it can't be broken down as a source of energy. Found in whole grains, fruit, and vegetables, fiber can be *soluble* (capable of being dissolved in water) or *insoluble* (meaning that it can't be dissolved). Fiber's main role is to maintain the digestive tract.

Although simple and complex carbs are metabolized somewhat differently, both supply the same number of calories per gram — 4. Carbohydrates should provide around 50 to 55 percent of your calories. (For more on how many total calories you should consume, see the section "A word about calories," later in this chapter.)

Protein

Protein is essential for the growth, maintenance, and repair of tissue. For example, the hemoglobin in the red blood cells, many hormones, and the antibodies that run the immune system are all made up of proteins. The best sources of protein are meat, poultry, seafood, dairy foods, and legumes.

Because protein is so important to keeping all your systems going, protein isn't tapped as an energy source in your body unless your carbohydrate and fat intakes are extremely low. Like carbs, protein supplies 4 calories per gram. Protein should provide about 20 percent of your calories.

Fat

Fat has become something of a dirty word, but, in fact, you need to eat a little fat every day. For one thing, four vitamins — A, D, E, and K — are fat-soluble, which means that they need fat to be absorbed. Also, dietary fat is necessary so that the body can make linoleic acid, which is needed for hormones, cell membranes, and skin health. And although carbohydrates are the chief source of energy, fats also supply a substantial number of the calories you burn.

Fats can be saturated, polyunsaturated, or monounsaturated.

- ✔ **Saturated fats,** generally speaking, come from animal foods, such as meat and dairy products (although coconut oil and palm kernel oil are also saturated). Solid at room temperature, saturated fats boost levels of *low-density lipoproteins,* or *LDL* (the "bad" cholesterol that contributes to heart disease), while lowering levels of *high-density lipoproteins,* or *HDL* (the "good" cholesterol that helps the body eliminate fat).

- ✔ **Polyunsaturated fats** come from plants. Examples include vegetable oils such as corn oil, which are liquid at room temperature. These fats don't raise levels of LDL, but they do decrease levels of HDL — making them a little better than saturated fats, but still not the greatest.

- ✔ **Monounsaturated fats** are also found in plants — examples include olive oil and canola oil. These fats are the healthiest because they raise blood levels of HDL, the good type of cholesterol that lowers the risk of heart disease. Remember, though, that even "healthy" fats are high in calories.

Fats are very concentrated sources of energy — a gram of fat packs 9 calories, more than twice as many as protein or carbohydrate. That's why keeping an eye on your fat intake is a good idea, because you can easily load up on a lot of calories with just a small portion of a fatty food. Although some people with heart disease or a family history of it should drastically lower their fat intakes, most people are best off when fat provides 25 to 30 percent of their calories.

The great debate: Butter versus margarine

Recently, trans fatty acids — also known as *trans fats* or *hydrogenated fats* — have been identified as a big risk factor for heart disease. *Hydrogenation* is a process that makes unsaturated fats — which are liquid at room temperature and prone to spoiling — harder and more resistant to spoilage. Hydrogenation is why margarines, especially stick margarines, are firm.

For a long time, researchers assumed that because the fats were actually unsaturated, they were as heart-healthy as liquid vegetable oils — and better for you than the saturated fat of butter. But research has shown that trans fats behave like saturated fats in the bloodstream, promoting plaque deposits in arteries. In fact, a Harvard study in late 1997, which followed a large group of nurses for more than 15 years, pronounced trans fats the biggest single dietary risk factor for heart disease in women.

The verdict isn't final, it's true, so you'd do well to limit your intake of both partially hydrogenated vegetable oils and butter.

Water

Few people think of water as a nutrient, and it's true that it doesn't deliver any calories. But you need more water than any other nutrient. It regulates virtually every physical process. Water accounts for 55 to 75 percent of your body weight, and it's essential for carrying nutrients to your cells and carrying waste products away. Water is also necessary for regulating body temperature, cushioning your joints, and (obviously) keeping everything moist.

Although a fair amount of water comes from food, most people don't drink enough water. Aim for a minimum of eight 8-ounce glasses a day, experts say.

Micronutrients

Vitamins and minerals are referred to as *micronutrients* because the daily amounts you need are quite small. But great things — like life and health — come in these small packages, and science is still learning about all the things that micronutrients do for you. ***Remember:*** It's not important to monitor how much of each of these individual elements you're getting. The important thing is to eat a balanced diet containing a wide variety of foods.

Beware of high doses of vitamins and minerals. Depending on the vitamin or mineral, a high dose can result in toxic levels in the body. To be on the safe side, talk with your doctor or a nutritionist before dosing yourself with large amounts of any vitamin or mineral. Also keep your doctor apprised of any supplements you're taking, because they can interfere with how medications work within the body.

Vitamin A

Vitamin A is unique in that it comes in both fat- and water-soluble forms. The fat-soluble form, called *retinol,* or preformed vitamin A, comes from eggs, organ meats, dairy foods, and fish liver oils. Water-soluble vitamin A is called *beta-carotene,* a "precursor" of vitamin A. Dark green, dark yellow, and orange vegetables, such as broccoli, carrots, squash, collards, and sweet potatoes, are rich sources of beta-carotene, as are apricots and peaches.

Vitamin A is essential to good vision; it keeps the tissues that line the mouth and all organs moist and healthy, and it strengthens the immune system. High intakes of beta-carotene, which is an antioxidant (as are vitamins C and E and the mineral selenium), have been connected to a reduced risk of some types of cancer, except in smokers, who have a higher risk of lung cancer.

TIP

Which are better: Foods or supplements?

One of the most important things to know about vitamins and minerals is that many of them have to work together. For example, your body can't use calcium properly unless your vitamin D levels are right, and vitamin C promotes the absorption of iron.

That's why it's best to get your nutrients from food rather than *supplements* — capsules or tablets that contain vitamins. Though it's generally safe to take supplements of single nutrients such as vitamin C, getting nutrients from food is more likely to keep you in balance.

Plus, you get all the other good things, such as protein and water, when you eat whole foods.

Tapping into this spectrum of nutrients is one of the main reasons dietitians say that people should eat a variety of foods. In this country, that's very easy to do. Supermarkets are bursting with literally tens of thousands of choices that let you sample heavily from a wide array of produce, grains, dairy foods, and lean meats and a huge range of flavors. Eating a variety of foods is not only good for you and your family — it's fun, too.

The B vitamins

The B vitamins — thiamin (B_1), riboflavin (B_2), niacin, pyridoxine (B_6), cobalamin (B_{12}), biotin, folic acid, and pantothenic acid — work together in many metabolic functions. However, each has individual characteristics and functions, and some, such as folic acid and niacin, have been found to be especially effective on certain conditions.

Thiamin, niacin, riboflavin, biotin, pantothenic acid, and vitamin B_6 all work together to convert food into energy. Thus they're essential to growth and development. These vitamins are also necessary in the process that creates red blood cells, hormones, and neurotransmitters. Vitamins B_6, B_{12}, and folic acid appear to play a bigger role in the nervous system than do the other Bs. Further, niacin is sometimes prescribed by doctors for patients who have high blood cholesterol. Vitamin B_6 has been touted as a cure for premenstrual syndrome and carpal tunnel disorder.

The recommended daily intake of folic acid was increased after it became apparent that folic acid can prevent neural tube birth defects. It also appears to play a role in preventing heart disease by holding down blood levels of a damaging substance known as *homocysteine*. Folic acid is one of the most common vitamin deficiencies in this country, but that should end soon because breads and other common grain-based foods are now fortified with it.

The B vitamins are water-soluble and are found in a wide range of foods. Many are found together in the same foods. In general, whole grains, meats, and beans are good sources. Breads and cereals are often fortified with B vitamins to replace those lost in processing.

JARGON ALERT

Antioxidants: Nutrients in white hats

Imagine that within the structure of your body, an oxidative reaction — one involving oxygen — occurs. Outside the body, the oxidative reaction causes butter to turn rancid and iron to rust. Inside, it spawns an enemy of a different sort: a *free radical*.

Think of the free radical as a molecular bad guy. He's chemically unstable, which forces him to steal electrons from other molecules. The theft damages these other molecules, turning them into free radicals as well. The dangers are great: Rampant free radicals are thought to contribute to heart disease, wrinkles, and even some forms of cancer. It's a sad tale. Who will save you?

Antioxidants to the rescue! Antioxidants, which include vitamins C and E, beta-carotene, and the mineral selenium, neutralize free radicals, making them harmless and stopping harmful reactions. Our heroes . . .

Some foods are especially good sources of individual B vitamins. For example, milk and dairy foods are the most important sources of riboflavin, providing half your intake; children and adults who don't eat dairy products are likely to be deficient. Folic acid is abundant in leafy green vegetables, avocados, and oranges, as well as in whole grains and beans. And vitamin B_{12} is found only in animal foods — meat, poultry, eggs, and dairy products. (*Vegans* — vegetarians who eat no animal products — have to take supplements of B_{12} to balance their diets.)

Vitamin C

Vitamin C is famous for warding off colds, but it's important for more than a healthy immune system. It helps form the connective tissue called *collagen* and forms and repairs red blood cells and the walls of the blood vessels. Vitamin C promotes skin healing and keeps gums healthy. Everyone knows that citrus fruits and juices are loaded with vitamin C, but broccoli, strawberries, and peppers are excellent sources, too.

Vitamin D

Most Americans don't have to worry about eating enough vitamin D because the body (miracle that it is) produces it when exposed to sunlight. And because vitamin D is a fat-soluble vitamin, you store excess amounts rather than excreting them. The main dietary source is fortified milk (other dairy foods such as yogurt and ice cream are not fortified), although eggs, margarine, and salmon provide small amounts.

Vitamin D is especially important for growing children because it is a necessary ingredient in the process of turning dietary calcium into bone. Older people need to watch their D intake, too, because their bodies are less efficient at making it, and because they are less likely to get out in the sun, especially in the winter.

Vitamin E

The most potent of the antioxidants, vitamin E mops up the toxic waste created by normal metabolism, elements called *free radicals.* Unchecked, free radicals do damage to cells that may lead to heart disease, cancer, and other degenerative diseases. Vitamin E also protects the tissues lining the respiratory system from pollutants.

Vitamin E is fat-soluble, and the best sources of it are fats — vegetable, nut, and seed oils such as sunflower, corn, safflower, and sesame seed. Wheat germ, spinach, and avocados also deliver very small amounts of vitamin E.

Minerals

Twenty-two minerals are needed for good health. Some are classified as *major,* which means that you have more than a teaspoon of each of them in your body; others are called *trace,* meaning that you have less than a teaspoon. But major minerals aren't more important to health than trace minerals — iron and zinc are counted among the trace minerals.

Calcium

Calcium is the most abundant mineral in the body because bones and teeth are mostly made up of it. But calcium is also very important in body fluids, where it helps regulate blood pressure, move muscles, transmit nerve messages, and maintain several other metabolic processes. Still, calcium's most important role is in building and maintaining bones and teeth, which makes it a critical nutrient.

The best sources of calcium are milk and other dairy foods; not only does milk contain high levels of calcium, but it also has vitamin D, protein, and phosphorus, which help turn calcium into bone. Some dark green, leafy vegetables are also good sources of calcium, and some processed foods, such as cereal, are enriched with it.

Magnesium

Magnesium is part of every major process in your body, including energy burning, nerve impulse transmission, and muscle contraction. Low intakes may contribute to heart disease and high blood pressure. Get your magnesium from bananas, peanuts (and peanut butter), milk, whole grains, and beans.

Phosphorus

Like magnesium, phosphorus has a role in every biologic function. It's the second most abundant mineral in your body, and it's impossible not to get enough, as it's found in nearly all kinds of foods. As a matter of fact, people who eat mostly meat, junk foods, and soft drinks and eat few vegetables and dairy foods may be getting too much phosphorus. An excess can cause bone loss and imbalances of calcium and magnesium.

Sodium, potassium, and chloride

These three minerals actually act as electrolytes in body fluids, and they work together to maintain fluid balance and pressure in your cells. They regulate blood pressure, heart rate, muscle contraction, nerve transmission, and acidity. Sodium and chloride are virtually never too low in the American diet; in fact, most people eat far too much of them, which some experts believe may cause high blood pressure. On the other hand, many people do not eat enough potassium, which is mostly found in produce, whole grains, and milk, as well as bananas.

Chromium

A trace mineral, chromium's chief function is as part of the insulin system that regulates blood sugar. Although chromium has been promoted as a weight-loss aid, no evidence proves that chromium supplements help you lose weight. However, indications are that a diet high in sugar depletes chromium. The best food sources are brewer's yeast, peas, whole grains, and eggs.

Copper

This trace mineral helps make *hemoglobin,* which carries oxygen in the red blood cells. Copper is also part of an antioxidant enzyme that may help prevent cancer. It contributes to growth; very low intakes of copper may play a role in the development of scoliosis. Copper is available from a wide variety of foods: whole grains, shellfish, nuts, legumes, poultry, and dark green, leafy vegetables.

Iron

Iron is necessary to make red blood cells, which transport oxygen through the blood to every cell in the body and then carry away the carbon dioxide that the cell makes when it uses the oxygen. This makes iron essential to every process in the body. Many people don't get enough iron; although they don't have obvious signs of anemia, they probably aren't functioning at their best. Low levels of iron have been linked with anemia, fatigue, rapid heartbeat, breathlessness, and inability to concentrate, among other things.

Children and women in their childbearing years need the most iron. Men and postmenopausal women need less iron. In fact, some experts suspect that excess iron in these people may cause heart disease.

It's best to get iron from foods — red meat, organ meats, and dark poultry meats provide the best-absorbed iron. Some plant foods also supply iron, as do iron-fortified cereals, but this form of iron (called *nonheme*) is not absorbed very well. You can boost the absorption by eating a vitamin C food with it.

Selenium

Selenium works as an antioxidant with vitamin E and also aids in cell growth. It probably plays a role in preventing cancer and heart disease;

these ailments are more common in areas of the world where little selenium is available. Whole grains, poultry, fish, and dairy foods provide selenium, although the amounts vary depending on the content of selenium in the soil where the food is produced.

Zinc

Zinc helps you taste your food and helps the body convert that food into energy. Zinc also plays a role in the immune system, in regulating cholesterol, and in healing wounds. Children who don't get enough zinc don't grow at the right rate.

Zinc is found in a wide variety of foods. Oysters, beef, pork and beef liver, lamb, crab, wheat germ, and *miso* (fermented soybean paste) are all good sources.

Other minerals

Other minerals are known to have a role in human health — sulfur, iodine, molybdenum, manganese, boron, fluoride, cobalt, vanadium, silicon, nickel, and tin — but either they're so abundant in food (sulfur, for example) that it's unlikely that anyone could be deficient, or so little is known about them that no daily intake recommendation has been set.

The way to make sure that you're getting enough of all these minerals is to eat a variety of foods every day — which, coincidentally, is the best way to make sure that you're getting *all* the nutrients you need.

Minding your 'mins and minerals

How much of each vitamin and mineral do you need? That's a tricky question. The U.S. government offers a list of *Recommended Dietary Allowances,* or RDAs, which indicates the amounts of nutrients that average men, women, and children need to prevent deficiency. Notice that we didn't say prevent *illness* in connection with RDAs. The RDAs are designed to make sure that everyone gets what they need, and not much more. In amounts *larger* than the RDAs, however, some vitamins and minerals — vitamin C, for example — are thought to help prevent disease, not just deficiency.

With this in mind, the U.S. government and the nutrition community are working to set new standards of healthy intake for nutrients. The standards will be called *Dietary Reference Intakes,* or DRIs. The DRIs include

- **Estimated Average Requirement (EAR):** The level estimated to be adequate for half the healthy people in an age or gender group.

- **Recommended Dietary Allowance (RDA):** The level estimated to meet the needs of as many as 97 percent of healthy people in an age or gender group.

✔ **Adequate Intake (AI):** The level estimated to reduce the risk of certain diseases rather than merely to prevent deficiency. The AI is used when there isn't enough scientific evidence to determine an EAR.

✔ **Tolerable Upper Intake Limit (UI):** The highest level of daily intake that is unlikely to cause problems.

Supplementing safely

Popping a vitamin is certainly much simpler than paying attention to your diet. But don't be tempted by the easy way out. Although supplements provide a kind of nutritional insurance, they're no substitute for getting the nutrients you need from foods. For one thing, supplements don't give you the other elements in foods, such as fiber, enzymes, and plant chemicals (such as *bioflavonoids*), that are known to contribute to good health. Also, many nutrients act *synergistically* — that is, they augment each other when eaten together.

Sometimes, though, taking a supplement is a good idea. For example, doctors usually advise pregnant and nursing women to take a supplement that is high in iron and folate. In fact, pregnancy and breast-feeding boost a woman's daily need for almost all nutrients, so the best insurance is a once-daily multivitamin and mineral pill formulated especially for pregnancy. And because kids can be so finicky about what they eat, many pediatricians suggest a multivitamin for children. Older adults may want to take calcium and vitamin D supplements.

Be sure to store children's vitamins well out of reach and in childproof containers. Most multis for kids look and taste like candy, but eating several of them at once puts a child at risk for iron poisoning.

Building meals with a pyramid

Now that you know the what and why of nutrition, you're ready for the how. Relax. It's not that hard.

Start by keeping a record of what your family eats for one week. That task may sound daunting, but the list doesn't have to be exhaustive. Don't worry about quantities; just jot down what you serve at each meal that you eat at home (don't forget about things such as butter, jelly, mayo, and beverages), and make it a point to catch up at dinner on what everyone had for lunch. Don't overlook snacks or in-front-of-the-TV munching.

Now take your seven-day list of foods and check it out against the Food Guide Pyramid. The pyramid, devised by the U.S. Department of Agriculture (USDA), gives guidelines for balancing your food choices throughout the day. The idea is to eat little of the foods at the top of the pyramid (fats, oils, and sweets) while basing your diet on those foods at the bottom (breads, cereals, rice, and pasta). These guidelines are consistent with the percentages that we mentioned in the "Macronutrients" section earlier in this chapter — they're just broken up into a pyramid to make them easier to understand. Figure 2-1 shows the Food Guide Pyramid.

- ✔ For the bread, cereal, rice, and pasta group, one serving equals 1 slice of bread, 1 ounce of ready-to-eat cereal, or $^1/_2$ cup of cooked cereal, rice, or pasta.

- ✔ For the fruit group, one serving equals 1 medium apple, banana, or orange; $^1/_2$ cup of chopped raw, cooked, or canned fruit; or $^3/_4$ cup of fruit juice.

- ✔ For the vegetable group, one serving equals 1 cup of raw, leafy vegetables; $^1/_2$ cup of other vegetables (cooked or chopped raw); or $^3/_4$ cup of vegetable juice.

- ✔ For the meat, poultry, fish, dry beans, eggs, and nuts group, one serving equals 2 to 3 ounces of cooked lean meat, fish, or poultry; 1 to $1^1/_2$ cups of cooked dry beans; 2 to 3 eggs; or 4 to 6 tablespoons of peanut butter.

- ✔ For the milk, yogurt, and cheese group, one serving equals 1 cup of milk or yogurt, $1^1/_2$ ounces of natural cheese, or 2 ounces of processed cheese.

- ✔ Fats, oils, and sweets should be used sparingly.

Although it's a bit broad and general, the pyramid is a good way to assess the variety and balance in your diet. We bet you'll find that you and your family meet the recommendations for the bread and cereal, meat, and milk groups while falling short in the mid-pyramid produce department. And if you're like most people, you don't eat "sparingly" from the fats, oils, and sweets block.

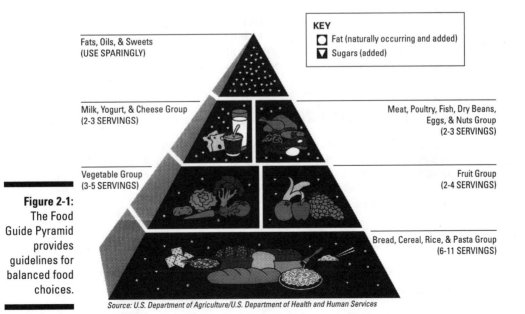

Figure 2-1:
The Food Guide Pyramid provides guidelines for balanced food choices.

KEY
- ◻ Fat (naturally occurring and added)
- ▼ Sugars (added)

Fats, Oils, & Sweets
(USE SPARINGLY)

Milk, Yogurt, & Cheese Group
(2-3 SERVINGS)

Meat, Poultry, Fish, Dry Beans, Eggs, & Nuts Group
(2-3 SERVINGS)

Vegetable Group
(3-5 SERVINGS)

Fruit Group
(2-4 SERVINGS)

Bread, Cereal, Rice, & Pasta Group
(6-11 SERVINGS)

Source: U.S. Department of Agriculture/U.S. Department of Health and Human Services

You also need to go past what you ate and look at *how* you ate it. Were the cereals whole grains, such as shredded wheat, bran flakes, or oat cereals? Or were they heavily processed, sugar-sweetened brands? White bread or whole wheat? Pasta drowning in cheese and margarine, or with vegetables and low-fat tomato sauce? Did you snack on greasy, salty crackers, chips, and other fun foods, or did you choose reduced-fat crackers, baked chips, and no-salt options?

After you figure out how what you've been eating compares to what you should have been eating, you may need to make some changes. When planning meals, keep the pyramid in mind, going heavy on starches and cereals and lighter on proteins. You'll also want to phase out high-fat dishes and substitute healthier fare gradually — going "cold turkey" and making large, unsustainable changes can lead to frustration and even failure.

Contrary to what many people believe, there's no such thing as a bad food. Sure, you should eat certain foods more — or less — often. But unless you have a medical condition such as diabetes or a real food allergy, nothing is strictly forbidden.

A word about calories

In all this talk about nutrients and food, don't forget about calories. A *calorie* is a unit used to measure energy — that is, energy supplied by food and also energy created with movement.

When you expend the same number of calories that you take in, your weight stays the same. If you eat more than you burn off, those calories are stored away in the fat cells for your body's future use. And if you burn off more than you eat, your fat cells release some of their stored energy, and you may lose a little weight. The average adult man or woman needs between 1,800 and 2,200 calories per day to maintain a healthy weight.

Feeding the family

Like their parents, kids on the average eat too much fat and saturated fat, too much sodium, and not enough fiber. Your efforts at improving your family's diet don't have to make special allowances for your children over age two — everyone will do well on the same good diet. That said, wise parents still need to keep an eye on their kids' plates.

Surveys indicate that many kids don't eat enough iron. Low iron intake, even if it isn't low enough to cause anemia, can sap energy and drain concentration in school. Serve iron-fortified cereals and breads daily (breakfast orange juice will boost the iron absorption) as well as lean red meat a few times a week to ensure your kids' iron status.

Never restrict fat in any child under the age of two. Babies' brains develop so fast in the first years that they need a steady infusion of energy, which is best provided by the extra calories from fat.

The topic of dietary fat restriction in kids over age two is controversial. The American Academy of Pediatrics somewhat half-heartedly endorsed the idea of limiting kids' fat intake to 30 percent of calories in the mid-1980s, but some experts say that there's no reason to assume that childhood diets influence the risk of heart disease in the adult years.

The prudent course appears to be to limit intake of saturated fats (from meat) and trans fatty acids (from snack foods, crackers, and stick marga-rine) for the entire family, while giving your kids, especially active and/or athletic kids, some leeway in their intake of unsaturated fats. Most active kids probably won't be hurt by getting as much as 40 percent of their calories from fat, again provided that most of it is unsaturated. For weight control in kids, restricting television watching (including video games) and encouraging activity is far better than restricting food, experts say.

Teenage girls and what they eat are problematic unto themselves. A very high percentage of adolescent girls who are of normal weight severely restrict their food intake, and many are prone to fad diets and fasting — practices that too often result in eating disorders. (See Chapter 14 for more information in that department.) Consequently, the average American teenage girl is deficient in several nutrients, most notably iron and calcium.

Although controlling how teenagers eat away from home is impossible, you can try to counter this tendency by offering a wide variety of low-fat foods, especially lean meat and dairy foods, at your own table. Parents, especially mothers, should communicate the attitude that appearance — notably the emaciated appearance of the fashion model — is less important than other aspects of life, including education, ambition, self-reliance, and individuality.

Shaping Up and Working Out

Baffled by the contradictory data that Americans are eating less fat and fewer calories but are fatter than ever, many experts lay the blame squarely on a sedentary lifestyle. Despite the proliferation of clothing and accessories that are meant to be used for sports and exercise, only about one-quarter of Americans exercise regularly. Meanwhile, video options multiply exponen-tially — cable, video games, and the Internet all conspire to keep people on their duffs more than ever. Although the best exercise may be pushing yourself away from the table, getting up from the TV or computer is just as good.

Being physically active pays such big dividends (physical, mental, and even social) that it should be a high priority for everyone. People who get regular exercise are fitter and trimmer; have much less risk of heart disease, diabetes, hypertension, and even some cancers; have stronger bones and muscles; tire less easily; are more flexible, agile, and less prone to injury; sleep better; and tend to feel better about themselves. In other words, exercise keeps you younger longer.

One of the most common excuses for not exercising is "I don't have the time." But if you stop thinking of exercise of only running or biking or lifting weights or going to aerobics classes, you find plenty of times to exercise throughout the day. Housework, gardening, and even hanging out the laundry expend between 200 and 300 calories per hour. And carving out half an hour every day for a brisk walk may be one of the best things you can do for your health.

Balancing your exercise gives you optimal results. A mix of aerobic exercise (walking, running, swimming — anything that gets your heart and breathing rates up), strength training (weight lifting or resistance workouts), and flexibility work (stretching) can keep you in tip-top form and health.

Before you start an exercise program, get the go-ahead from your doctor — especially if you haven't been active in a while.

Aerobicizing

Aerobic exercise is any movement that lifts your heart and respiratory rates. Experts recommend getting at least 30 minutes of aerobic exercise at least three days a week. The best workout raises the heart and breathing rates to a target range and keeps them there for at least 20 minutes.

To find out your target heart rate, subtract your age from 220 and take 70 percent of that number. This is your ideal pulse rate during exercise. In some cases, this won't work. Try the "talk test" instead — exercise to the point where you can carry on a conversation while exercising, for 30 minutes, with no loss of breath.

If you haven't been active, walking is the best aerobic exercise to start with; you can vary your pace or the terrain you cover to either push yourself or give yourself a breather. Walking is also unlikely to cause injuries. Other aerobic options include jogging, swimming, cycling, and cross-country skiing. But you don't need to pick just one activity and stick with it. Variety, they say, is the spice of life, so change your routine regularly to ensure that you won't get bored. And don't limit yourself to traditional exercise, either. Raking leaves, window washing, dog walking — it's all exercise as long as it gets your heart pumping and your body moving.

Training for strength

Strength training isn't just for body builders and pro football players. Lifting weights challenges your muscles, and they respond by becoming firmer and stronger. If you want to stay trim and close to a healthy weight, muscle is the key. Lean muscle tissue is much better at burning calories than fatty tissue is. For most people, starting a program of light weight lifting will probably result in more energy and better-fitting clothes, if not out-and-out weight loss.

Strong muscles protect you from injury, too — a fact that is especially helpful for older adults who may have fragile bones. Several years ago, a study of people in their 80s and 90s showed that lifting light weights a few times a week gave even these very elderly people more strength and agility, lowered their blood pressure, and lifted their spirits.

Like aerobics, strength training takes many forms. *Free weights* — sets of bars and individual weights — can be mixed and matched according to your needs. Weight machines are another option. Designed with padded seats and pulley systems, these machines offer standard exercises without loose parts that you might drop on your foot or trip over, so they're generally safer than free weights. Another choice is *resistance bands* — rubber straps that you can loop around your arms and legs and pull against. But all you really need is some resistance to challenge those muscles — even soup cans and water bottles work.

Flexing for fitness

Gentle stretching is an essential part of physical fitness — just as essential as strength training or aerobics. Yet most people forget about flexibility, jumping into their fitness routines without so much as touching their toes. That's unfortunate, because stretching preserves flexibility and range of muscle movement, and it helps ensure that you won't suffer nasty cramps or pulls during exercise.

Give yourself time for stretching at both "ends" of your regimen, for warm-up and cool-down. It's best to stretch after you've done some exercise — never stretch "cold" muscles. Stretch only until you feel a slight pull, not pain. Hold the stretch for 20 to 30 seconds. **Remember:** The key to safe stretching is to move slowly and gently.

Shedding Pounds

A healthy diet and regular exercise are the foundation of any successful weight-loss program. Refuse to be wowed by specialty diets or wonder products that promise a quick fix to weight problems. The formula is simple: Eat fewer calories and work out more, and the pounds will come off.

How do you know whether it's time to take off a few pounds? Check your height and age in Table 2-1 to see whether you fall within suggested guidelines for a healthy weight.

Moderate cutbacks in calorie intake promote weight loss. However, don't starve yourself. Not only is this method not healthy, but it also slows the body's metabolism, causing it to conserve the fat that you want to lose.

Before you embark on a weight-loss plan, talk with your doctor. If you've been ill or you're out of shape, get a complete physical before picking up your sneakers, just to be on the safe side. Your practitioner should know you and your habits and can offer advice that you can use to tailor your exercise program and make it more efficient.

Table 2-1	Age-Adapted Healthy Weights for Men and Women				
	Age				
	20-29	*30-39*	*40-49*	*50-59*	*60-69*
4'10"	84-111	92-119	99-127	107-135	115-142
4'11"	87-115	95-123	103-131	111-139	119-147
5'0"	90-119	98-127	106-135	114-143	123-152
5'1"	93-123	101-131	110-140	118-148	127-157
5'2"	96-127	105-136	113-144	122-153	131-163
5'3"	99-131	108-140	117-149	126-158	135-168
5'4"	102-135	112-145	121-154	130-163	140-173
5'5"	106-140	115-149	125-159	134-168	144-179
5'6"	109-144	119-154	129-164	138-174	148-184
5'7"	112-148	122-159	133-169	143-179	153-190
5'8"	116-153	126-163	137-174	147-184	158-196
5'9"	119-157	130-168	141-179	151-190	162-201
5'10"	122-162	134-173	145-184	156-195	167-207
5'11"	126-167	137-178	149-190	160-201	172-213
6'0"	129-171	141-183	153-195	165-207	177-219
6'1"	133-176	145-188	157-200	169-213	182-225
6'2"	137-181	149-194	162-206	174-219	187-232
6'3"	141-186	153-199	166-212	179-225	192-238
6'4"	144-191	157-205	171-218	184-231	197-244

Height

Source: National Institutes of Health

Taming Tension

Some days, trying to handle your stress is just one more stressor. But knowing how to calm down is important because stress can do a major number on your physical and mental health. High anxiety causes everything from insomnia to migraines to respiratory ailments to heart disease.

The reasons that stress can hurt your health lie with stress hormones and with an ancient gut reaction. Back in prehistoric days, when our ancestors were confronted with a stressor, it was usually one that could seriously and immediately hurt them, such as a saber-toothed tiger. In such situations, they did all they could do — fight back or run away.

Gradually, an automatic response to stress evolved. In the face of stress, the body automatically releases stress hormones such as *epinephrine* (also called *adrenaline*) and *cortisol*. These hormones prime the body for a confrontation by raising heart and breathing rates and increasing muscle tension. They also divert blood and nutrients from systems such as the immune and digestive systems that are not necessary in the event of an emergency. This is known as the *fight or flight response.*

Nowadays, most people don't have to run from saber-toothed tigers. But that doesn't stop the hormones from flooding in — and worse, you can't take the physical action that helps them dissipate. The result is lingering tension, heightened blood pressure, a depressed immune system, and poor digestive function.

So you have to learn to short-circuit your stress response. There are a number of ways to do so, ranging from relaxation techniques you can do on the spot to living in a way that minimizes your stressors and allows you to be healthy enough to handle the ones you can't avoid.

Relax on the spot

When you really relax, your brain releases *endorphins,* substances that make you feel good. You can call up your endorphins quickly by practicing a number of relaxation techniques:

- ✔ **Deep breathing:** Take long, slow, deep breaths, filling and emptying your lungs completely with each one. Inhale deeply through your nose and blow out slowly but fully through your mouth.

- ✔ **Meditation:** In a quiet place, close your eyes and concentrate on a single word (called a *mantra*) while ignoring all external stimuli.

- ✔ **Progressive muscle relaxation:** In a quiet place and in a reclining position, systematically contract and relax each of your muscles, from your toes to your head.

✔ **Visualization therapy:** Close your eyes and imagine a pleasant situation or place. Or imagine your stress as a physical object, such as a bag of garbage, and picture yourself throwing it away.

The more often you practice these techniques, the easier it will be for you to relax where and when you want. Your body becomes attuned to the relaxation response and lets goes of stress more readily.

Live for lower stress

Nowadays, a multitude of books and tapes purport to tell you how to simplify your life. Although these books and tapes tend to be simplistic (pardon the expression), plenty of things can be said for living in a way that cuts down on your stress. One of the keys to managing stress is to control the things you can and to let go of the things you can't.

✔ **Set priorities and stick with them.** Decide what you must do, when you must do those things, and how to schedule enough time to do them. Then arrange other tasks around those must-dos.

✔ **Get onto a schedule.** Doing some things at the same time, whether it's daily, weekly, or monthly, means that they get done. Getting into a routine saves time and stress.

✔ **Delegate and learn to let go.** Give your spouse, kids, coworkers, or whomever some responsibilities that they can handle. And then let them take care of those responsibilities.

✔ **Just say no.** Many people are involved in clubs, committees, and projects that they have little or no interest in or commitment to. Stick with a few activities that are meaningful and let the rest go.

✔ **Stop trying to keep so well-informed.** More news and data is floating around than ever, and most of it has no relevance to your daily life.

✔ **Take time for yourself, and encourage your family to set quiet times.** Try to get everyone to agree to a few set hours a week with no TV, telephone, radio, music, or computer interference.

✔ **Learn to live with a bit less.** Many people really are working to support their stuff. Doing without some stuff that probably winds up in a closet anyway may let you get out of the rat race, at least once in a while.

Chapter 3

Prevention Prowess

. . . .

In This Chapter

▶ Knowing the value of prevention

▶ Screening for everyone: Men, women, children, and seniors

▶ Looking into your family's medical history

▶ Checking your medical records

. . . .

*W*hen it comes to health, prevention takes a number of forms, both public and personal. City sanitation measures are prevention. Wearing a helmet when riding your bike is prevention. Fastening your seat belt on the turnpike is prevention. But accidents aside, can prevention really make you healthier? You bet. One University of California at Los Angeles study looked at the habits of 7,000 men and women, taking into account factors such as smoking, drinking, being physically inactive, and having poor sleep habits. The research revealed that a 45-year-old man with fewer than four negative factors would live 11 years longer than a similar man with more than four bad habits. Women experienced smaller, but still significant, gains.

Maintaining your health is far easier than trying to restore it after an illness. Unfortunately, too many Americans fail to take this commonsense notion to heart. Physicians often neglect prevention as well by not counseling patients on the dangers of smoking and the benefits of regular exercise, or by ignoring recommendations on routine screening examinations. And unfortunately, treating certain conditions — heart disease, for example — may actually be cheaper than preventing them in the first place.

These facts should give you the motivation to make prevention a priority in your family. In this chapter, we give you the information you need to boost your family's health. Here, you can find out how to earn your family that pound of cure.

Maintaining Your Miracle Machine

The key to maintaining health is heading off problems before they occur. How can you detect problems? By going to your doctor for regular checkups and keeping to a schedule of specific preventive tests, known as health screenings.

The recommended screenings vary among men, women, children, and seniors, so we break them up here according to those categories to make life easier. Keep in mind, though, that these recommendations aren't set in stone. Everyone has different needs, and your doctor should tailor a screening schedule to meet them. Plus, doctors, leading medical groups, and government agencies often disagree on which screenings are necessary and when.

Screening all around

Despite obvious differences between the male and female anatomies, a body is a body. So it's easy to understand that several routine tests are appropriate for both men and women.

Basic physical

Every three years for healthy adults under age 40, every two years from 40 to 50, and every year after 50.

Physicals aren't bad. First, the doctor asks a series of questions about your lifestyle, occupation, and current and past health problems. This information is known as your *medical history.* A thorough history is often the key to diagnosing risks and problems, so answer all the questions carefully and honestly.

After taking your history, the doctor checks your eyes, ears, and skin (including the appearance of any moles or other lesions), the lining of your mouth and throat, and your height and weight, and performs the familiar whack-on-the-knee reflex test.

And no physical would be complete without a few standard screening tests. Be aware that considerable controversy exists among some medical groups and government agencies as to what constitute "standard" screening tests. Be sure to discuss this with your medical practitioner.

- ✔ **Urinalysis** (every three years until age 40, every two years from 40 to 50, and every year after 50): The point is to watch out for diabetes, urinary tract infections, hormonal imbalances, liver conditions, and gallbladder health.

✔ **Blood pressure** (at least once per year according to the American Heart Association, but most practitioners take your blood pressure at every visit): To measure blood pressure, a nurse wraps a blood pressure cuff around your upper arm, pumps it up to temporarily squeeze shut the main artery in your arm, and then slowly deflates the cuff, while listening with a stethoscope for distinctive sounds made by your blood as it rushes back into your arm.

The nurse listens for two sounds that match the pressure when the heart is pumping _(systolic pressure)_ and when your heart is relaxed _(diastolic pressure)._ These two numbers, especially the diastolic, or lower of the pressures, are important because they predict blood pressure–related complications such as heart attacks. You can buy a blood pressure cuff and take your own blood pressure at home (some models even have pulse as well as blood pressure readouts, but take time to make sure that you're on the same page as your nurse and doctor regarding which sounds match which blood pressure measurements). By most accounts, a reading in the range of 120-129 systolic over 80-84 diastolic is "normal," but you'd be hard pressed to find anybody with exactly 120/80 pressure, or with exactly 120/80 all the time.

✔ **Blood tests** (every three years until age 40, every two years from 40 to 50, and every year after 50): A thorough test includes a complete blood cell count (CBC), a cholesterol test, a more complete test called a _blood chemistry survey,_ and sometimes a test for HIV, the virus that causes AIDS (depending on your answers in the history part of the exam).

✔ **Tuberculosis test** (every five years): At one time, tuberculosis was very rare. However, a resurgence of the disease is striking the United States. To test for the disease, a doctor injects a small amount of purified protein derivative under the skin. If TB is present, the area becomes red and irritated within 72 hours. A follow-up visit is necessary to check the results of the test.

Chest X-ray

Every year for smokers. (Note, though, that some experts do not believe this annual screening to be beneficial.)

If you're still puffing away, you need to have an annual chest X-ray to look for lung damage and lung cancer. But you could save yourself the trouble — and simply save yourself — by quitting.

Colorectal cancer screening

Experts disagree on frequency of screening for colorectal (or colon and rectal) cancer, but generally recommend annual testing after age 50. Adults at risk of colon and rectal cancer, including people with strong family or personal history of colon and rectal disease, should be screened earlier and more often.

Screening for colorectal cancer includes two tests. In the fecal occult blood test, you provide a stool sample for your doctor, who tests it for blood. Blood in the stool indicates that cancer may be present. The other test, a sigmoidoscopy, is more invasive. In this test, a flexible or inflexible scope is inserted into the rectum. Through the scope, your doctor can see whether cancer or other diseases are affecting the lower part of the colon.

Electrocardiogram (ECG or EKG)

Every three years after age 30 if your doctor thinks that you're at risk for heart disease; every three to four years after 50 if you're not at risk. Some doctors suggest that you get a baseline ECG test at age 40 to compare to later results.

An ECG involves electrodes pasted to your chest that, believe it or not, actually pick up your heart's electrical activity right through your skin. The heart is a big muscle, and the way your nerve impulses travel through it reveals a lot about how good a job it's doing. If you can step back from the situation, the electronics freak in you may find this test pretty cool.

Men, it's time to bite the bullet

When it comes to prevention, the worst offenders are men. We all know guys who say, "We limp to the medicine chest in this family, buddy." And it's not just a stereotype: Medical research shows that men are more uncomfortable with physicians than women are, and that they're less likely to keep to a schedule for preventive health.

Unfortunately, the "strong and silent" approach to health becomes a risky toss of the dice as men get older. Consider that many conditions — such as high blood pressure, high cholesterol, heart disease, diabetes, and cancer — often don't cause noticeable symptoms until they have put you at serious risk. In fact, many experts think that this phobia about doctors may explain why men don't live as long as women — an average 72 years for men versus 79 for women.

The following sections summarize the screenings that men should make an effort to get.

Digital rectal examination (DRE)

Every year after age 40, although many doctors perform the test on patients at an earlier age.

The doctor's going to do what? Yes, guys, get over it. In a DRE, the doctor dons a glove, lubricates it, and then inserts a finger into the lower part of the rectum (see Figure 3-1). This exam picks up any problems with your prostate gland, including prostate cancer and benign prostatic hyperplasia,

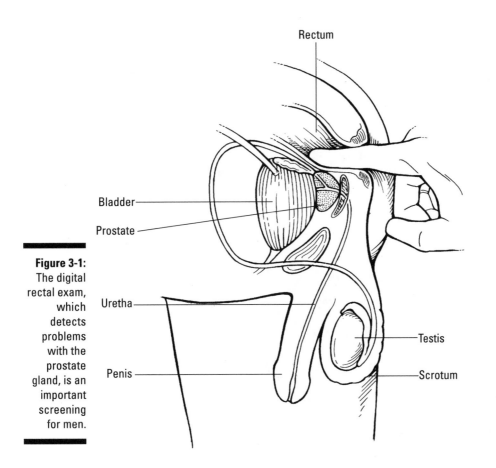

Rectum

Bladder

Prostate

Uretha

Penis

Testis

Scrotum

Figure 3-1:
The digital
rectal exam,
which
detects
problems
with the
prostate
gland, is an
important
screening
for men.

or enlarged prostate. This test probably does more to keep squeamish men from getting physicals than any other, but realize that it causes minimal discomfort and is over in a minute or less.

Prostate-specific antigen test

Annually after age 50.

To check for signs of prostate cancer, your doctor may perform a simple blood test called the *prostate-specific antigen (PSA) test*. The test measures the amount of prostate-specific antigen in your blood. High levels of this substance may indicate cancer.

Not all doctors agree about the course of action to take with a positive result on the PSA because roughly a third of the time it either misses the disease or says that a person who doesn't have it has it. Talk with your physician about this test, and also see Chapter 16 for more information about prostate disease and this controversy.

Testicular examination

Annually by a professional, along with monthly self-examinations, starting in adulthood.

Although it accounts for only 1 percent of all cancers in American men, testicular cancer is the most common cancer in men between the ages of 15 and 34. Many doctors perform the exam during an annual physical, and experts recommend self-examination monthly. Self-examination increases the chance that the disease is caught early, when it's most curable. Figure 3-2 shows the correct method for performing a testicular self-exam.

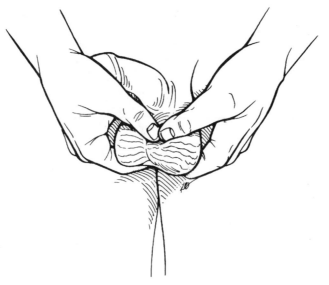

Figure 3-2: Men should perform a testicular self-exam monthly.

To perform a testicular self-exam, or TSE, do the following:

- ✔ Look for any swelling on the surface of the scrotum while standing before a mirror.

- ✔ Gently examine each testicle by placing your index and middle fingers underneath the testicle and your thumbs on top. Roll the testicle between your thumbs and fingers, feeling for any abnormal lumps. Do not confuse the epididymis (the cord within the testicle that transports sperm) with a lump.

- ✔ If you feel anything unusual, visit your doctor as soon as possible. Lumps occur for reasons other than cancer (for example, infection), but only a professional can make a diagnosis.

Women, keep up the good work

When it comes to health care, women are generally in charge. From the teenage years, women begin to learn their way around the medical system, thanks to concerns about menstruation, birth control, and pregnancy. The education continues as women take the roles of partners, wives, and mothers.

Prevention, of course, matters very much to women, so make sure that you get what you need. Don't limit your contact with your doctor to a mere phone call when your birth control prescription runs out. The following sections cover a few of the basic screenings that you should get, and when you should get them.

Gynecological exam

Annually after age 18 and for women who are sexually active.

The gynecological exam usually includes a pelvic examination, a Pap test, and a breast examination:

✔ **Pelvic exam:** In a pelvic exam, the practitioner inserts a duck-billed device called a *speculum* into the vagina. When the speculum is opened, the walls of the vagina are spread apart, allowing the doctor to check for signs of infection and view the *cervix,* the opening of the *uterus,* or the womb. With a swab or brush, the doctor takes samples of the mucus covering the cervix to check for infection and also does a Pap test.

After removing the speculum, the practitioner inserts two gloved fingers into the vagina and places the other hand on the abdomen. The doctor then feels the uterus and *ovaries,* the organs that produce female hormones and eggs, checking for any abnormalities. The doctor may also insert a finger into the rectum to check for problems.

✔ **Pap test:** A Pap test (named after its inventor, Dr. George Papanicolaou, and sometimes called a Pap smear) is nothing more than a special way of sampling cells from the cervix for an early detection of changes that could turn into cancer. During the pelvic examination, the gynecologist uses a swab or small brush (the latter has been found to be more effective) to collect cells, which are then examined under a microscope. An abnormal result means that some cells may be showing changes that could lead to cancer or that cancerous cells are already present. But don't panic: Noncancerous conditions, such as vaginal infections, sometimes produce abnormal results as well. Figure 3-3 shows how a practitioner performs a Pap test.

Some women who get a clean bill of health from a Pap test three times in a row may be able to get the test less frequently.

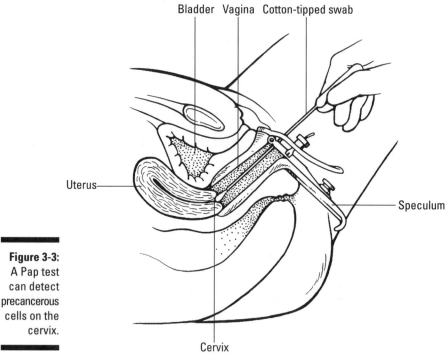

Bladder Vagina Cotton-tipped swab

Uterus

Speculum

Figure 3-3:
A Pap test
can detect
precancerous
cells on the
cervix.

Cervix

JARGON ALERT

Following up a Pap test

A colposcopy and a biopsy are performed as follow-ups to an abnormal Pap test in some cases. A colposcopy sounds a little scary, but it's actually just the use of a magnifying scope to view areas of the cervix up-close. Through the scope, practitioners can see areas they'd like to sample.

After an area is located, a biopsy is done. In a biopsy, a small amount of tissue is removed to be tested for abnormal cells. Through biopsy, practitioners can tell whether cancer is present and, if so, how advanced it is.

✔ **Breast exam:** For this test, you lie on your back and extend one arm above your head. The practitioner gently feels the breast and armpit for any abnormal lumps. Then you switch arms, and the practitioner examines the other breast.

But don't leave the breast exam up to your doctor — perform it yourself on a monthly basis. Figure 3-4 shows the correct method for a breast self-exam. (You can do the self-exam while in the shower if you wish.) A breast exam is your first line of defense against breast cancer. In fact, about 80 percent of breast cancers are detected through women checking their breasts themselves. The value of breast self-examination can't be stressed enough. When caught early, breast cancer can be cured. When caught late, you can die. Enough said.

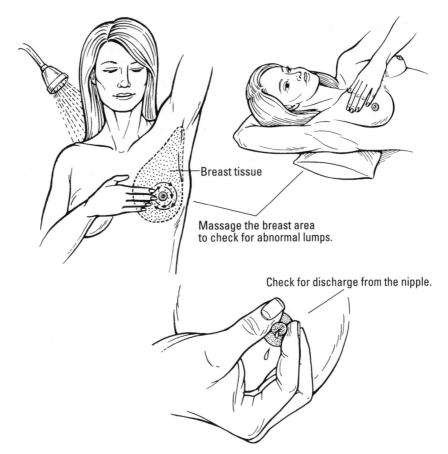

Breast tissue

Massage the breast area
to check for abnormal lumps.

Check for discharge from the nipple.

Figure 3-4:
Doing a
monthly
breast self-
exam may
help you
detect signs
of breast
cancer early.

HEALTH AT HOME

Examining your breasts at home

Try to remember to do this exam at the same time every month because your breasts can change throughout your menstrual cycle. You can also do this test in the shower — the water and soap make it easier for fingers to slide over the skin. To perform a breast self-exam, says the American Cancer Society, do the following. See your doctor immediately if you notice anything unusual during the exam.

✔ Lie down, place a pillow under your right shoulder, and stretch your right arm over your head. Use the three middle fingers of your left hand to feel the right breast for any lumps or thickening. Press hard enough to know what the breast feels like. Repeat the process for the other breast.

A pattern helps make sure that you don't miss an area. You can move your fingers in straight rows across the breast, start at the center and spiral outward, or start from the center and radiate outward in a star pattern.

✔ After checking for lumps, examine the nipples for any changes and squeeze them gently. Tell your practitioner of any irregularities or discharge.

✔ Finally, stand in front of a mirror and look for any dimpling or swelling in the breasts. Check with your hands at your sides and then raise your arms above your head and check again.

Many women skip the self-exam because the idea of doing it makes them worry about breast cancer — not a welcome thought. Try to think of the exam as a way to stay healthy and catch any molehills before they turn into mountains.

Mammogram

Annually for women over age 50 and for women at risk of breast cancer. Women ages 40 to 49 should decide with their practitioners whether to have a mammogram.

A mammogram uses X-rays of the breast to detect breast cancer. A technician places your breast between two flat plates, which are then gently squeezed together as the X-ray picture is taken. In terms of comfort, it may not be a barrel of laughs, but it's worth it if you value your health.

A *radiologist,* an expert in deciphering X-rays, interprets the results of a mammogram according to the appearance of the image. A cancerous tumor tends to have irregular edges, for example, whereas a benign one usually has well-defined edges. Know, however, that a mammogram is not a diagnosis of cancer. Images on X-rays are not always what they appear, and because the picture is judged by an individual, results are somewhat subjective.

Diagnosis of cancer can be done only through a breast biopsy, a procedure that removes a small amount of tissue for lab tests. The biopsy can take the form of a small surgical operation or can be done with a hollow needle that samples a smaller amount of tissue.

Experts are unable to agree on when women between the ages of 40 and 49 who don't have a risk for breast cancer should begin to have regular mammograms. (Cancer is hard to detect in younger women because the breast tissue is denser. As a result, the younger you are, the greater the chance you will be misdiagnosed and have to undergo an unnecessary biopsy.) Your decision on mammography should be based on your personal needs, however, so talk over the issue with your practitioner.

Children: Looking toward a lifetime

Chapter 13 provides a lot of detail on keeping your kids healthy, but we want to stress just a few tips about regular health testing specifically for children.

Metabolic screening

Immediately after birth.

By law, your child will be checked for certain disorders of the body's chemistry called metabolic disorders — for example, *phenylketonuria* (PKU), an inherited disease that interferes with the body's ability to eliminate substances found in many foods. Parents should know as soon as possible about such conditions so that, as in the case of PKU, they can make sure the child avoids consuming the problem substance in the first place.

Routine visits

Well-baby visits every two to three months in the first two years of life, with annual examinations each year after age 2.

During a routine visit, your child's height, weight, head circumference, and blood pressure are measured and recorded. The doctor checks for normal reflex development, muscle and skin tone, and overall appearance. The doctor also observes the child's breathing and evaluates the lungs by using a stethoscope. The doctor also asks you questions about the child's sleeping and eating habits and other behaviors.

What new parent hasn't agonized over whether a child is gaining enough weight in the first few months? For reassurance, pop into your doctor's office for a spot-check of weight. Most practices won't require a prior appointment.

Routine visits are important because they

- ✔ Forge a relationship between you, your doctor, and your child, without the stress of illness as a backdrop.
- ✔ Help children become comfortable with doctors; because they're not sick at the visits, they don't associate the doctor with pain.

✔ Give you an opportunity to ask questions and boost your confidence as a parent.

✔ Provide normal, baseline measurements of your child against which to compare abnormal findings during illness.

Hemoglobin test

At 9 months of age.

The American Academy of Pediatrics suggests that children get a finger-prick blood test to determine hemoglobin level. *Hemoglobin* is a molecule in the red blood cells that helps the blood carry oxygen.

This procedure tests for *anemia,* a condition that occurs most commonly from a lack of iron. Anemia is more prevalent in children under 1 year than you may expect. Anemia in children interferes with their proper development.

Although you may see that formula and cereal are fortified with iron, the baby's body cannot absorb this type of iron as easily as the type found in breast milk. And even mother's milk by itself may not provide enough iron in all cases. Depending on the mix of formula, solids, breast milk, and other foods that you give your baby, there's always the chance that the baby may not have received an adequate amount of iron.

Lead test

At 9 months of age.

You should ask that your child's first blood lead level test be performed at 9 months, even though some practitioners will want to give the test only to kids living in older houses. The problem with skipping the test is that, if yours is like most families today, you have patched together a mix of baby-sitting, day care, and other child care providers, all in different buildings. Knowing whether lead-based paint has been used in all these different structures is impossible. To play it safe, ask for the test.

Vision and hearing tests

At 3 years of age.

The American Academy of Pediatrics recommends that your child receive his or her first standardized tests of hearing and vision at age 3. Before that, subjective tests will do. If 3 years old sounds early, remember that hearing and vision problems can be confused with learning problems, and your child could needlessly experience serious developmental problems if he or she can't see or hear well.

If something's wrong

If a checkup uncovers a problem, ask the following questions:

✔ What's the exact name of my child's illness?

✔ What causes it?

✔ How long does it last?

✔ Is it infectious? Can my child go to day care or school?

✔ What should we be doing at home to make the child better?

✔ If it gets worse, what symptoms should I look out for?

✔ Should we schedule a follow-up visit now?

✔ What can we do to prevent it in the future?

Seniors: Staying young at heart

We can't stress strongly enough that age does not equal disease. Granted, many people do face more health problems as they grow older, but that doesn't mean that they're inevitable or that you have to take them lying down. What's more, it doesn't mean that you should neglect prevention. Whatever the adage says, it's not all downhill from here.

Stick to your preventive schedule much as you have in the past, but be sure to speak with your doctor about exceptions and additions to your plan. For example, if you've had regular Pap tests throughout your life and have not experienced any abnormalities, you may be able to forgo that test. If colon and rectal cancer runs in your family, preventive screening may need to be stepped up a bit. Everyone is unique, and the older you become, the more your care will need to be individualized to suit your needs.

Find a practitioner who specializes in *geriatrics* — treatment of the elderly. These doctors, who sometimes subspecialize in heart disease or cancer treatment, have additional training that puts them in tune with seniors' needs. Contact the American Geriatric Society at 212-308-1414 to find a geriatric specialist in your area.

That said, consider these additional preventive screenings that are recommended for older adults.

Vision and hearing tests

A doctor uses standard testing to test your eyes and ears. Unfortunately, the senses of hearing and sight often deteriorate with aging — but again, you don't have to accept it. Regular testing can help catch problems early, before they put you out of action.

Influenza and pneumonia vaccinations

As an older adult, you're more vulnerable to the flu and the complications that it can cause. To prevent problems, the Centers for Disease Control and Prevention recommends an annual flu vaccine and pneumonia vaccine for everyone over the age of 65.

Nutrition tests

Physicians should monitor nutrition as well. Surprisingly, some older adults have trouble getting enough vitamins and minerals. Some men and women find it hard to get out to buy food, and others have problems with their teeth and gums. Seniors with memory problems may simply forget meals. (See Chapter 2 for more on nutrition.)

Polypharmacy

No, *polypharmacy* is not the name of the latest drugstore chain. That's what experts call the problem of the complicated mix of over-the-counter and prescription drugs that many older people take. As a preventive measure, a doctor should sit down with you regularly and go over the medications that you're taking to ensure your good health.

Why is this step necessary for seniors? Because the kidneys and the liver become less effective at ridding your body of toxins with age, it's especially important that your doctor know all the medicines you're taking. They can interact harmfully and may even cause a problem that would require a visit to the doctor.

Digging Up Your Family History

We're not talking about skeletons in the closet here, but about medical history. Why dig into your family's medical past? Because, to borrow a cliché, to be forewarned is to be forearmed in your quest to keep your family healthy. Many health conditions are passed down from generation to generation. And knowing what you're up against can help you prevent and anticipate certain health problems.

Family history comes into play in two ways when it comes to health. Genetic conditions may occur because of problems with the genetic material passed on by parents. In addition, a number of other conditions — such as heart disease, diabetes, and cancer — also tend to run in families, although they're not directly linked to gene abnormalities. Such problems are called *familial conditions*.

Pooling your genes

First, a genetics lesson. We know that your eyes glazed over when your junior high biology teacher started babbling about Gregor Mendel, his pea plants, and the wonderful history of genetics. But now it's time to pay attention.

Everybody on this planet started from a single fertilized egg made up of an egg cell from the woman and a sperm cell from the man. What's remarkable is that a single fertilized cell contains the complete blueprint for a person. The information of this blueprint comes from chromosomes, genetic material made up of *DNA,* or *deoxyribonucleic acid.* Every cell contains 46 chromosomes arranged in 23 pairs. Half of the chromosomes are inherited from the mother and half from the father.

Now, this genetic blueprint can have problems: Little bits of genetic information can get thrown out of whack, which can result in a health disorder. Or an abnormal chromosome may be inherited from one or both parents. Parents may not even know that an abnormal gene is present because the characteristics of certain genes (called *dominant genes*) can overshadow others (called *recessive genes*). If a child ends up with a pair of recessive genes, however, that overshadowed trait comes to the surface.

Some genetic traits cause serious disease. Wouldn't you want to know as soon as possible? That's what genetic testing is for. If you're concerned about the possibility of a genetic condition (for example, you may know of something that runs in your family), you can have your chromosomes analyzed *before* conceiving a child to anticipate the odds of certain genetic problems. Ask your doctor for more information about getting tested.

Combating familial disease

Check into your family's disease history by starting with your parents and siblings and then moving farther out on the limbs of the family tree. If a disease occurred early in a relative's life, or if you see it popping up in several places, that may be a warning sign that you're at risk for a similar condition. Table 3-1 lists some common inherited conditions.

Table 3-1	**Preventing Inherited Conditions**
Problem	*Screening*
Breast cancer	Yearly mammogram beginning at about age 35, plus regular self-exams
Cervical and vaginal cancer	Yearly Pap test and pelvic exam

(continued)

Table 3-1 *(continued)*

Problem	Screening
Colon cancer	Yearly test for blood in the stool, plus follow-up blood tests and physical examinations
Cystic fibrosis	Regular tests of lung dysfunction, stool, and sweat of infants and young children who may have inherited it
Diabetes	Regular blood sugar tests and urinalysis
Glaucoma	Glaucoma exam at age 40
Heart disease (heart attack, clogged arteries, stroke)	Regular blood pressure, serum cholesterol, and triglyceride tests; ECG test; and exercise-tolerance test
Leukemia	Complete blood count, chromosome analysis, and bone marrow biopsy
Lung cancer	Yearly chest X-ray and sputum (lung mucus) test beginning at age 50, NSE blood test
Oral cancer	Yearly dental exam, plus biopsy of suspicious tissue
Osteoporosis	Bone-density test before menopause
Ovarian cancer, cysts, and tumors	Yearly pelvic exam, ultrasound, and CA 125 blood test
Pancreatic cancer	CA 19-9 blood test
Polycystic kidney disease, kidney tumors	Urinalysis, ultrasound, and CAT scan
Prostate cancer	Digital rectal exam and PSA blood test
Stomach cancer	Endoscopic exam
Testicular cancer	AFP blood test, regular self-exam, and ultrasound
Uterine cancer	Endometrial biopsy

Enlist your doctor in your fight against familial disease. For many conditions, lifestyle changes, such as changes in the amount you exercise or eat, can reduce risk. Your doctor can also make sure that you get the proper screening tests to catch any problems early on, when they're most easily treated and cured. However, not every screening test is 100 percent accurate. *False-positive results* (which say that you have a disease when you don't) and *false-negative results* (which give you a clean bill of health when you have a problem) are common. Because many medical procedures are inherently risky, you shouldn't charge off and get serious treatment, such as an operation or chemotherapy, on the basis of limited testing. Instead, ask for repeat testing or a different type of test to confirm initial results.

Asking your parents about your medical history

Following are some of the specific questions with which you should ply your parents and other relatives — all in the name of health (yours and theirs!):

✔ **What are your health problems?** Ask for details about your parents' medical histories. Find out what medical conditions they had, at what age they developed those conditions, and how they were handled.

✔ **What was your parents' health like?** Ask for the same information about your maternal and paternal grandparents (if you can't ask your grandparents directly). Going back another generation can help define links further and alert you to potential problems. And while you're at it, be nosy about your aunts, uncles, and any other close relatives, too.

✔ **What about mental disorders?** Don't limit your quiz to questions about purely physical ailments. A number of mental conditions — depression and schizophrenia, to name a couple — sometimes have a family link.

✔ **Do any genetic diseases run in our family?** Hemophilia (a blood disorder) and muscular dystrophy (a degenerative muscle disease) are examples of genetic diseases. Ask about grandparents, aunts, uncles, and cousins. Get everyone in on the information exchange.

✔ **What sort of health did the women in our family have?** The answer to this question can alert you to potential health problems that you could face. For example, cervical cancer — one of the most serious cancers for females — can run in families. The normal risk of this disease is about 1 woman in 70, or 1.4 percent; however, if two or more first-degree relatives (a mother or a sister) have it, your risk jumps to 50 percent.

✔ **Mom, did you use DES while you were pregnant?** DES is a synthetic estrogen that was prescribed between 1941 and 1971. Millions of women took the drug, which was thought to help prevent miscarriages. The drug proved ineffective and, even worse, was found to have adverse effects on the reproductive, immune, and cardiovascular systems of the fetuses being carried by women taking the drug.

✔ **What were my vital statistics at birth?** Find out the date and time of your birth, your weight, your length, and your APGAR score (the results of a test that rates the general health of a newborn by examining heart rate, respiratory effort, muscle tone, response to a tube in the nostril, and color). If your parents can't give you specific information, at least find out your general condition at birth.

✔ **What was my health like when I was a child?** Find out which childhood conditions you suffered (chicken pox, measles, mumps, and so on), as well as whether you had any allergies or special health problems. Also ask about immunization. If you missed some shots as a child, you may be vulnerable to those same conditions now.

✓ **What were the names of your doctors? What were the names of mine?** The names of these physicians may come in handy if you need to track down medical records from long ago.

✓ **What is our family's background like in terms of lifestyle and environment?** A family may share health problems not because of a hereditary link but because of common lifestyles and environments. For example, if your family traditions include rich foods, you may find that many family members are overweight. Families who regularly vacation in sunny spots or who live along the equator may be more prone to skin cancer. To supplement your family's medical history, take notes on where they lived, their lifestyles, and any habits that catch your eye.

Checking Your Medical Records

Keeping track of your family's medical records is a key to prevention. A written record documents basic medical information (height, weight, blood pressure, cholesterol levels, and drug allergies), personal history (any health conditions and their treatments), family history (a record of diseases that may run in your family), preventive screening records, immunizations, and all the little details of health that may escape you through the years.

You can see why such a record would be handy if a health condition arose — all that information at your fingertips gives you more control over your health and can be crucial in making treatment decisions. Emergency situations also call for quick recall on matters such as blood type and prescription drug use.

You may assume that your doctor or hospital has all your pertinent medical information should you need it, but this is unfortunately not always the case. Fewer than half the states in the U.S. have laws guaranteeing consumers the right to their medical records. And many consumers who have requested copies of the records have found inaccuracies and problems in the pages.

In addition, medical records kept by practitioners are often incomplete. You may move several times in your lifetime and change physicians each time. Your different doctors may not keep each other informed of your treatment. Too often, an attempt to piece together a medical history becomes a futile search through old bills and insurance records — not something you want to be doing when a crisis occurs.

Putting together a medical record

For each family member, record the following information:

- Emergency phone numbers (police/fire/ambulance, poison control center, doctors, and other practitioners)
- Conditions or diseases that run in the family
- Vital statistics (blood types, heights, weights, cholesterol levels, blood pressure, and immunization records for children and adults)
- Personal medical histories (medical problems and treatments)
- Preventive screenings and results
- Known allergies, allergy symptoms, and treatments
- Hospital and laboratory records
- Gynecological and prenatal records for women
- Over-the-counter and prescription medications used
- Vision and hearing test results

Obtaining medical records

Don't just rely on your memory in putting together your record. Be sure to get copies of medical records from the professionals and facilities that have treated you and your family. These records complement your family record. Obtaining the records also gives you a chance to make sure that they're accurate.

For your reference, the 24 states that allow you direct access to your medical records (and those of your children) are Alaska, Arkansas, California, Colorado, Connecticut, Florida, Georgia, Hawaii, Indiana, Louisiana, Maryland, Michigan, Minnesota, Montana, Nevada, New Hampshire, New Jersey, New York, Oklahoma, South Dakota, Virginia, Washington, West Virginia, and Wisconsin. In Maine, Massachusetts, and Texas, your doctor has the option of giving you just a summary of your records.

What if your state isn't among the ones that allow direct access? Don't despair. States without the access law aren't prohibiting access — just remaining silent on the issue. Many medical practices will respond to a written request for records even if no state law calls for their release. Offer to pay a reasonable per page copying fee — up to 50 cents per page, for example. If you run into a roadblock, ask the office manager to put the denial in writing.

Obtaining veterans' medical records

If you were treated by the military or a Veterans Administration hospital, your right to see your hospital records is guaranteed by the federal Freedom of Information Act. This includes military hospitals, Veterans Administration hospitals, and prison hospitals. If you're on active duty, write to the facility at your post or a previous duty station. If you are retired or not on active duty, write to the National Archives Record Center, 9700 Page, St. Louis, MO 63132. Include your military identification number, branch of service, and dates of service.

Accessing the Medical Information Bureau (MIB)

Ever have the feeling that an organization is out there keeping tabs on you without your knowledge? Well, when it comes to health, such an organization exists: the Medical Information Bureau, or MIB.

The Medical Information Bureau provides information about individuals to insurance companies. How do they get that information? From health insurance forms you've filled out. Over the years, the details of your health are forwarded to the MIB by your insurance company and entered into its database.

Insurance companies use the information supplied by the MIB to determine whether they will insure you, so you must make sure that your file is accurate. If your file erroneously states that you have cancer, for example, you may be denied insurance or charged exorbitant rates for coverage.

In the past, the MIB's files were closed to consumers. However, the MIB will now disclose your records to you for an $8 fee. To request your record, write to Medical Information Bureau, P. O. Box 105, Essex Station, Boston, MA 02112, or call the MIB at 617-329-4500 and ask for a copy of the form "Request for Disclosure of MIB Record Information."

Part II
Health Begins at Home

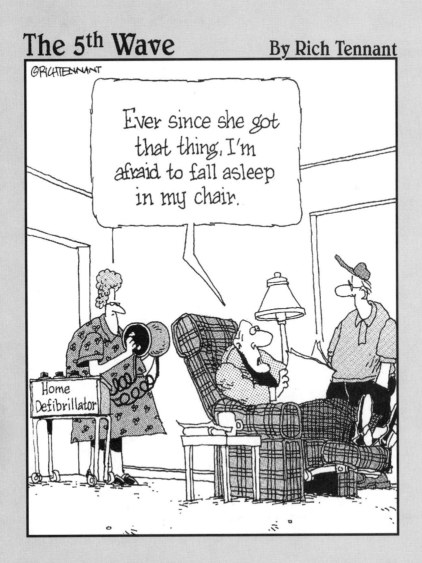

The 5th Wave   By Rich Tennant

@RICHTENNANT

Ever since she got that thing, I'm afraid to fall asleep in my chair.

Home Defibrillator

In this part . . .

The Boy Scout motto is "Be Prepared," and that's just what we want you to be. This part helps you make sure that your home is prepared for minor first aid and emergencies. We tell you what to keep in your medicine chest, what *not* to keep in your medicine chest, and when to call for help. Scout's honor, this is important stuff!

Chapter 4

Being Prepared

• •

In This Chapter

▶ Keeping basic medical supplies on hand

▶ Troubleshooting with home remedies

▶ Childproofing your home

▶ Discovering hidden dangers: Radon and carbon monoxide

• •

*H*ealth begins at home. Sure, your family practitioners are there — we hope — when you need them, but for the most part, you're going to be preventing and dealing with everyday health problems on your own turf. And whether you realize it or not, you're probably quite capable of handling your family's health care needs. In fact, estimates say that a whopping 80 percent of all health care is self-care!

If this sounds like a lot of responsibility, realize that you're probably better equipped than you think. On a day-to-day basis, you may take care of minor medical problems (skinned knees and headaches), regulate your family's nutrition ("Finish your vegetables or no dessert!"), and protect everyone from accidents and injuries. Whether you've treated a twisted ankle with ice or prepared for major surgery, participating in self-care activities is something you've done.

This chapter can help you become more prepared by telling you what to stock in your medicine cabinet, giving you the knowledge to monitor signs and symptoms, and helping you develop the ability to treat a wide range of injuries and illnesses with some common home remedies — plus a little common sense. For information about emergency care, check out Chapter 5.

Stocking Your Medicine Cabinet

Nine basic items should be in everyone's medicine cabinet:

> ✔ **Pain relievers such as aspirin or aspirin substitutes:** Keep in mind that aspirin should not be given to children under age 18 because of its association with Reye's syndrome.

- ✔ **Syrup of ipecac, used to induce vomiting:** Ipecac is good to have on hand, but never use it without your doctor's advice — it may do more harm than good in certain circumstances.

- ✔ **Antacid:** For gastrointestinal distress.

- ✔ **Antidiarrheal medication**

- ✔ **Petroleum jelly:** For soothing some minor skin conditions, softening the skin, and protecting wound dressings.

- ✔ **Laxatives**

- ✔ **Salt:** A natural antiseptic.

- ✔ **Thermometer:** If you have kids under age 3, have a rectal thermometer on hand as well as an oral one.

- ✔ **First aid kit containing antibiotic ointment, hydrogen peroxide, an ice pack, gauze, adhesive and gauze pads, bandages, cotton and cotton-tipped swabs, hydrocortisone cream, scissors, soap, tissues, tweezers, and a first-aid manual:** Every first-aid area should also include a list of essential phone numbers in case of emergency: local police, fire, and ambulance, poison control center, and family physician.

Your medicine cabinet should not be easily accessible to children or in an area where the temperature fluctuates. See Chapter 11 for specifics on storing medications.

Childproofing Your Home

Accident-free homes do not exist. Tragically, accidents are the leading cause of death among children, causing one of every two fatalities. Whether your child is young, with no sense of danger, or old enough to deliberately experiment with the hazards around your home, take steps to make your home a safer environment for your child.

Eyeglasses, garage doors, airbags — even the cords on the blinds in your living room — are hazards for kids given the right circumstances. Because so many potential dangers lurk all around you, listing every child safety guideline is impossible — you'd be looking at information about topics ranging from car seats and sports equipment to choking hazards and playground games. As you know, kids get into anything and everything — and you can't anticipate every circumstance that may befall them. (That's why they're called "accidents.") But still, you have to try.

For a complete overview of child safety — we can't say it all here — we recommend that you check out your local library for books and magazine articles on the subject. Don't forget to look in magazines designed for parents — they're especially attuned to these issues.

In the meantime, the following sections give you an idea of some of the potential problem areas that you and your kids may encounter in the home.

Taking baby steps to prevention

Babies are rarely out of a parent's sight and thankfully don't have the run of the house. Still, you should take a few precautions to ensure your infant's safety.

Take the crib, for example — the one place your baby spends time without your looking on. To be safe, a crib should have no sharp edges and a locking mechanism to keep the sides in place. The distance from the top of the rail to the mattress should be at least 26 inches when the mattress is at its lowest level. The mattress should fit snugly, and bumper pads should be in place to protect the baby from banging against the sides. A pillow is unnecessary and should not be used.

If you're using a family heirloom or a second-hand crib, make sure that it's up to date on safety requirements. An old crib may be painted with a lead-based paint, which is poisonous if consumed, or the slats on its sides may be too far apart, posing a choking hazard.

These additional tips will help keep your baby safe:

- ✔ Keep plastic bags away from your baby. Young children can suffocate while playing with plastic bags.
- ✔ Select only fireproof blankets and pajamas.
- ✔ If you place a mobile over the crib, make sure that it is secure and out of baby's reach.
- ✔ Toys in the crib should be large and soft — no sharp edges! Avoid stuffed animals or other toys with buttons or parts that can be swallowed.
- ✔ Check how low to the floor or crib — and the reach of a child — cords from curtains or blinds hang down. Cords pose a choking or hanging risk.

Taking care of toddlers

After kids find their feet, there's no stopping them. When your child begins to have access to your entire home, you need to take extra safety measures.

First, you need to restrict access for your child. Place baby gates at the tops and bottoms of staircases, and lock or guard windows that may be accessible to your child. After you've got your child toddling in just a few rooms, eliminate the hazards. Cover unused electrical outlets with those inexpensive covers available at most hardware stores, and cut off access to dangerous substances such as cleaning products, insecticides, matches, and medications. (See the section "Storing toxic products" for more tips.) Keep these items out of reach, or install childproof locks on cabinets. Keep an eye out for less-obvious hazards, too. For example, some plants can be toxic, so keep them up high, away from your child.

In the kitchen, keep pot handles pointed toward the stove so that they can't be grabbed or bumped into, and don't use cloths or mats that your child can easily pull off the table. Never leave a hot beverage near the edge of a table, and don't drink hot stuff with your kid on your lap. Even tap water can be a hazard — 160-degree water can scald a child. Keep the thermostat on your water heater between 120 and 125 degrees Fahrenheit.

In the bathroom, restrict access to cupboards and the medicine cabinet. Keep the lid down on the toilet seat, too. As unlikely as it seems, a few inches of water pose a drowning hazard. Finally, never leave your infant unattended in the bathtub, no matter how little water is present.

Playing safely outdoors

You've taken care of the inside of the house. Now take a look at the yard.

- ✔ Locate your child's outdoor play area where you can monitor activities from inside your home.
- ✔ Put play equipment on grass, wood chips, sand, or other soft surfaces to reduce the risk of injury from falls.
- ✔ Make sure that equipment is anchored to avoid tipping.
- ✔ Make sure that equipment is safe and in good condition: Sand rough wood to avoid slivers, file metal smooth to avoid scrapes, and discard equipment that is fragile or worn out.
- ✔ Establish ground rules: one person on the swing at a time; hold on with both hands, no standing or kneeling allowed.

Storing toxic products

Keeping your home environment safe requires a little extra effort, but doing so decreases your risk of accidents due to potentially toxic household items.

In the kitchen:

- ✔ Keep your kitchen knives and matches stored out of the reach of children.
- ✔ Be careful to keep grease and drippings away from open flames.
- ✔ Never leave small children unattended in your kitchen.

   ✔ Store cleaning fluids and other chemicals in a high or locked cabinet.

   ✔ Keep drawers and cupboards closed.

   ✔ Be sure that all poisons are stored safely and clearly marked.

In the bathroom:

   ✔ Keep all medicines out of the reach of children.

   ✔ Avoid discarding razor blades, hypodermic needles (for insulin and other shots), and other potentially dangerous goods in wastebaskets to which your child has access.

   ✔ Dispose of all expired medicines safely.

In the basement, garage, and utility room:

   ✔ Keep cleaning fluids, paints, additives, fuels, and oils labeled and well out of the reach of children.

   ✔ Never reuse food containers to store toxic liquids — a child may take a sip from a soda bottle that now contains paint thinner or some other poison.

Seniors and safety

Children aren't the only members of a household who are vulnerable to accidents: Seniors are at risk, too. Poor vision, limited mobility, and health problems can contribute to accidents in older people, so it's important to think of them when giving your house a once-over for safety.

Think about lighting, for one thing. Are your halls and stairwells well-lit, and can you turn the lights on and off from either end of the hall? Do you have exterior lights at all entrances to make coming and going easier? You may want to invest in flashlights and night-lights — and maybe line the walls with luminescent tape — to prevent nighttime accidents.

Because a fall can be devastating to an older adult, you want to "fall-proof," as well. Make sure that the stairs have handrails — you can even install them in the shower and tub. Rooms should be uncluttered, with low-pile carpeting or slip-resistant area rugs. Arrange the furniture to create unobstructed pathways through the house.

Finally, think about burns and other emergencies. Some seniors are vulnerable to burns because they've lost sensitivity to heat and cold; when they touch a hot object, they may not feel enough to pull away until serious damage has been done. Make sure that your stove has lights to indicate when it's on, and adjust the water temperature in your house to prevent scalding. Keep flammable items, such as paper towels and dishcloths, away from the stovetop, too. Also post emergency numbers in large letters next to phones — and see that the phones themselves have large numbers on them.

Preventing Food Poisoning

Diarrhea, stomach cramps, nausea, and a few hours of discomfort: If you think that's all food poisoning adds up to, you're dead wrong. Although a healthy adult's system may be able to fight off an unwanted bug with minor symptoms, children and seniors are very vulnerable to the bacteria that cause food poisoning. If poisoning occurs and you don't seek emergency care immediately, you may face a life-or-death situation.

When your kids order a burger at a fast-food restaurant, you probably worry that they may be getting a little something "extra." Odds are, however, that when food poisoning strikes your family, it will be at home in your kitchen. Some of the very things that Mom taught you about food preparation could lead to big trouble. To minimize your family's risks, keep these tips in mind:

- Store uncooked meats away from other foods, and never rinse raw meat off in the sink before cooking.

- Make sure that your refrigerator temperature stays at a constant 40 degrees Fahrenheit and your freezer below 0 degrees Fahrenheit.

- Wash your hands, cooking utensils, and cutting boards frequently. Antibacterial soaps, as well as bleach, may help prevent contamination.

- Thaw frozen food in the refrigerator, not on the counter.

- Wash all produce, even cantaloupes and other fruits with rinds that you don't eat. The bacteria that cause food poisoning aren't limited to meat products.

- Don't undercook meat or poultry.

- Cool cooked food quickly before storing it in the refrigerator. Break it up into smaller portions to speed the cooling process.

- Eat leftovers promptly.

- Disinfect your sink drain, pipes, and garbage disposal with a weak bleach and water solution.

- Air-dry your dishes. Towel drying can spread germs.

Want to reduce your risk of infection all around? Kill those germs! Wash your hands several times a day, before eating or handling food, and after coming into contact with someone who may be ill. Lather up with warm water and an antibacterial soap and wash for about 20 seconds before rinsing for the best effects.

Spotting Invisible Hazards

Don't have enough to think about? Then consider this: Radon and carbon monoxide are odorless, invisible gases that may lead to disease and death if not detected in time. How to stop them? Read on.

Reacting to radon

Most people are not exposed to enough radon to have it seriously harm their health. However, evidence shows that prolonged exposure may lead to lung cancer and related health problems. Children may be at a higher risk than adults from indoor radon because, at their smaller size, they receive a higher dose per unit of exposure.

Radon can enter your home through cracks and crevices, loose joints, water pipes, sewer pipes, basement drains, exposed earth, or any opening. The Environmental Protection Agency (EPA) estimates that up to 8 million homes may have radon levels that exceed current allowable limits and that require corrective action. This means that you have about a 10 percent chance of your home containing a significant amount of radon.

So if you can't smell it, taste it, or see it, how do you know if it's there? Several inexpensive ($15 to $40) and easy-to-use kits are available to measure the level of radon present in your home. If testing your home reveals radon levels of 4 picocuries per liter of air or higher, the EPA recommends that you take corrective action. Removing radon can be done at a minimal expense and inconvenience.

Sniffing out carbon monoxide

Carbon monoxide causes more deaths in the United States each year than any other toxin. The gas is produced when natural gas, coal, or other fuels aren't burned completely or adequately ventilated by appliances such as gas dryers and furnaces.

Although the effects of radon gas build up over a lifetime, carbon monoxide kills quickly. A few minutes of exposure trigger symptoms such as headache, dizziness, drowsiness, rapid breathing, chest pain, nausea, and a red skin color. Further exposure leads to convulsions, unconsciousness, and heart and respiratory failure. Breathing an air concentration of a mere 0.05 percent of the gas can be fatal within a half-hour.

To prevent carbon monoxide poisoning, have your furnace inspected annually, and use heaters and barbecue grills in well-ventilated areas. Don't heat up your car in a closed garage, especially if the garage is attached to the house.

Also, invest in an early-warning system. Carbon monoxide detectors, which sound an alarm when they detect the gas, are relatively inexpensive, and studies show them to be highly effective in preventing poisoning from the gas. The alarm is designed to give you enough warning time to open windows and shut down appliances that may be generating the gas.

Home Remedies

Ever wonder whether Granny Clampett was on to something? Granted, the home remedies that she used on *The Beverly Hillbillies* — from 'possum tail to eye of newt — were pretty outrageous, but her character may have reflected what we always suspected: that Grandmother's home remedies were usually pretty effective. Why else would they be passed on from generation to generation?

Recently, a trend toward natural, basic treatments (in lieu of drugs and chemicals) has been growing. In addition to being less costly than doctor visits, these time-tested treatments are at times much safer than drugs and carry less danger of side effects. (Bear in mind that in some cases, you'll need to resort to OTC medications, but most of the remedies listed here are natural.)

Treating 25 common ills

Home remedies — using products that are easily found in the marketplace, indeed also found in typical household use — are the cornerstone of self-care. However, if you have any question or doubt about a product, mixture, or application, do not attempt self-care. Consult a first-aid or self-care guide or a medical practitioner for additional information.

Athlete's foot

Dab the infected area with vinegar morning, night, and throughout the day if your schedule permits. Vitamin E oil applied to the infected area is an additional remedy that many people find helpful (although some people are sensitive to it and should avoid putting it on their skin). Over-the-counter preparations specially formulated for athlete's foot are available as well.

Bee stings

Quickly apply meat tenderizer. It contains papain, which helps break down the proteins found in insect venom. ***Very important:*** Remove the stinger by scraping across the sting with a knife or other firm object — do not use your fingers to remove the stinger because you could accidentally squeeze the venom sack, releasing more venom into the wound. Take an antihistamine to reduce pain and swelling, and apply an ice pack to further reduce swelling. Elevate the body part if possible.

Boils

Hot compresses can help bring a boil to a natural head, allowing it to rupture and drain. Poultices, a favorite Pennsylvania Dutch folk remedy, are made from either warm milk and flour or bread crumbs and honey. The warm mixture is spread between layers of soft fabric and placed over the boil. Applying vitamin E directly to the boil is also recommended (although some people are sensitive to it and should not put it on their skin).

Bruises

To help avoid a nasty bruise when you've been bumped hard, immediately apply an ice pack wrapped in a towel to the area. This constricts the blood vessels and reduces the swelling. If no ice is available, a pack of frozen vegetables will do. Use the ice pack as long as it is comfortable.

Burns and sunburns

Calamine lotion can be used for subnurn and minor thermal (heat) burns that do not result in blisters. The same is true of aloe vera (the juice from the aloe plant).

Chicken pox

An oatmeal bath often relieves the itching that accompanies chicken pox. First, cook 1 to 2 cups of oatmeal and put it into a cloth bag made from two thicknesses of an old sheet. Float this bag in a tub of warm water, swishing it around until the water becomes silky. Let your child play in the water, making sure that the water covers all the sores.

Common cold

Flavored zinc lozenges have become very popular for use in preventing or lessening the severity of the common cold. Vitamin C is helpful in preventing a cold, but after a cold is established, garlic tea is a good remedy. Boil 4 cups of water and remove from the heat. Add freshly crushed garlic cloves to the water and let the mixture steep. Drink it while it's quite hot. Adding crushed garlic to a vaporizer may also relieve the nasal congestion that's often associated with a head cold.

Constipation

A high-fiber diet is known to be of vital importance to digestion. Make sure that your daily intake includes foods such as peas, beans, potatoes, carrots, whole-wheat bread, other whole-grain products, dried and fresh fruits, nuts, berries, and seeds. Bran is a concentrated form of fiber; include it in your diet, and drink plenty of water.

Cracked skin

Cracked skin often responds to zinc supplements. Experts suggest that a person take 10 milligrams, three times a day. It may take a month or more before you see results. Another remedy is vitamin E oil (although some people are sensitive to it and should not put it on their skin). A few drops rubbed into cracked skin each day often bring results within a week.

Cuts and scrapes

Cuts and many other minor skin injuries heal faster when they are closed. Covering a cut also helps prevent infection. Petroleum jelly helps protect skin surfaces by providing a physical barrier to further harm or irritation and making the wound area less painful.

Dandruff

More than one home remedy exists for dandruff. You can try applying one or two capfuls of apple cider vinegar to your scalp after a shower. Next, take a small portion of castor oil, rub it vigorously into your scalp, and then comb your hair.

Diaper rash

Both liquid lecithin and vitamin E oil are reportedly effective when commercial ointments and cornstarch fail to work. (Some people, though, are sensitive to topical vitamin E and should not put it on their skin.)

Headaches

Vitamin B_6 (pyridoxine) at a recommended dosage of 100 milligrams a day has been reported to help relieve migraine headaches. For sinus headaches, you can try taking niacin three times a day for a total of 100 milligrams.

Hemorrhoids

If your case is severe, see your doctor. For less-severe cases, rutin tablets, a bioflavonoid found in health food stores, may help ease the pain and swelling. Rutin is found naturally in buckwheat, oranges, and lemons, but not in sufficient amounts to provide rapid relief. Sitz baths can also be used to relieve the discomfort and pain of hemorrhoids, as well as to speed healing. A high-fiber diet has been known to prevent and even help relieve some hemorrhoids.

Hives

Take an over-the-counter antihistamine, but be sure to read the label first. Some antihistamines cause drowsiness, making it inadvisable to drive or operate large machinery after taking them. If shortness of breath occurs, get yourself to the nearest emergency room.

Indigestion

One simple cause of indigestion is eating too much. Smoking also can add to the problem. But if neither overeating nor smoking is the culprit, simple remedies are available. Try drinking mint tea to aid in digestion. Papaya enzymes (available at health food stores) also can help.

Leg cramps

If you suffer from chronic, nighttime leg cramps, taking dolomite and bonemeal orally before bedtime has been known to help. Sometimes bone-meal alone brings relief. If you have recurring leg cramps, you may be deficient in potassium. Adding foods such as bananas, oranges, potatoes, and tomatoes to your diet may provide the potassium you require.

Mosquito bites

Apply ice to the bite. The ice may help reduce swelling and inflammation. Or dissolve 1 tablespoon of Epsom salts in a quart of water, chill, and then place on the bite with a cloth.

Poison ivy, poison oak, or poison sumac

Immediately rinse the affected area with rubbing alcohol followed by water. Wash your clothing to deactivate poison ivy's itch-causing urishol oil. If you break out in a rash, try any of the following: calamine lotion, zinc oxide, witch hazel, baking soda, or Burow's solution (aluminum acetate).

The best way to deal with the rash that these plants cause is to avoid the plants in the first place! Figure 4-1 shows you what to steer clear of.

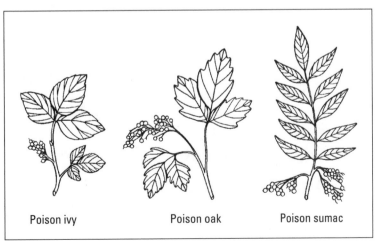

Figure 4-1:
Poison ivy, poison oak, and poison sumac can cause an itchy rash.

Poison ivy   Poison oak   Poison sumac

Shingles

Increase your intake of vitamins C and E. Liberally apply vitamin E oil to the sores (although some people are sensitive to it and should not put it on their skin).

Sore throat

Severe sore throats should be examined by a doctor to rule out strep infections. For common sore throats, however, several types of hot teas and gargles are recommended. One tea recipe calls for hot water, honey, lemon, and a dash of red pepper. One gargle cure calls for $1/4$ cup of vinegar in 1 cup of water, with a dash each of black pepper and salt. Heat the mixture before gargling.

Swimmer's ear

A few drops of warm vinegar in the ear canal can restore its proper pH balance (a measure of acidity or alkalinity) and prevent the growth of the bacteria that are responsible for the infection.

Toothache

Oil of clove can provide some anesthetic relief. Apply a drop or so directly onto the painful tooth, or dab a small amount on a cotton ball and place it next to the ache.

Warts

Try rubbing liberal amounts of vitamin E oil on the affected area (although some people are sensitive to it and should not put it on their skin). You may also want to take garlic-parsley tablets to relieve warts.

Yeast infections

Lactobacillus acidophilus, which is found in yogurts that contain "live" cultures, can help eliminate yeast infections. A similar recommendation is to eat plain yogurt, combined with acidophilus pills, available at health food stores. For troublesome cases, apply plain acidophilus yogurt directly into the vagina.

Using common home remedies that you have at your fingertips

You probably have the following common household products on hand, and they can be used to relieve some everyday ailments.

Acetaminophen: A painkiller and fever reducer for children and for people allergic to aspirin.

Alcohol (rubbing): A mild topical antiseptic or germ killer. Alcohol cools and soothes certain cases of irritated skin.

Ammonia: Used as "smelling salts" for fainting. A whiff of ammonia from an open container held under the victim's nose can bring a person out of unconsciousness. Ammonia also can be used to neutralize insect bites.

Baking soda: When scantily applied, a soothing treatment for sunburn to reduce pain, itching, and inflammation.

Benzalkonium chloride: A detergent-type cleanser and disinfectant for treating wounds.

Boric acid: A weak germ and fungus killer used as a dusting powder.

Calamine lotion: Used to treat rashes, sunburns, and other minor heat burns that don't result in blisters.

Chloride of lime (bleaching powder): A disinfectant, not to be used in direct contact with a wound. (You can wash soiled items in it.)

Egg white: Used as a *demuculent* (a substance that soothes or protects irritated mucous membranes) to soothe the stomach and retard the absorption of some poisons. Before using in suspected cases of poisoning, call your local poison control center, which will instruct you in how — if at all — to administer it.

Epsom salts: A soothing treatment for wounds when dissolved in water. Also used to make wet dressings for wounds.

Flour: When made into a thin paste, used as a demuculent to soothe the stomach and retard the absorption of some poisons.

Hydrogen peroxide: A germ killer when it comes into direct contact with bacteria. Follow directions on the product.

Milk: Used as a demuculent to soothe the stomach and retard absorption of some poisons.

Milk of magnesia: A substitute for magnesium oxide (see *Universal antidote*). Milk of magnesia is also used in small doses as an antacid for stomach upset and as a laxative for constipation.

Petroleum jelly (Vaseline): A skin softener and protective ointment used on wound dressings.

Powdered (dry) mustard: Used as an *emetic* (something that induces vomiting). Dissolve 1 to 3 teaspoons in a glass of warm water. Before using in suspected cases of poisoning, call your local poison control center, which will instruct you in how — if at all — to administer it.

Salt (table salt): Used as an emetic to induce vomiting. Dissolve 2 teaspoons in a glass of warm water. Before using in suspected cases of poisoning, call your local poison control center, which will instruct you in how — if at all — to administer it. (You can use clean seawater if you need an emetic or wound cleaner near an ocean beach.)

Soap suds (not detergents): Used as an antidote for poisoning by certain metal compounds, such as mercuric chloride. Before using in suspected cases of poisoning, call your local poison control center, which will instruct you in how — if at all — to administer it. Soap and clean water can also be used to cleanse wounds.

Starch, cooked: When made into a thin paste, used as a demuculent to soothe the stomach and retard the absorption of poison. Before using in suspected cases of poisoning, call your local poison control center, which will instruct you in how — if at all — to administer it.

Universal antidote: You can make an antidote for poisoning when the poison cannot be identified by mixing $1/2$ ounce of activated charcoal, $1/4$ ounce of magnesium oxide, and $1/4$ ounce of tannic acid in a glass of water.

Vinegar: Recommended treatment for a number of problems, including jellyfish stings, sunburns, and yeast infections. To help neutralize jellyfish stings, splash vinegar over the affected areas. For sunburns, mix 1 cup of white vinegar in a bathtub of cool water and soak. While over-the-counter premixed vinegar solutions are available for yeast infections, the home-mixed concoction for douching is lukewarm vinegar and water: 4 teaspoons of vinegar to 1 pint of water is a standard recipe. Vinegar is also used to treat alkali burns and to relieve swimmer's ear.

Chapter 5

Handling Home Emergencies

. . . .

In This Chapter

▶ Gathering the tools you need to administer first aid

▶ Dealing with common injuries and emergencies

▶ Calling for help

. . . .

*Y*ou spend most of your time at home. You go there to feel safe. Unfortunately, home is also the place where you are most likely to get hurt. More than 22,000 home fatalities occur each year from falls, poisonings, choking, fires, shootings, burns, and drownings. That's reason enough for alarm, but don't panic. Although it's impossible to anticipate every injury in the home — especially with children around — you can easily equip yourself to handle emergencies when they arise.

Preparing for Family First Aid

Now's the time to prepare for the day when someone gets hurt in your house. You need a first-aid kit that you can locate quickly. It should contain

- ✔ Large and small bandages
- ✔ Sterile gauze pads
- ✔ Adhesive tape
- ✔ Hydrogen peroxide
- ✔ Scissors
- ✔ A sterile set of tweezers
- ✔ Moist towelettes
- ✔ Latex gloves
- ✔ Face barrier for rescue breathing
- ✔ Ice packs
- ✔ Smelling salts
- ✔ Syrup of ipecac or activated charcoal

The last thing you want to do when you're in the middle of an emergency is to stop and look up a phone number. But you won't have to stumble around looking for the right phone number if you post the numbers for the poison control center, ambulance, fire department, and doctor by all the phones in your house.

Calling for Help

Are you unsure whether your emergency warrants a call to the emergency service system? Here are the circumstances that *always* warrant a call to 911 or your emergency service:

- ✔ Someone has fallen and can't get up.
- ✔ Someone is slurring words.
- ✔ You think that someone is having a seizure.
- ✔ You suspect that someone has swallowed poison.
- ✔ Someone can't breathe.
- ✔ You suspect a drug overdose.
- ✔ Someone has persistent chest pain.
- ✔ A serious head, neck, or back injury has occurred (for example, the person is unable to move or is in great pain).
- ✔ Someone is coughing up or throwing up blood.

Making the call

More than 50 percent of the United States is now covered by the 911 emergency medical services system that links homes like yours to a network of trained emergency personnel, such as dispatchers, emergency medical technicians, nurses, doctors, and fire, police, and ambulance personnel.

When you call 911, your first contact is with the dispatcher, who will ask you many questions. Stay on the line and slowly answer them all, beginning with where you're calling from, what happened, and what condition the person is in. Tell the dispatcher what you have done to assist the victim, and listen to the instructions the dispatcher gives you for further care until trained personnel arrive on the scene.

Is it always wise to call 911?

Dispatching for 911 is a lot more sophisticated than it used to be. Dispatchers who receive 911 calls often work behind computer terminals that display the street address of the caller. This is known as *enhanced 911*.

However, some rural communities may be too small to support the service, which is usually financed through tax dollars or surcharges on phone bills. When people who live in such communities call 911, they are usually patched through to a local telephone company operator, who then calls the appropriate police, fire, or ambulance crew.

Find out now whether true 911 service is available in your community. If it isn't, the operator has to make an extra phone call, and that could mean losing valuable seconds or minutes. You can avoid this problem by getting the direct phone numbers for the local police, fire, and ambulance services and keeping them handy near all telephones.

Encountering Common Emergencies

The most common household injuries and emergencies are falls, burns, drownings, and accidental poisonings. How should you handle them? In almost every case, the rule to follow in an emergency is to first call for help, whether it's 911 or your local ambulance or emergency service. After help is on the way, put your first aid know-how to work.

Before we embark on a tour of the specifics of emergency first aid, know that two procedures are used for many different problems: *rescue breathing* (also known as mouth-to-mouth resuscitation) and *cardiopulmonary resuscitation* (CPR). We mention these procedures throughout this chapter, so we'll describe them up front.

✔ **Rescue breathing:** Rescue breathing is what we used to call mouth-to-mouth resuscitation. Use a face barrier when performing this procedure. Pinch the victim's nostrils shut and cover the person's mouth with your mouth while you slowly breathe two full breaths into it. If the person has a pulse but is not breathing, keep breathing for the person every five seconds. Don't stop until the person begins to breathe or until help arrives.

✔ **CPR:** Cardiopulmonary resuscitation combines rescue breathing (mouth-to-mouth resuscitation) with chest compressions that get the blood circulating. To perform CPR correctly, you need expert training. Certification classes — which take only three hours to complete — are available from the American Heart Association, the Red Cross, and local hospitals and health centers. Considering that you could save a life, the three hours of training are well worth your time.

Three basic steps, known as the ABCs, come into play with CPR:

A is for airway: Open the person's airway by tilting the head back and moving the chin forward (see Figure 5-1). This position moves the person's tongue and epiglottis — the two most common airway obstructions — out of the way.

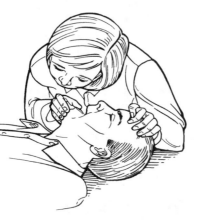

Figure 5-1: Open the airway by tilting the head back and moving the chin forward.

B is for breathing: Breathe for the person by pinching the nose closed and placing your mouth over his or her mouth, as shown in Figure 5-2. Slowly breathe two full breaths, lasting about 1.5 seconds each, into the victim's mouth. Repeat until the person begins to breathe or until help arrives.

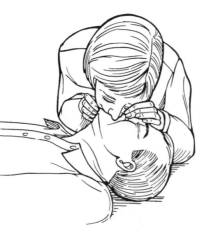

Figure 5-2: Pinch the nose closed and breathe two full breaths into the victim's mouth.

C is for circulation: Intersperse rescue breathing with chest compressions if the person's heart is not beating. Chest compressions maintain blood flow to the lungs, brain, and other major organs. To compress the chest, kneel beside the person with your knees touching one of the shoulders. Your own shoulders should be straight and square. Find the spot where the lower ribs and sternum meet — it feels like a notch, and you may even be able to locate it through light clothing. Place the heel of your hand slightly above the spot, with your fingers extended away from your body. Put your other hand on top of the first. Using the heel of your bottom hand, press down on the sternum about 2 inches and then release. Repeat in cycles of 15 compressions and two breaths. (See Figure 5-3.) After four complete cycles, check to see whether the victim has regained a pulse. Continue as necessary.

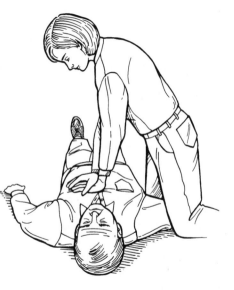

Figure 5-3: Compress the chest, repeating in cycles of 15 compressions.

CPR for children and infants is slightly different than for adults. Use only one hand to perform CPR on an infant or child. For an infant, place two fingers one finger width below the baby's nipple and press down five times. Breathe once into the baby's mouth, and then repeat cycles of five compressions and one breath as necessary. To perform CPR on a child, place the heel of one hand on the lower half of the child's sternum and the other hand on the head. Do five compressions followed by one breath, and repeat as necessary.

Accidental poisonings

Homes are filled with hundreds of products that are poisonous if ingested, touched, or inhaled. Toilet bowl and oven cleaners, auto windshield washer solutions, mouthwashes, and pesticides are all poisonous if not handled properly. Other common poisons include vitamins, aspirin, alcoholic beverages, gasoline, paint thinner, and even some plants.

The typical victim of an accidental home poisoning is a child between the ages of 1 and 6. The most likely setting for an accidental poisoning of a child to occur is in the kitchen between the hours of 4 p.m. and 6 p.m., when Mom and Dad are focusing on dinner. Household cleaners are frequently left in the open in the kitchen, or mealtime medications are within easy reach on the kitchen table. Likewise, the bathroom, with its irresistible medicine cabinet, is number two on the list of spots where children are likely to encounter poisons.

Recognizing the signs of a poisoning is key to getting help quickly and ensuring the victim's recovery. Poison may be involved when someone suddenly becomes ill, loses consciousness, has visible burn marks, has breath that smells like chemicals, vomits, or has difficulty breathing. Headaches, fever, chills, stomach pain, dizziness, a painful and swollen throat, and loss of appetite are also possible indications of poisoning.

If you suspect that someone in your household has ingested poison, get help fast. Keep the number for the poison control center by your telephone, and be prepared to tell the following to the person who answers the phone:

- Who took the poison and how old he or she is
- What the poison is (have the label handy) and how much poison you believe was ingested
- What the person's present condition is: Is he or she unconscious or having trouble breathing? Does he or she have a pulse?

The poison control center expert will tell you what to do. Depending on the poison involved, the authority may suggest that you give the person syrup of ipecac or activated charcoal to induce vomiting, or he or she may tell you to stick your finger down the victim's throat. If the victim is conscious, the poison control center expert may suggest that you give the victim a glass of milk or water. Follow the poison control expert's advice carefully. If detergent, cleaner, gasoline, or kerosene has been ingested, for example, you do *not* want to make the victim vomit.

Other comfort measures that you can take while waiting for emergency medical assistance to arrive are loosening the person's clothing, placing the person on his or her side or face down, and keeping the person's head lower than his or her body.

Amputation

Accidental amputation can be your worst nightmare. It can happen during a moment of carelessness when a family member is mowing the lawn, fiddling with the snowblower, or using a power tool. Staying calm under these circumstances is difficult — but know that what you do may prevent disaster.

Start by calling 911. Then follow the advice for heavy bleeding listed later in this chapter. After controlling the bleeding (here comes the grisly part), wrap the amputated part in a towel or piece of gauze and place it in a waterproof plastic bag. Surround the plastic bag with lots of ice and make sure that it gets to the hospital with the victim. In many cases, severed body parts can be successfully reattached in surgery.

Asthma attacks and anaphylactic shock

If someone in your family has allergies or suffers from asthma, seemingly innocent things can cause life-threatening situations in no time flat. An allergic reaction to shellfish, nuts, medication, insect bites, or dog or cat dander can send an affected individual into anaphylactic shock. Anaphylactic shock causes the body's airways to narrow, the heart to race, and blood pressure to drop suddenly.

Anaphylactic shock is marked by

✔ Swollen eyes, face, or tongue

✔ Difficulty swallowing

✔ Dizziness

✔ General feelings of weakness

✔ A pounding heart

✔ Itching and hives

If a family member goes into anaphylactic shock, call 911 immediately. If the person has an emergency kit containing *epinephrine* (a hormone that opens breathing passages and helps return the heart rate to normal), follow the directions to inject the medication; then seek emergency care.

Today, automatic injectors are available to deliver a life-saving dose of epinephrine. If you or a family member has severe allergies or asthma, keep one on hand in case of emergency. Protect it, though, in a carrying case (an opaque toothbrush case works well), and periodically check the expiration date.

Bleeding

Even an ordinary nosebleed can be pretty scary for an adult, let alone a child and concerned parents. If a nosebleed develops suddenly, pinch the nose just under the bony ridge and keep the nostrils closed tightly for five to ten minutes. Keep the head upright. If the bleeding doesn't stop after that, seek medical attention.

Heavy bleeding is an entirely different — and much more serious — story. If the injured person is unconscious or is losing a lot of blood, call 911 immediately. If he or she is breathing but the bleeding will not stop, use a clean cloth to apply pressure directly on the wound. If blood soaks through the dressing, place another piece of cloth on top of the first — don't remove the first one — and continue applying pressure. Elevate a bleeding leg or arm that isn't broken so that it is above the heart. When the bleeding stops, bandage the wound, taking care not to make it too tight.

Look for signs of shock such as clammy skin and listlessness. If those symptoms are present, keep the person warm and elevate the feet. Exception to this rule: If the person is unconscious, has trouble breathing, has an injured chest or head, or appears to be in shock, call 911 and do not elevate the feet.

Do not use a tourniquet unless you have exhausted every other means of stopping the bleeding. To make a tourniquet, place a piece of cloth around the limb between the wound and the heart and, using a stick, twist the cloth until it becomes just tight enough to cut off the flow of blood. Tie the tourniquet in place or continue to hold it until help arrives.

Broken bones

It can be a tumble from a favorite tree house or a topple from a rickety ladder while cleaning the rainspouts. Even a minor fall or push at just the right angle can be enough to break a bone, as strong as bones are. For kids and adults, breaks are pretty common. So what do you do about them?

First things first: If the person is unconscious, call 911 right away.

A broken bone may be obvious — it may look funny or be bent at an odd angle. Other indications that a bone may be broken are pain and swelling. Often, a person with a broken bone is unable to place weight on it or move it at all. Until medical attention is available, splint the injury by using a rolled-up towel or newspaper, a pillow, or a piece of wood, as shown in Figure 5-4. As much as possible, keep the injured limb still while arranging the splint.

Burns

Burns are categorized by severity and labeled first-, second-, or third-degree. *First-degree burns* are minor, affecting only the skin. Most sunburns, in fact, are a type of first-degree burn. *Second-degree burns* affect deeper layers of the skin and result in pain, swelling, and sometimes blistering. *Third-degree burns* — the worst kind — damage the skin as well as underlying tissue and organs. Such burns appear white or charred. Electric shocks, burning

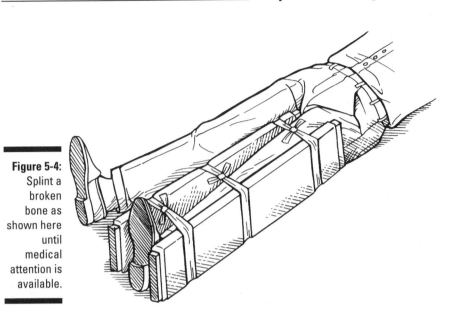

Figure 5-4: Splint a broken bone as shown here until medical attention is available.

clothes, and severe fires usually cause these serious burns. All burns greater than first-degree generally should be evaluated by a physician to prevent complications, particularly infections.

You may have to deal with three types of burns in your household: burns caused by fire and scalding, burns caused by electricity, and burns caused by chemicals.

For a broken . . .

Ankle or foot: Use a pillow to make a tight splint. Place an ice bag over the injury, placing a cloth between the ice and the skin.

Elbow, collarbone, or shoulder: Support the injured part in a sling that you tie to the body. Being sure not to touch the skin, place a cloth and then an ice bag rolled in a towel over the injury.

Lower leg: Use a rolled-up newspaper or magazine or a piece of wood for a splint, and build in some padding by using a cloth or pillow. After securing the splint, place an ice bag over the injury, but not directly on the skin. (Place a cloth over the skin first.)

Wrist or arm: Use a rolled-up newspaper, magazine, or piece of wood to make a tied splint, securing it with a soft or cushiony tie. Place the arm in a sling tied to the body. Place an ice bag over the area, separating the ice and the skin with a cloth.

Upper leg, hip, or pelvis: Call 911 or the medical emergency number in your community. Do not move the person, and do not attempt to fashion a splint.

Burns from fire or scalding

For a heat burn that is not particularly serious, such as a first-degree burn in which the skin turns red and the victim feels some pain, apply a cool compress or cool water to the area. Don't slather on butter and ointment like your grandmother always told you — they actually trap heat and can lead to infection.

If someone is actually on fire or has been splashed by hot liquids, your first job is to stop the burning. That may mean getting the person to "stop, drop, and roll" (remember your grade-school training?) to put out the flames — or you can use water or an extinguisher.

After calling 911 or a doctor (if you suspect that the burn is greater than first-degree), make sure that the person is breathing. Open his or her airway by laying the person on his or her back, carefully tilting the head back and lifting the chin slightly. If the person isn't breathing, perform rescue breathing, as described at the beginning of the chapter. If the person has no pulse, start CPR (if you've been trained), also described at the beginning of the chapter.

Elevate the victim's legs and use a clean sheet to cover the victim's body. Do not disturb the burned area by applying ointments or breaking blisters.

Electrical burns

Here's another tough one. Before coming to the aid of a victim with electrical burns, first turn off the electricity in the house. Your gut instinct may be to rush right over to the person, but fight it. Otherwise, you might come in contact with the current and put yourself out of commission, which helps no one.

In most homes, the circuit breaker box is in the basement or garage. In smaller homes, the breaker box is typically found in a closet near the kitchen. Open the door to the breaker box and throw the large black toggle switch on top, being careful not to touch anything else in the box. In older homes with fuse boxes, the main fuse block or "disconnect" has to be pulled out of the box. Open the door and look for a small steel insert with a handle near the top of the fuse box.

Before an emergency sends you to your fuse box, be sure that you know exactly where it is and how to open it and tinker with the breaker switches.

After the power is off, remove the person from the source of the current. Make certain that the person has a pulse and is breathing. If you find no pulse, perform CPR (or call 911 if you're not trained in CPR). If you find a pulse but no breathing, perform rescue breathing. Both techniques are explained earlier in the chapter.

Chemical burns

Get the chemical off the person's body as quickly as possible. Do so by taking off his or her clothes and placing the victim in the shower for a minimum of 30 minutes. If no shower is available or if the person is not conscious, a hose or buckets of water will do. Be careful to wash the chemical out of the eyes and off the skin as soon as possible. If the person has no pulse or is not breathing, perform CPR and rescue breathing as described earlier in the chapter.

Elevate the victim's legs and use a clean sheet to cover the person's body. Do not disturb the burned area by applying ointments or breaking blisters.

Choking

How can you tell if someone is choking? The best way is to ask! If the person can't talk, breathe, or cough, he or she is choking. If the person is coughing and clearly uncomfortable, he or she is probably okay, and slapping the person on the back or putting your fingers down his or her throat would probably create even more discomfort.

The best way to dislodge the food or object that is making a person choke is to perform the Heimlich maneuver. This lifesaving procedure is simple enough that just about any adult can perform it. Have someone call 911 (or the medical emergency number in your community) while you are doing the maneuver. Follow these steps, and refer to Figure 5-5:

1. **Stand behind the person who is choking and place your hands around his or her waist.**

2. **Make a fist with one hand and place your thumb just above the person's belly button. Wrap your other hand around the fist.**

3. **Thrust upward. Repeat at least four times.**

   Check to see how the person is doing after each thrust. Has the blockage been expelled? If the person is still choking, repeat the upward thrusts until the blockage is expelled or until the victim loses consciousness. Should that occur, phone 911 immediately.

Drowning

A family doesn't need to own a swimming pool to experience an at-home drowning. A drowning can happen in just a few seconds if a young child is left alone in the bathtub or even near an open toilet or bucket. Here's what to do if a drowning occurs at your house:

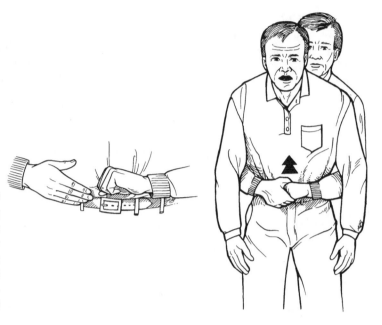

Figure 5-5:
The Heimlich
maneuver
can save a
person who's
choking.

1. Remove the person from the water.

2. Do nothing if he or she is breathing, talking, or coughing.

3. Call 911 if the person is unconscious.

4. Lay the victim on his or her back and gently tilt back the head. Slightly lift the chin to open the airway. Use all your senses to determine whether the person is breathing.

5. If you don't detect breathing, pinch the nostrils closed and place your mouth over the victim's mouth. Breathe into the mouth and watch to see whether the victim's chest rises and falls. Repeat.

6. If the chest does not rise and fall, try once more to reopen the airway. Tilt the person's head back and lift the chin again. Give two more full breaths. Check for a pulse if the chest does rise and fall.

The person's airway may be blocked if your second attempt does not produce a rising and falling chest. To release the blockage, straddle the person's legs and place the bottom of your hand just above the navel. Put your other hand on top of the first, with your fingers pointed toward the victim's nose. If you push your hands upward into the stomach, perhaps as many as five times, you may be able to bring up the blockage. Carefully roll the person onto his or her side if water or vomit comes up. Next, clear out his or her mouth by putting your index finger inside and swirling it around at the base of the tongue.

After removing the blockage, you can resume rescue breathing, watching again for the rise and fall of the chest. Place two or three fingers on the side of the neck near the Adam's apple, or at the outer edge of the left wrist, and feel for a pulse. If you find a pulse but the person has not resumed breathing, continue breathing for him or her until emergency medical help arrives.

Drug overdoses

It's a fact of life that some children — and adults, too — will experiment with drugs, so parents should recognize the signs of possible drug use. You should be concerned if your child shows a marked change in appetite, mood, and sleep habits, or exhibits confusion, isolation from friends, and secretive behavior.

A person experiencing a drug overdose is likely to

- Breathe abnormally.
- Have a high or low body temperature.
- Display poor coordination.
- Perspire freely.
- Experience hallucinations.
- Become very sleepy.

A person who is experiencing a drug overdose needs immediate medical help. Call the poison control center, 911, or your physician. If the person is unconscious, check his or her airway, breathing, and pulse. If the person is not breathing and has no pulse, perform CPR (if you've been trained).

Eye injuries

Whether caused by a blow or a foreign object, eye injuries can be extremely painful and worrisome. If a family member has a foreign object — such as a wood or metal splinter — embedded in his or her eye, has a cut on an eye or eyelid, has gotten a harsh chemical in an eye, or has received a severe blow to the eye, seek immediate emergency medical help.

Black eye

Even a common black eye can be distressing, especially if it's your child who has one. To treat it, immediately put a cold compress over the affected eye. The compress minimizes the amount of puffiness and "black and blue" discoloration that the injury will leave.

If it's a child's eye, you may want to give acetaminophen for the pain. Adults can also take acetaminophen but may want to stay away from aspirin; it can cause more bleeding and, consequently, more bruising. Follow up with a warm compress.

Foreign body in the eye

Never try to remove a foreign object from the eye — doing so can cause further damage. Instead, cover the affected eye with a clean object, such as a paper cup. Use tape to keep the object in place, but don't let the tape touch the eye. To prevent the injured eye from moving, cover the good eye with a clean bandage, too.

Blow to the eye

When an eye has absorbed a strong blow, close it and lightly place an ice compress over the injured area. Have the person lie down with his or her eyes closed until help arrives.

Cuts to the eye and surrounding area

Call 911 and then carefully cover both eyes with sterile gauze held in place by tape. Have the person lie on his or her back with eyes closed until help arrives.

Chemical irritants in the eye

When a chemical accidentally enters the eye, flush the eye with water as soon as possible. After calling 911 or contacting a medical professional, follow these steps for the best way to flush the eye:

1. **Have the person lie down with his or her head to the side so that the good eye is higher than the affected eye. Hold the affected eye open.**

2. **Using warm water from a clean container, pour generous amounts of water into the eye for about 30 minutes.**

   To determine exactly how long you should flush the eyes, follow the instructions given by the 911 dispatcher or medical professional whom you have contacted.

3. **Without touching the eye, use sterile cloth and tape to create a loose bandage.**

If both eyes have been exposed to chemicals, you may treat them both at once or take turns flushing them.

 If you are alone with the victim, it may be more convenient to fill the sink or a container with warm water and have the person lean over into it headfirst. After his or her face is underwater, ask the victim to open and close his or her eyelids to flush the eyes.

Neck, back, and head injuries

Tap the victim gently on the shoulder. Call 911 immediately if the person cannot respond when you ask whether he or she is okay. Don't move the victim unless it is absolutely necessary. If the person is not breathing or has no pulse, perform CPR or rescue breathing as appropriate, if you've been trained.

Place rolled-up towels on both sides of the head to keep the person's head and neck from moving. Keep the towels from being displaced by placing something heavy next to them, such as books or sandbags. Immobilize the rest of the person's body by surrounding it with rolled-up towels that have been stabilized.

Part III

You Can Get There from Here: Navigating the Medical Landscape

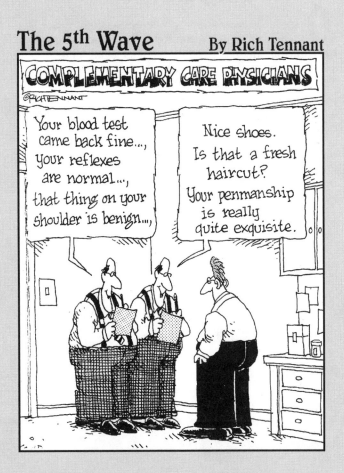

In this part . . .

Don't let anyone tell you different — health care is a business like any other field. You have to make decisions about where to do business, what kinds of services you'll use, and how to pay for those services. This part helps you make choices about conventional practitioners, complementary care, and insurance plans. You want to make these choices with your best business head.

Chapter 6

Finding the Perfect Practitioner

● ●

In This Chapter

▶ Understanding your options in practitioners

▶ Finding your ideal doctors

▶ Forging a healthy doctor/patient relationship

● ●

*T*hings used to be quite simple. You (or your spouse or your kids) got sick. You visited your friendly neighborhood doctor — the same doctor whom you could turn to for every medical situation. And chances were, you all saw the same doctor through the years until he or she retired and another, younger doctor stepped in.

Today, choosing a doctor — and staying with one — is not so easy. The process is filled with questions for both you and the prospective doctor, but the right choice can save your health — and your money. After all, bad medical care costs a lot more than good care and takes its toll on your family's health as well.

Knowing Your Options

Years ago, most doctors were *generalists* — doctors with well-rounded training, able to deliver babies, set broken bones, and perform surgeries. Television's kindly Marcus Welby represented the old-time general practitioner who moved confidently from examining room to operating room to patients' living rooms, providing care for entire families.

But general practitioners are no longer the only doctors who provide *primary care* — that is, care for all your run-of-the-mill, general needs. Primary care is provided even by a number of professionals who are not doctors at all. Today, the number of all-around general practitioners has declined, while *specialists* — doctors with advanced training in specific fields — proliferate. Although the trend toward specialization certainly opens up your options, it also makes choosing a practitioner for your family that much harder.

Primary care practitioners

Physicians are the most common practitioners of primary care. Today, adults have three types of primary care physicians to choose from:

- ✓ **General practitioners:** These physicians have completed medical school and have had only one year of internship experience. They go into practice after one year of residency. Although they're dwindling in numbers, G.P.s usually can treat a range of medical problems.

- ✓ **Family practitioners:** Recognized by the American Medical Association since 1969 as specialists in family medicine, F.P.s complete a three-year residency that includes certain aspects of internal medicine, gynecology, minor surgery, obstetrics, pediatrics, behavioral science, and preventive medicine.

- ✓ **Internists:** Like family practitioners, internists complete a three-year residency and pass a comprehensive exam. Unlike family practitioners, their training focuses more in depth on the adult organ system, consisting of diagnosis and management of gastrointestinal, liver, kidney, and heart problems.

The world of medicine is changing rapidly these days, and new and different types of health care professionals are making themselves available. In addition to physicians, nurse practitioners and physician assistants may provide primary care.

- ✓ **Nurse practitioners** (or N.P.s) are registered nurses who have completed an approved graduate program beyond nursing school or the baccalaureate degree. Many nurse practitioners also have completed clinical training in a specialty, such as pediatrics, family health, geriatric health, or obstetrics and gynecology. Nurses with these credentials are recognized as *advance-practice,* or *specialist,* nurses.

  Nurse practitioners can be found in doctors' offices, outpatient clinics, emergency rooms, health centers, and, in some states, their own freestanding clinics. In most states, however, N.P.s must practice with a physician's supervision. State regulations also dictate whether N.P.s are able to write prescriptions independently or under doctor supervision. Your state department of health should be able to tell you the regulations for N.P.s in your area.

- ✓ **Physician assistants** (or P.A.s) are educated in a general medical program and are qualified to perform between 75 and 80 percent of the duties that physicians perform. A P.A. usually goes through two years of training involving many medical school courses. Most programs offer a bachelor's degree, although master's degree programs are increasingly common.

Most states require P.A.s to pass a national certifying test after graduation. Those who have passed the test may use the credentials P.A.-C., which stands for Physician Assistant-Certified. P.A.s may specialize in areas such as pediatrics and gynecology.

State law dictates what P.A.s can and cannot do. Usually, P.A.s must practice under the supervision of a licensed physician. Your state department of health should be able to give you details on P.A.s in your area.

Women, men, children, and seniors can also seek primary care from practitioners with specialized training. A woman can seek primary care from an *obstetrician-gynecologist (ob-gyn),* a specialist in the female reproductive system, pregnancy, and childbirth. *Urologists* are specialists who primarily treat men's reproductive health, but they also see women with urological complaints. A child's specialist is the *pediatrician,* who can serve as a primary care doctor. Seniors have the option of seeing a *geriatric specialist* or *geriatrician* for primary care.

In addition to choosing whether to go to a general practitioner, family practitioner, internist, nurse practitioner, physician assistant, or specialist, you have the choice between M.D.s and D.O.s. A physician with a degree in *allopathic* medicine is known as a medical doctor, or M.D. A physician with a degree in *osteopathic* medicine is called a doctor of osteopathy, or D.O. Sounds complicated, but except for a notable difference in philosophy and, to a lesser extent, practice habits, D.O.s and M.D.s are essentially the same.

✔ **Allopathy** (which is more common in the United States) is founded on scientific principles in which diseases are treated with lifestyle changes or medications to counteract what's going on within the body. An allopathic physician begins with a medical history and then conducts an examination and diagnostic tests, which may include blood tests, X-rays, and ultrasound. After determining a diagnosis, the allopath may administer medications or use such treatments as chemotherapy, surgery, and ionizing radiation.

Nurses and names

Many different types of nurses walk the halls of doctors' offices and hospitals, but the two you're most likely to encounter are *registered nurses* (or R.N.s) and *licensed practical nurses* (or L.P.N.s).

R.N.s are at the top of the ladder as far as education goes. They usually have a baccalaureate degree from a four-year college nursing program and sometimes a master's degree. Some R.N.s take further education to specialize in a particular field. On the other hand, L.P.N.s can go into practice after only a year of nursing school — although many do have more training and experience.

✔ **Osteopathy** is a sometimes-forgotten branch of mainstream medical care. Even with tens of thousands of practitioners in the United States alone, osteopathy is still overshadowed by allopathic medicine and its half-million practitioners, and in part ignored as a result of the public perception that the M.D. is the sole torchbearer for traditional medicine. An osteopathic physician, or D.O., sees the body as a interrelated system. Doctors of osteopathic medicine are recognized physicians and surgeons who stress the unity of all body systems. The practitioners are called osteopaths because they emphasize the role of bones, muscles, and joints — the musculoskeletal system — in a person's well-being. They also emphasize holistic medicine, proper nutrition, and environmental factors and view manipulation or palpation as a less-intrusive aid to diagnosing and treating various illnesses.

Specialists

A *specialist* is a doctor who concentrates on a specific body system, age group, or disorder.

Some specialists — for example, pediatricians for children and gynecologists for women — offer primary care, providing for everyday health care needs such as colds, flu, and headaches. However, most people rely on specialists to provide a special brand of care. Heart patients, for example, seek out *cardiologists* — experts in heart health. A person with arthritis may visit a *rheumatologist* for specialized attention. Your primary care practitioner can help you determine which type of specialist can provide the care you need.

A doctor who has taken extra training in his or her field often chooses to become *board certified*. To obtain board certification, a doctor must hold a valid medical license, complete the required number of years of residency (usually two or three), and pass a rigorous exam administered by a specialty board. Some physicians continue on to become subspecialists. For example, maternal and fetal medicine is a subspecialty of gynecology.

A doctor who passes the board exam is given the status *Diplomate*. Most board-certified doctors become members of their specialty's society. Any doctor who meets the membership requirements is a *Fellow* of the society and may use the designation.

In its most basic sense, board certification indicates that a physician has completed a course of study in accordance with the established educational standards of one or more of the 24 member boards of the American Board of Medical Specialties.

Board certification has been called a minimum standard of excellence and nothing more. Paper certification does not produce professional excellence. On the other hand, board certification is a good sign that a doctor is up to date on the procedures, theories, and success-failure rates in the specialty.

Many people don't know this, but a licensed doctor can hang out a shingle advertising any specialty *without having any training in that specialty.* A doctor can open a practice — say in psychiatry, obstetrics, or even neurosurgery — without having any training in that field. Be on your guard.

How can you determine whether a physician is a board-certified specialist or subspecialist? You can call the American Board of Medical Specialties at 800-776-CERT to verify board certification status for any allopathic physician. For osteopaths, contact the American Osteopathic Association at 800-621-1773.

Or you can find out at the library whether an allopath is board certified; the *Official ABMS Directory of Board-Certified Medical Specialists* contains a listing of board-certified physicians. The directory lists all the ABMS board-certified specialists in the country who chose to be included. The listings cover state, specialty, education, training, and membership in professional organizations of their specialty. You can use this book to obtain two other important facts about doctors:

- Where they did their residency training (Did they practice at a major university hospital or a community hospital?)

- How long they have been practicing as doctors, based on their residency training (Are they fresh out of school or over age 70?)

Seeking the Right Practitioner

Don't wait until you have a medical problem or, worse yet, a medical emergency to find a practitioner. Not always the best choices, spur-of-the-moment decisions can be costly, too, in terms of money *and* health.

Knowing what you need

The more thought and effort you put into finding a qualified doctor, the better off you'll be. To boost your chances of success, ask your family a few questions to pinpoint their needs and attitudes:

- Do we want a doctor who serves as a constant resource, or one who primarily provides care only during illness?

- Do we want a doctor who explains the pros and cons and asks for our decisions, or one who makes the medical choices for the family?

✔ What sort of physician or practitioner do we want? Allopath? Osteopath? Specialist? Nurse practitioner or physician assistant?

✔ If we changed family doctors in the past, why? What should this new doctor do differently?

✔ Do we require certain features to fit our lifestyles? For example, are weekend and evening appointments a must? Must the office be near public transportation?

✔ Is cost a factor? Does our insurance cover care from this practitioner? If a health maintenance organization is involved, must the practitioner participate?

✔ Does anyone in our family have special health care needs that must be addressed?

✔ Do we have any preferences for male or female, young or old, solo or group practitioners?

Gathering referrals

Begin your search by getting a few good recommendations, also called *referrals,* from family members, friends, and neighbors. Word of mouth is still one of the best methods of finding out which doctors are taking new patients and what others think of these doctors. Remember the old adage: "If you want to find a good doctor, ask a nurse."

As you start to look for your ideal doctor, don't forget to check these promising resources:

✔ A physician referral service operated by the local medical society

✔ Newspaper advertisements of practitioners opening new practices

✔ Your company's human resources office

✔ Your health insurance company (Depending on your insurance, you may be able to seek care only from certain practitioners.)

✔ The phone book

✔ Nurses or other medical professionals

✔ Senior centers

Getting acquainted

Doctor-shopping should include an all-important get-acquainted visit to your prospective physician. You've never been on a get-acquainted visit before? Well, in today's competitive market, the more consumer-oriented doctors are more than happy to schedule a 10- to 15-minute introductory appointment to "sell" themselves to you. If the doctor refuses, go to the next one on your list.

Fifteen minutes is probably all you'll get, but if you're prepared, you'll be surprised just how much you can learn about the doctor and his or her staff if you ask the right questions.

When you meet the doctor, concentrate on credentials — medical degree, board certification, and other specialized or postgraduate education — and hospital affiliations. If the doctor is not on the staff of any hospital, he or she may not be able to serve you when you need him or her most. Also find out about basics such as office hours and whom to call if you have an emergency when the office is closed. Find out whether the doctor will take calls for questions and whether such consultations carry a fee.

Ask about the doctor's fee schedule and payment plans. A doctor who will willingly discuss fees is more likely to be open about other aspects of your medical care. Find out about insurance coverage as well. If you're on Medicare, ask whether the doctor accepts assignment. If not, ask whether the doctor will accept your case — it's negotiable.

Pay particular attention to the doctor's manner. Does the doctor's personality seem agreeable to you? Are questions answered in an honest, forthright manner? Remember that you may be trusting this doctor to treat you and your family for years to come, so you want a good match.

When you visit, you also want to notice the following things:

- ✔ Is the practice solo or group? If more than one doctor is on staff, do you have any guarantee that you'll be treated by the one you're meeting with? You may want to meet all of them!

- ✔ Does the office appear neat and clean? Patient-friendly? Are the magazines current?

- ✔ Do sick and well patients have separate waiting rooms?

- ✔ Does the staff maintain a professional, friendly attitude?

- ✔ Was your appointment kept on time? Is the waiting room full of people, indicating a backed-up schedule?

Forming a partnership

The doctor/patient relationship should be a partnership based on trust and mutual respect. Your doctor should understand that *you* are responsible for your family's health and that *you* are in control.

Make sure that the doctor you choose gives you the credit you deserve by explaining difficult health issues, keeping you informed of your family's health, and including you in diagnosis and treatment decisions. And if something doesn't please you, speak up! Doctors aren't the high-and-mighty experts that they sometimes think they are — they're there to serve your needs and the needs of your family.

In 1983, the People's Medical Society created the Code of Practice as a statement that we believe each doctor should subscribe to. Ask your doctor to review it and tell you whether he or she will apply it to your care.

The People's Medical Society Code of Practice

I will assist you in finding information resources, support groups, and health care providers to help you maintain and improve your health. When you seek my care for specific problems, I will abide by the following Code of Practice:

Office procedures

1. I will post or provide a printed schedule of my fees for office visits, procedures, tests, and surgery, and provide itemized bills.

2. I will provide certain hours each week when I will be available for nonemergency telephone consultation.

3. I will schedule appointments to allow the necessary time to see you with minimal waiting. I will promptly report test results to you and return phone calls.

4. I will allow and encourage you to bring a friend or relative into the examining room with you.

5. I will facilitate your getting your medical and hospital records, and will provide you with copies of your test results.

Choice in diagnosis and treatment

6. I will let you know your prognosis, including whether your condition is terminal or will cause disability or pain, and will explain why I believe further diagnostic activity or treatment is necessary.

7. I will discuss with you diagnostic, treatment, and medication options for your particular problem (including the option of no treatment), and describe in understandable terms the risk of each

alternative, the chances of success, the possibility of pain, the effect on your functioning, the number of visits each would entail, and the cost of each alternative.

8. I will describe my qualifications to perform the proposed diagnostic measures or treatments.

9. I will let you know of organizations, support groups, and medical and lay publications that can assist you in understanding, monitoring, and treating your problem.

10. I will not proceed until you are satisfied that you understand the benefits and risks of each alternative and I have your agreement on a particular course of action.

Calling Off Your Doctor

For the sake of your family's health, you need to ensure that your physician is giving you the best care for your dollar. You want a doctor who treats your family with respect and makes you an equal partner in your own health care.

Signs that you could be doing better include

- ✔ Overcrowded waiting rooms
- ✔ Excessive waiting time
- ✔ Hurried appointments
- ✔ Difficulty getting in touch with your practitioner
- ✔ Lack of communication
- ✔ Fee increases
- ✔ Difficulty accessing medical records

You may wonder how to go about "breaking up" with your practitioner — or if your practitioner can dump you as well. According to the law, your relationship with a doctor is a legal one. After it is established, it can be ended only by one of four conditions:

- ✔ Both parties agree to end the relationship.
- ✔ The patient ends it.
- ✔ The practitioner is no longer needed.
- ✔ The practitioner gives reasonable notice that he or she is withdrawing from the relationship.

Choosing a dentist with a smile

Choosing a dentist is very much like choosing a physician or other practitioner. To track down a dentist who may suit you, start by gathering referrals, think about what you're looking for in a dentist, and then arrange for a get-acquainted meeting to see who fits the bill.

In addition to the questions we list regarding physicians, take into account a few other considerations unique to dentists:

✔ Do we want a dentist who is prevention-oriented and who provides information about steps that our family can take at home to lessen the need for dental therapy?

✔ Does anyone in the family have a medical condition, such as diabetes or heart disease, that could affect oral health or that requires special monitoring during dental care?

✔ How do we plan to pay for care? Do we have access to dental insurance? What are its provisions for coverage? If we belong to an HMO or other managed care plan, how does the choice of dentist affect coverage?

Chapter 7

Investigating Complementary Care

- -

In This Chapter

▶ Sizing up complementary therapies

▶ Looking for a practitioner

▶ Knowing your options: An overview of what's available

- -

*C*omplementary, or *alternative,* medicine is nothing new. A hundred years ago, your great-grandparents treated their families' ills with remedies passed down from previous generations. Country doctors made house calls during times of illness. Movement and massage were used. Medicine contained mostly organic and herbal substances.

But after World War II, the medical world began to change. Families came to rely more heavily on their general practitioner for medicine and advice and left grandmothers' remedies behind. Touch, once a mainstay of treatment, was used almost exclusively for diagnostic purposes. As technology advanced, new synthetic drugs were created to mimic the chemicals found in nature. High-tech diagnostic tests and treatments were developed, changing the nature of medical care and causing health care costs to rise.

What goes around comes around, so it's no surprise that traditional remedies are back in style. As health expenses climb and the health care system becomes more complicated and difficult to use, you may find yourself looking for alternatives to the high-cost, high-tech medical industry.

Understanding Complementary Medicine

Complementary medicine is a label given to therapies that do not fall within mainstream medicine in the United States — therapies such as acupuncture, massage, herbalism, and yoga. At one time, these therapies were termed "alternative" therapies because they were alternatives to so-called regular medical care, and most medical professionals considered them inappropriate for use in treating illness.

However, in recent years, a few mainstream medical doctors have begun speaking out in support of the use of some of these therapies, and researchers have started to study their effectiveness. As these alternatives have become more accepted by traditional medicine, they have earned the label "complementary" — implying that they should be used side by side with, not instead of, "regular" medical treatments.

The signs of complementary medicine's popularity are everywhere. Medical practices in progressive areas are offering these therapies in their offices or referring patients to outside practitioners. Some major hospitals have units that offer complementary therapies in conjunction with regular treatment. The National Institutes of Health have even published a statement declaring acupuncture effective for some medical conditions — a move that brings more credibility than ever to complementary medicine.

Bringing Therapies Home

You can bring traditional medicine home to your family just by picking up some cough syrup at the drugstore. What about complementary therapies? Chances are good that they're already at home in your life.

Okay, maybe you don't whip out the acupuncture needles at the first sign of illness, but you may ask your better half for a neck rub after a long day at the office — one form of massage therapy. A steamy soak after a tough racquetball game eases sore muscles, but it's more than a hot bath: You're practicing hydrotherapy by making use of the healing powers of water. And you probably don't think of singing your child to sleep as sound therapy — the use of music to relax, calm, and heal — but it is.

Beyond these basics, complementary therapy is, by nature, well suited to home use. Although some forms of such therapies require specialized training and office visits, you can pick up others simply by reading a book or watching a video. This means no costly office visits — the techniques are at your fingertips. Complementary therapies (with some exceptions) also tend to have fewer side effects than traditional treatments, which makes them ideal for children and older people. In fact, some therapies are so safe that amateurs can practice them with little risk.

Athough some therapies are relatively harmless, many have *contra-indications,* or situations in which they may be dangerous to use. Pregnancy, heart disease, diabetes, high blood pressure, and many other conditions may preclude the use of a complementary therapy. For example, using Traditional Chinese Medicine while pregnant may trigger early labor. Some herbs spark heart attacks. *Apitherapy,* or bee venom therapy, can be deadly to those with allergies to bee stings. For these reasons, always consult a qualified practitioner when experimenting with complementary therapies.

What is holistic health?

In your search for complementary care, you may encounter the term *holistic* (sometimes spelled *wholistic*) *health.* Holistic health is based on the idea that everything, from your lifestyle, diet, and the way you think to your work environment, contributes to your balance of health. When practitioners describe themselves as holistic, they usually mean that they look at you as an overall person and examine how you live.

A headache is a good example. Suppose you get headaches once or twice a week. Headaches are known to be caused by any number of things, including stress, muscle tension, allergies, brain tumors, hormonal imbalances, and eyestrain. Rather than just prescribing the latest headache reliever, a holistic practitioner will try to determine the source of the headaches by taking into account your personal situation. Are you eating something that you're allergic to? Is a situation at home causing you stress? Do you work with computers or around loud equipment that may cause headaches?

More important, don't play doctor. After you read up on a therapy, practicing what you've learned is tempting. But some people treat symptoms without sufficient knowledge of treatment options. For chronic or acute problems, get a qualified diagnosis before deciding on a treatment.

In some cases, complementary therapies, such as herbs and homeopathy, are excellent as first aid. However, don't substitute biofeedback for bandages in serious circumstances. Always see a medical practitioner or go to the emergency room if a bone is broken or in cases of severe trauma or accidents. Mainstream medicine excels in this area.

Also, always inform your regular doctor of what complementary therapies you're using, and keep your complementary practitioner up-to-date on what your doctor is doing for you. Doing so ensures that the treatments prescribed will complement each other for the best results. In a worst-case scenario, your complementary therapy and traditional therapy may clash in what's called a *negative interaction* — for example, your asthma medication may be rendered useless by an herbal therapy, or the exercises you're practicing may raise your blood pressure.

Finally, if a therapy does not work within the specified time frame, stop the treatment and seek other options.

Using Complementary Medicine

When first exploring complementary medicine, figure out your reasons for seeking a complementary therapy. Are you looking to incorporate a therapy into your lifestyle, or do you want to treat a particular condition? What do you hope to get out of it? Relaxation? Healing? A new philosophy?

Take a look at your reasons, and then do a little research. In the section "Exploring Complementary Options," later in this chapter, we provide a brief overview of some of the most common complementary therapies. Make a list of the ones that seem to fit your needs, and then make a trip to the library and hit the books for more information. Internet sites and complementary therapy organizations are also good sources of information.

After you've figured out which therapy you're going to try, you need to find a practitioner. Look to these resources for help:

- ✔ Ask your friends and coworkers to refer you to someone they know.
- ✔ Look in the phone book under the therapy you want to try. If it isn't listed, check under "Therapeutic Massage." The therapist may be able to refer you to a practitioner who specializes in the therapy you want.
- ✔ Ask your medical practitioner if he or she can refer you to someone.
- ✔ Call an organization that specializes in the therapy you're interested in. Many groups provide referrals to local practitioners or may be able to point you in the right direction.

Paying for a complement

Complementary therapies tend to cost less than mainstream treatments. Even so, they may end up costing you more because most insurance companies do not reimburse for complementary treatments. Find out whether your insurance company provides coverage for a complementary therapy *before* being treated to avoid being caught with unanticipated expenses.

This policy of noncoverage is beginning to change, however, as complementary medicine becomes more accepted by mainstream practitioners. Therapies that are supported by scientific research and positive results are more likely to be covered than untested options. Insurers are also more likely to cover therapies that license and certify their practitioners. Demand also plays a role: If enough people request a therapy, an insurance company may include it in its benefits package.

Hydrotherapy, for example, is often paid for when used as physical therapy. Chiropractic treatments are sometimes paid for as well. Experts predict that acupuncture will soon be covered due to its recognition by the National Institutes of Health.

Questioning complementary practitioners

Ask prospective practitioners the following questions to find out more about their practices, philosophies, and experience. Use the answers to assess their quality and compatibility with your needs.

✔ Do you specialize in this complementary therapy? Do you work in other fields as well?

✔ What percentage of your practice is devoted to this therapy?

✔ Where were you trained? Do you have certification in this field?

✔ Does this state require licensing for this therapy? Are you licensed?

✔ Have you had experience with my diagnosis?

Searching for quality

As with any other service, the maxim "Buyer, beware" comes to mind. Most of these complementary therapies are not regulated, and knowing who is qualified can be difficult. What's more, your family doctor may not have sufficient training in these areas to assist you in your search.

Licensing and *certification* are two criteria that you can use to evaluate practitioners in certain fields:

✔ **Licensing** refers to state requirements for practitioners, which a practitioner must meet before he or she can practice in that state. For example, in Arizona, a homeopathic physician must be licensed in order to practice. However, in states where licensing is not required, homeopathic physicians can practice without meeting any requirements.

✔ **Certification** is awarded to a practitioner after he or she has completed a specific program of study. Many organizations and schools that train complementary practitioners offer certification programs. Unlike licensing, certification is not required by law in order to practice. But you can use it to help determine whether a practitioner is qualified.

Exploring Complementary Options

What follows is a sampling of the most commonly used therapies, along with a brief description of each therapy. Keep in mind that the way these therapies are practiced tends to vary because they're not standardized in the same way that traditional medicine is. Different groups may perform techniques differently or use different therapies to treat different ailments.

Acupuncture

Feeling out of sync? Traditional Chinese Medicine (TCM), which has been practiced for thousands of years, is a whole health care system that works to keep the body's systems and energy in balance. TCM balances and cultivates *chi,* the life force or energy that flows throughout the body. Chi flows through 12 major *meridians,* the "energy highways" of the body. According to Chinese tenets, illness results when congestion (like a traffic jam) or a blockage (like an accident) occurs on these highways. And just like a highway, each meridian has its own pulse or speed limit.

Acupuncture is one of the most well-known and widely practiced TCM therapies in the United States. In acupuncture, thin needles are inserted just below the skin at predetermined points along a meridian to correct the flow of chi. If you're afraid of needles, don't worry — acupuncture looks worse than it is. You may feel a little prick when the needles are inserted, but that's about all.

Asthma, nausea, stroke, addictions, and chronic pain are among the conditions that may be treated with acupuncture. The acupuncturist decides where to place the needles based on your physical appearance, symptoms, and the feel of your meridian pulses.

More and more insurance companies are covering acupuncture since the National Institutes of Health announced that the therapy is effective for treating a number of conditions, including postoperative pain and nausea. Be sure to ask your company whether you're covered before seeking treatment.

Some states limit the practice of acupuncture to licensed physicians. Others require acupuncturists to become certified and licensed.

Aromatherapy

Concentrated plant products called *essential oils* are the basis of *aromatherapy,* which uses scent to promote relaxation and alleviate symptoms and conditions. The oils can be diluted with water, applied to the skin, or heated to release their scents. Experts believe that aromatherapy works by stimulating the parts of the brain that control emotions, triggering feelings of happiness, calmness, or alertness.

Aromatherapy is used to treat aches, allergies, arthritis, mood swings, headaches, and menstrual and menopausal symptoms, among other conditions.

Aromatherapists are also available to provide treatment. Licensing is not required to date, and a certification program is currently being developed.

Ayurvedic medicine

Ayurvedic medicine is an ancient Indian system of medicine that employs a comprehensive system of lifestyle habits and natural medicine to treat and prevent disease. This therapy is governed by five elements (earth, fire, water, air, and ether) within the body. Diseases are thought to be caused by imbalances among these five elements. The elements combine in the body to make up your "humor," or personality type, which can be *vata, pitta,* or *kapha.*

- ✔ **Vata:** Thin; dry skin; prominent features; prone to nervous disorders and anxiety-related conditions
- ✔ **Pitta:** Medium build; ruddy or fair complexion; short-tempered; prone to acne, ulcers, and heartburn
- ✔ **Kapha:** Heavyset; thick and wavy hair; pale skin; slow to anger; prone to allergies, sinus infections, obesity, and high cholesterol

Arthritis, chronic fatigue syndrome, digestive disorders, menopausal symptoms, tension, and stress-related conditions may be helped with ayurvedic medicine. Because diagnosis using this therapy is complex, it may be difficult to use it at home, although you can incorporate its philosophies into everyday life.

Ayruvedic physicians, also called *vaidyas,* treat ailments based on personality type and other factors, including the illness presented. Certification programs are available for vaidyas. Licensing is not required, although many of those who practice ayurvedic medicine are mainstream medical practitioners.

Chiropractic

Like many other therapies, *chiropractic* began as the result of a chance occurrence. In 1895, a man named Daniel David Palmer manipulated the spine of a deaf man. After the adjustment, the man was able to hear! Palmer came to the conclusion that the condition of the spinal vertebrae affects health, especially that of the nervous system.

Chiropractors are categorized according to two schools: the "straight" school and the "mixed" school. Straight chiropractors limit their practice to traditional spinal manipulation. Mixed chiropractors supplement spinal manipulation with therapies such as heat, ultrasound, traction, vitamins, minerals, and exercise. Members of the mixed school may also have training in homeopathy, naturopathy (a healing art that emphasizes the body's natural healing forces), applied kinesiology (which tests the strength of specific muscles to determine where chiropractic adjustments are needed), and acupuncture.

Chiropractic may help arthritis, asthma, back pain, neck pain, carpal tunnel syndrome, headache, sprains, sports injuries, and related conditions. A visit to a chiropractor includes a physical and, usually, an X-ray examination of your spinal column to see whether it is aligned properly. If the spine is out of alignment, the chiropractor gently pushes on the vertebrae to encourage them to move into place.

A spinal or joint adjustment should be made only by a trained chiropractor. An adjustment made by anyone who doesn't understand the mechanics of the body's structure can damage the spine.

A chiropractor receives a college degree followed by five years of chiropractic training before earning the degree of Doctor of Chiropractic (D.C.). Chiropractors also can become accredited upon completing further education. All states have laws regarding the licensing and practice of chiropractic.

Herbalism

The use and study of plants to heal is known as *herbalism, botanical medicine, phytotherapy,* or *phytomedicine.* Herbalism began thousands of years ago; plants were the first medicines. In fact, the word *drug* comes from the German word *droge,* meaning "to dry" — which is how the plants were prepared for use. Many experts speculate that ancient people observed the plants that sick animals ate and then tried them out themselves when they were under the weather.

Herbalism is used to treat a wide range of conditions, including allergies, anxiety, colds, digestive disorders, stress, sore muscles, and menopausal and premenstrual symptoms. Herbs can be found in many different forms, from fresh greens to capsules and tablets to dried leaves. Some are ingested, and others are applied to the skin. The combinations of dosages, forms, and uses are endless, so you can see why it's a good idea to consult an *herbalist* (one who practices herbalism) to find out what sort of herbs suit your condition best. The sidebar "Herbal remedies at a glance" gives you an idea of the types of herbs used to treat various conditions.

Training programs for herbalists differ greatly. Academic programs, correspondence courses, residencies, and apprenticeship programs all teach herbal medicine. Certification is available for herbalists. Although the U.S. Food and Drug Administration does not allow therapeutic information to be printed on the labels of herbs, no other state laws or licensing stipulations govern herbalism at this time.

Herbs may be natural, but they are powerful and should be treated with respect. Although many herbs have fewer side effects than drugs, some kinds interact with medications or cause medical problems. For example, some types of herbs may cause miscarriage. Others can affect heart rate and

HEALTH AT HOME

Herbal remedies at a glance

Hundreds of herbs in hundreds of forms line the walls of health food stores. To help point you in the right direction, here's a quick run-down of some common conditions and the herbs used to treat them. Just remember to talk with your doctor and an herbalist before treating yourself to avoid any dangerous side effects.

Anxiety: Peppermint, valerian

Arthritis: Evening primrose oil, goldenrod

Bronchitis: Licorice, echinacea, garlic

Chicken pox: Aloe, chamomile

Common cold: Echinacea, sage, ginger, goldenseal

Fatigue: Ginseng, echinacea, goldenseal, licorice

Indigestion: Chamomile, peppermint

Insomnia: Chamomile, sage, valerian

Prostate troubles: Nettles, saw palmetto

blood pressure. For these reasons, talk to an herbalist _and_ your physician before treating yourself with herbs. Both practitioners should be kept abreast of your condition, your treatments, and your progress.

Homeopathy

Homeopathy treats illness by using safe, natural substances that stimulate the body's own healing processes, at the same time avoiding harmful side effects. It is based on the theory that "like cures like" — that what creates symptoms in a healthy person will cure a sick person with the same symptoms.

Homeopathic remedies can be helpful for teething, nausea, headaches, and skin irritations, and may be used as first aid treatment in nonemergency situations. Remedies come in liquid or tablet form and are taken by mouth. In homeopathy, your symptoms dictate your treatment, because a list of symptoms is used to locate the appropriate remedy. Remedies should be used one at a time for effectiveness, say those who practice homeopathy. The therapy is considered safe for home care because little or no trace of the active substance can be found in the remedy. However, long-term use may cause a worsening of some conditions.

TIP

Determining which remedy to use may be difficult. If you are inexperienced or develop a number of symptoms, consult a homeopathic practitioner. Remember that self-treatment with homeopathy should be done only on a short-term basis. If the treatment doesn't help, seek assistance from a trained professional.

Those who practice homeopathy are known as *homeopaths* or *homeopathic physicians.* They are trained extensively in conventional medicine as well as in homeopathy and oftentimes are mainstream medical practitioners. Some states license homeopathic physicians, and certification is available.

Mind-body techniques

Many complementary care therapies focus on the connection between mind and body: If your mind is well, your body will be well, too. Here are a few common mind-body techniques:

- ✔ **Biofeedback** is a healing art that uses the conscious mind to control the functions of the involuntary or autonomic nervous system, which controls breathing, heart rate, and body temperature.

  Used to treat anxiety and panic attacks, attention deficit disorder, and a number of other conditions, biofeedback involves gaining control of your body. In biofeedback, you learn to will your body to change a function — perhaps you raise your body temperature or slow your heart rate. A device called a *monitor* is used during training. The monitor beeps at intervals, in tune with your pulse or electrical muscle signals, for example. Through concentration, you attempt to slow the beeping to relax. After you develop your skills, you are able to do it on your own without equipment.

  Certification is available for biofeedback therapists. Licensing is not required, although some licensed practitioners employ the therapy in their practices.

- ✔ **Hypnotherapy** induces a state of advanced relaxation and focused concentration in order to promote healing. The therapy plants positive statements called *affirmations* into the subconscious mind by bypassing the conscious (or waking) mind.

  Anxiety, addictions, and fears can be treated using hypnotherapy. It's also used to help stress disorders, addictive habits, asthma, high blood pressure, and migraine headaches.

  Certification is available for practitioners of hypnotherapy, which often include physicians and other health professionals. Licensing is not required.

- ✔ **Tai chi,** actually a form of martial arts, is a series of gentle movements that are used to balance and enhance chi (energy) in the body. These movements are free-flowing and graceful, involving shifting your weight from one foot to the other. As you shift your weight and move your body, you stimulate and create chi.

  People who practice tai chi claim that it's good for relaxation, long life, and flexibility. It's generally not used for a specific condition but for overall wellness.

Tai chi classes are available in many major cities and are appropriate for all ages. Most instructors are trained within a particular school of tai chi. No national certification is available because each school is different, and licensing is not available.

✔ **Yoga** is a 6,000-year-old Indian system consisting of a series of stretches that are meant to unite the body, mind, and spirit to achieve self-realization. Practiced in the United States today, yoga is performed primarily in learning to concentrate and in improving self-discipline, reducing stress, and increasing flexibility.

Yoga is used to treat symptoms of anxiety, arthritis, addiction, insomnia, diabetes, and many other conditions. No standards for certification are in place for yoga instructors, and licensing is not required.

Reflexology

You could call *reflexology* "acupressure for the feet" because it is based on the idea that the feet and hands are mirrors of the entire body. *Reflexologists* (practitioners of reflexology) work the hands and feet to stimulate or calm areas that correspond with other parts of the body. Figure 7-1 shows a reflexology chart for the bottom of the foot.

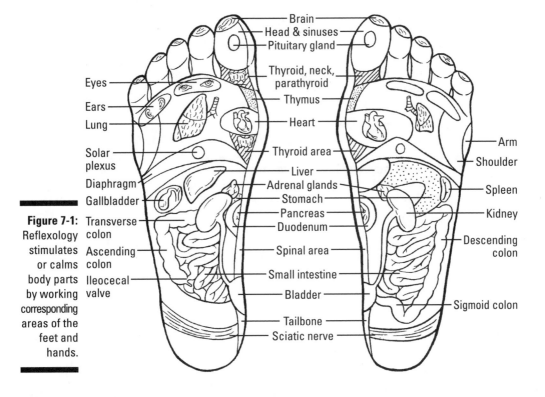

Figure 7-1: Reflexology stimulates or calms body parts by working corresponding areas of the feet and hands.

Brain
Head & sinuses
Pituitary gland
Thyroid, neck, parathyroid
Thymus
Heart
Thyroid area
Liver
Adrenal glands
Stomach
Pancreas
Duodenum
Spinal area
Small intestine
Bladder
Tailbone
Sciatic nerve

Eyes
Ears
Lung
Solar plexus
Diaphragm
Gallbladder
Transverse colon
Ascending colon
Ileocecal valve

Arm
Shoulder
Spleen
Kidney
Descending colon
Sigmoid colon

Foot reflexology is practiced more often than hand reflexology. In foot reflexology, pain in the foot can be an indication of an imbalance in the corresponding part of the body. Another aspect of foot reflexology is the existence of deposits in the feet that reflexologists call *crystals*. Reflexologists believe that crystals block the function of the nerve and energy impulses. They apply pressure to the crystals to break them up, which reopens the nerve and energy flows.

Studies have found reflexology to be helpful with diabetes, chronic constipation, headaches, backaches, and PMS (premenstrual syndrome). Reflexology can be used at home and is easy to learn. Many books and videos are available on the subject.

Certification is available for this therapy. Some states and cities have licensing restrictions for reflexologists.

Beware the reflexologist who suggests that you need to purchase special gadgets to practice the therapy. Such gizmos aren't necessary to obtain successful outcomes with reflexology.

Therapeutic massage

Therapeutic massage involves the use of the hands to work the muscles and connective tissues of the body to promote healing. Massage releases physical and emotional tensions, improves circulation, and provides relief from minor aches and pains. Two common types of therapeutic massage are

- **Holistic massage,** which looks at the body as a whole. The massage takes a more integrated approach, making sure that your entire body feels connected.
- **Swedish massage,** developed by Per Henrik Ling, which uses vibration and friction on the muscles to relieve tension and tone the body.

Of course, massage is easily used in the home — and plenty of books are available on the subject. (You can even find books on massaging your pets!) Certification is available for massage therapists, and some states require licensing.

Chapter 8

Insuring Family Health

- -

In This Chapter

▶ Finding out about fee-for-service

▶ Understanding managed care

▶ Exploring Medicare

▶ Choosing plans and practitioners

- -

*W*ith the cost of health care spiraling at a rate several times that of inflation, you'd better pay close attention to the health care insurance plans available to you and your family.

The advent of different types of health care plans has brought with it a host of acronyms — HMO, PPO, POS, and ERISA, just to name a few. And with plans designed to lower the cost of care to the employer, the employee, the government, and the insurance company, the amount of information you have to know quickly becomes overwhelming. Fee-for-service plans, managed care options, point-of-service providers, health maintenance organizations — all these terms have become familiar in the last few years. This chapter explains what they mean to you.

Paying for What You Get: Fee-for-Service

To understand traditional fee-for-service medical plans, take their name literally. They are simply insurance programs that pay a fee for a service. Such plans reimburse you or your doctor for services rendered.

Definitions aside, these plans don't stay so simple. They usually require a deductible and a copayment for each type of coverage under the plan. The *deductible* is the amount of the service charge that you must pay before the insurance company makes its payment. The *copayment* is a percentage of the covered service that you are required to pay. For example, for a service covered by your plan, you may have a $100 deductible and a 20 percent copayment. So if the doctor charges $500, you pay the first $100 (the deductible) and 20 percent of the remaining $400 (the copayment) for a total of $180.

Don't worry. You can opt for safeguards, called *stop-loss limits,* to keep copayments from breaking the bank. A stop-loss limit is an upper limit on the amount of copayment that you are required to pay. It goes into effect after the total copayment (often about $1,000) is met during a normal calendar year. An upper limit on the total payments that the insurance plan will pay may also exist, such as $1 million over a lifetime.

Your company's *schedule of benefits* spells out what's covered and what's not. In this document, you can find information about such points as the number of days of hospital treatment that will be covered, the deductibles and copayments required, and any other limits of coverage. Read your plan profile carefully to determine what your plan requires in order to provide services (for example, a second opinion or prior approval of admission) and what it will pay in these cases.

Understanding fee-for-service components

Traditional medical insurance plans contain three main types of coverage: hospital insurance, medical/surgical insurance, and major medical insurance. All three are required in order to secure full coverage for you and your family.

- ✔ **Hospital insurance** under a traditional health plan covers inpatient and outpatient charges for emergency and nonemergency services.

- ✔ **Medical/surgical insurance** covers charges in the hospital for doctors' visits, surgical services, physician fees, medications, X-rays, laboratory testing, anesthesia, and other specialist treatments. Some office procedures, office visits, and outpatient treatments or surgeries also are covered under this portion of the insurance plan. Medical/surgical insurance is usually included with hospital insurance and sold as a package program.

- ✔ **Major medical insurance** covers charges that do not fit into the preceding categories. All charges for doctors' office visits that do not relate to hospital care, laboratory testing charges, medications, and treatment for accidents or illness are covered under this type of plan.

A plan that includes all three types of coverage is often known as a *comprehensive health plan.* Comprehensive health plans are package arrangements in which hospital, surgical, and major medical insurance are sold together to provide total coverage for you and your family. Blue Cross/Blue Shield, which requires both the "Blues" to provide complete coverage, is a good example of this type of plan. These plans cover most types of medical services, with the exception of some elective types of surgery or treatments that are not required for the health of the patient.

Considering some consumer caveats

Because doctors are paid according to the procedures they perform, some say that traditional fee-for-service insurance encourages doctors to recommend unnecessary procedures to boost their profits. A few extra tests or a more expensive treatment, and a doctor rakes in the bucks. For you as a consumer, this tendency poses two problems:

- ✔ Even though you don't personally shell out for such procedures, your insurance company does — and repays the favor with higher premiums in the long run.

- ✔ Your personal health, as well as your pocketbook, is at stake. We've said it before, and we'll say it again: Every time you undergo a procedure, whether minor or major, you're at risk. You have no reason to face that risk unnecessarily just because your doctor is getting greedy.

We're not saying that fee-for-service is inherently bad or that your practitioner is evil. We're just pointing out that a financial incentive does exist. To protect yourself, ask plenty of questions about all procedures, including whether they are truly necessary. If you're in doubt, get a second opinion — a wise move no matter what type of insurance you have. (See Chapter 10 for specifics on avoiding unnecessary procedures.)

Knowing Your Options for Family Care

One of the fastest-growing areas of the health care field today is the trend toward *managed health care.* Under a managed care plan — you'll find a few different types — you are usually required to seek medical care from providers (for example, a physician or hospital) specifically designated by the plan in order to receive full coverage for those services. In return, these providers are required to accept payment by the managed care company as payment in full, meaning that you aren't billed for any additional costs, except for incidentals such as telephone charges during a hospital stay.

Therefore, if you're in managed care, you probably aren't able to go to any doctor you choose and still have coverage. If a doctor, even one who's made house calls to your home for years, isn't on your managed care company's list of providers, chances are good that you'll have to foot the bill yourself if you see that doctor. This lack of freedom is widely thought to be the biggest drawback of managed care, although certain plans are trying to change that stigma by offering consumer "out-of-network" options.

Plenty of variations exist on the theme of managed care, from the health maintenance organization (HMO) to the preferred provider organization (PPO), and more are developing all the time. When choosing a managed care option, take into account your personal situation, and make sure that all your questions are answered before you sign on the dotted line. And be aware that managed care plans apply for accreditation with one of three national organizations: the National Committee for Quality Assurance, the Joint Commission on Accreditation of Healthcare Organizations, or the American Accreditation Healthcare Commission. Accreditation is a voluntary process in which the plan pays a fee to the accrediting group for the "honor" of undergoing the process of evaluation.

Health maintenance organizations

Health maintenance organizations, or HMOs, provide insurance coverage within a system of HMO-approved physicians and facilities.

As an HMO member, you must choose a single primary care physician from a list of approved doctors provided by the plan. This primary care physician is often called a *gatekeeper* because you must go through this practitioner to obtain medical care. When you make an office visit, your primary care doctor may treat you personally or may refer you to a specialist or a hospital or facility. Even if you know what you want — suppose that you need to see your cardiologist — you must get your primary care doctor's approval before proceeding, or the HMO may not cover any care provided by the specialist. HMOs even require gatekeeper approval in many emergency circumstances, within reason, before they'll pay.

Find out the procedure and criteria your HMO demands for an emergency *before* one arises. Most plans take into account that you won't have time to contact your primary care doctor en route to the emergency room, but many have rules regarding how long you can wait after receiving care before calling your doctor. HMOs also put restrictions on what constitutes an emergency. If you make an emergency visit for a problem that the HMO thinks could have waited, you may be responsible for the cost.

Low copayments, often as little as $5 or $10, coupled with few or no out-of-pocket expenses and little paperwork, are the winning features of HMOs, especially for families. Prescription drugs also are covered with a similarly low copayment, and extras such as eyeglasses and hearing aids may be covered, too. In a traditional fee-for-service plan, you may end up paying up front for doctor visits, services, and medications, only to have to file a load of forms to get reimbursed.

Also, because the doctors are paid a set fee regardless of how much care you need, it's in the best financial interest of the practitioners and the HMO to keep you as healthy as possible. To this end, HMOs, unlike traditional fee-for-service plans, offer you a variety of benefits:

✔ **One-stop shopping:** You can easily obtain all your health care needs by using the providers within the HMO network. The HMO provides coordination of care because your primary care physician directs all referrals and makes sure that you receive the proper care without possible dangerous conflicts (such as two different doctors prescribing for you medications that conflict with each other).

✔ **Preventive health care:** Routine "well" visits and screening tests may reduce your need for health care by staving off illness before it starts or by catching a disease in its earliest stages. Traditional health care plans often don't support this option.

✔ **Wellness programs:** HMOs often provide workshops and literature on diet, exercise, and other topics to keep you and your family healthy. HMOs may also allow for counseling in such areas as losing weight or quitting smoking.

✔ **Health education:** An HMO may help keep you advised of important news in the health care field.

Now for the disadvantages: The limited choice of physicians approved by an HMO can be a drawback, and a limited number of physicians may be available for referrals for specialized care. HMO plans also have higher monthly payments (considered prepayments for services) as compared to traditional insurance plans. If you seek treatment by a physician outside the plan, those services may not be covered or may be only partially covered, depending on the plan.

Preferred provider organizations

A preferred provider organization, or PPO, is similar to an HMO in that it offers a limited number of physicians or facilities where you can obtain service with full coverage. However, a PPO does not tie your care to a single primary care gatekeeper. In a PPO, services will be paid for according to the plan schedule as long as you stay with the approved doctors, specialists, or facilities on the plan's list.

PPOs have a copayment factor, similar to traditional health plans, and also may require you to pay for the difference between the physician's or facility's actual charge and the amount that the plan schedule believes is a reasonable payment. Again, services provided by a doctor or facility outside the plan, except in some emergency situations, receive a much lower percentage of payment, or possibly no payment, from the PPO.

Point-of-service plans

A point-of-service plan is an option for many HMO or PPO members. It allows visits to both participating and nonparticipating providers, but with different levels of coverage. Quite simply, you pay more for any services that you obtain from a provider outside the approved list. Although such a plan offers great flexibility, the percentage of service fees payable by you may increase dramatically for services rendered by providers outside the approved list.

Employer plans

Many companies contract with large insurance corporations for coverage for their employees. However, some employers have *self-insured plans:* health care programs that they design and pay for themselves.

In these plans, each employer is free to decide without regard to legal mandate what type of coverage it will extend to employees. For example, employer plans are exempt from the Employee Retirement Income Security Act (ERISA), which mandates that certain benefits (maternity, pediatric wellness, and so on) be provided when more traditional insurance plans are offered to employees.

Employer plans are funded by the employer up to a certain dollar amount per employee, which may be subject to change from year to year. For example, an employer may state that it will cover appropriate medical expenses up to $2,000 per year for each employee, after which an outside insurance plan takes over. Employers protect themselves from unlimited liability by carrying the equivalent of a major medical policy to cover expenses over a certain dollar amount.

Making Sense of Medicare

Medicare is, by definition, the federal insurance plan that covers individuals who are age 65 and older, who are permanently and totally disabled, or who have end-stage renal (kidney) disease.

The Social Security Administration (SSA) is responsible for processing applications for Medicare from their offices around the country. If you have any questions about Medicare — and chances are good that you will — address your questions to the SSA.

Medicare, Part A

Part A of Medicare, which is free to applicants who meet the eligibility requirements, deals with hospital insurance and helps pay for hospital stays and care in a skilled nursing home or from a home health agency.

You pay a deductible of $768 (per the Department of Health and Human Services as of January 1, 1999) for services provided under Part A for a hospital stay of up to 60 days. For inpatient stays over 60 days and up to 90 days, you pay an additional deductible of $192 per day, and for stays over 90 days up to a total of 150 days, you pay a deductible of $384 per day. After 150 days, you are responsible for all costs. For skilled nursing care or inpatient treatment, the deductible is $96 per day after the first 20 days of care up to 100 days. After 100 days, you are responsible for all costs.

Medicare, Part B

Part B of Medicare, which has a premium set by federal guidelines ($45.50 per month as of January 1, 1999), covers physician fees, outpatient hospital services, and medical supplies and services. You have a copayment require-ment of 20 percent after a $100 deductible, plus any additional charge above the amount charged by the provider as approved by Medicare.

Medicare supplemental policies that cover the additional expenses and deductibles not paid by Medicare are available from private insurers.

Becoming eligible for Medicare

To be fully eligible for Medicare, you must meet the following requirements:

- You have worked a minimum of 40 quarters, or a total of 10 years, in jobs covered under the Social Security Act, or you are covered under the Railroad Retirement Act. Applicants who have not worked the full 40 quarters can apply for benefits but are required to pay a premium based on the number of quarters worked.

- You are a citizen of the United States, either by birth or by naturaliza-tion, or an alien admitted for permanent residence who has lived in the United States for at least five years.

A person who has not fulfilled the work requirement alone may be eligible for coverage on the record of someone else who is covered. For example, spouses are eligible if they are 65 or older and if their spouse is insured. Widows and widowers are covered if they were married to their spouse for at least one year prior to the death of that spouse and are over 65. Divorced persons are eligible if they were married to the covered person for at least ten years and have not remarried. Mothers of covered children are eligible if they are over 65. Parents of children eligible for Social Security who were receiving at least half of their support from the child at the time of the child's death or disability are eligible when they reach age 65.

Signing up for Medicare

Being 65 or older does not mean automatic enrollment in Medicare. If you are in doubt, make application when you turn 65. The worst that can happen is that you'll find out your application has already been taken care of.

A "window of opportunity" exists for Medicare enrollment. In order to have Medicare effective as of your 65th birthday, you can apply any time within three months of turning 65. If you apply more than three months after your 65th birthday, Medicare becomes effective on the date of application. This may leave you with a period of no coverage, because most private insurance plans stop on your 65th birthday.

A few different situations exist regarding enrollment:

- ✔ If you are already receiving benefits under Social Security or Railroad Retirement benefits, you are automatically enrolled for Parts A and B of Medicare when you reach age 65. You should receive your insurance card three to four months prior to your 65th birthday. However, the card is not effective until that birthday. If you receive no card and you are eligible for benefits, a hospital or other provider can bill under your Social Security number. You can obtain a Temporary Notice of Medicare Eligibility in these instances from the Social Security office.

- ✔ If you are 65 or older and are applying for Social Security benefits, you are automatically enrolled in Medicare as part of the process. The card is sent to you in the mail. If you are found eligible for Social Security, you are automatically eligible for Medicare.

- ✔ Individuals with end-stage renal (kidney) disease are automatically enrolled if they are receiving Social Security disability benefits. If not, they must apply for coverage under Medicare.

- ✔ If you have not applied for Social Security or Railroad Retirement benefits before age 65, you must file an application to enroll in Medicare. Notification that you are now eligible to receive these benefits, which was formerly sent automatically, has been dropped as a cost-cutting measure. If you have any doubts regarding your eligibility for Medicare or Social Security, contact your local Social Security office for clarification of your status.

You don't need to worry about having your Social Security card on you if you need a sudden trip to the doctor's office or hospital. Just give the providers your Social Security number — they can bill with that.

SAVVY CONSUMER

Full payment may not mean full payment!

You checked out your health insurance plan, deciphered the payment program, figured out the proper deductibles and copayment, and even know how to file the paperwork for a claim. Your plan says that you will receive full payment for inpatient charges in case of inpatient treatment if previously approved by the company. One hundred percent of the charge will be paid, right?

Not necessarily.

Additional charges not covered by the insurance policy often surface. These fees occur when your provider charges more for the service than your insurer believes is "usual, reasonable, or customary" (UCR). Insurers determine UCR figures by looking at similar services in the same geographic region. In these instances, the amount above the approved charge as reviewed by the insurer is your responsibility.

This situation often occurs for Medicare charges when the provider is not an assigned provider. Assigned providers are required to accept Medicare's payment as payment in full. However, if your provider doesn't accept assignment, no such requirement exists. So after you pay the appropriate deductible and your copayment, you could be responsible for a portion of the charge if the provider charges more than Medicare is willing to pay.

In some instances, you can appeal the charge to Medicare, and if they feel that an additional allowance is justified, you may receive a larger payment. An appeal to the physician to see whether he or she is willing to lower the fee in this instance may help as well. But after you go through these procedures, whatever is left of the charges is your responsibility. So read your bill carefully and make sure that you understand all the charges, as well as whether they are being paid in full.

Opting for a Medicare HMO

In 1985, the Health Care Financing Administration made available the first Medicare HMOs as an option for Medicare beneficiaries and retiring employees who already belonged to HMOs.

The Medicare HMO plan provides all the Medicare services and some additional services, usually including a deductible for hospital and skilled-nursing services and a deductible and copayment for physician services in hospital and office settings, diagnostic and rehabilitation services, prescription drugs, hearing aids, and eyeglasses.

You must meet the following criteria to enroll in a Medicare HMO plan:

- You must be enrolled in both Part A and Part B of Medicare.
- You can join only an HMO that has a contract with Medicare, not just any HMO.

✔ You must live in the service area of the HMO — in other words, the geographical area from which the HMO is licensed to enroll members.

✔ You must enroll during the HMO's open enrollment period. Some HMOs limit the period during which you can sign up to certain months of the year. You can drop out of the HMO at any time by notifying the HMO in writing on the form that it requires for this purpose. It's common for the drop-out request to be received by the tenth day of the month in order to be effective by the end of the month. If the request is received after the tenth day, it is not effective until the first day of the second month following the request. In the meantime, you still have coverage under the HMO program.

Covering the gaps

Because Medicare does not cover all the charges that you incur while either in the hospital or in the physician's office, a new type of insurance policy has appeared for the consumer: *Medicare supplemental policies,* also known as *Medigap policies.* Several types of insurance relating to Medicare coverage are offered; however, only one type is a true Medicare supplemental plan.

A Medigap is designed to pick up those expenses that Medicare does not cover, such as Part A and Part B deductibles and copayments. These policies are coordinated with Medicare and do not duplicate Medicare coverage. All insurance companies that sell supplemental plans must comply with the new federal standards for supplemental coverage. Companies are required to offer a core component of basic coverage and may offer up to nine additional plans with expanded coverage to cover items such as at-home recovery, foreign travel, excess physician charges (for nonparticipating physicians), prescription drugs, and preventive services.

Finding a Compatible Practitioner

Some insurance plans, most recently HMO and PPO plans, restrict which physicians or facilities you can use to obtain full payment for services. In the same way, not all physicians or facilities accept all types of insurance.

Heed the following advice before choosing a physician:

✔ **Ask what insurance coverage is accepted.** Many hospitals and clinics also have policies as to what type of insurance coverage they accept. If you receive treatment from a physician or facility without checking on its insurance policies, you may find yourself with a sizable out-of-pocket expense for medical services.

✔ **Get a list of providers.** Many physicians accept large insurance carriers, such as Blue Cross/Blue Shield, and large insurance company plans, such as CIGNA or Prudential. These plans can provide you with the names of providers who accept their insurance.

Insurance from smaller companies may not be as readily accepted by providers, which means that you, the patient, are responsible for the costs and for submitting them for reimbursement from your insurance plan. Contact a representative of your insurance plan to obtain a listing of providers who will accept your insurance for payment.

For Medicare plans, you can find a list of practitioners who accept this type of payment through your local Social Security office. HMOs, by nature, provide a listing of participating physicians and facilities.

✔ **Find out whether your physician, hospital, or clinic will accept your insurance company's benefits as payment in full.** Even if a physician or hospital accepts the insurance, the insurance may not fully cover the cost of the services provided. In that case, the difference between the total amount and the amount covered by insurance (including your copayment) is your responsibility.

✔ **For Medicare charges, ask whether your provider accepts Medicare assignment.** If assignment is accepted, the Medicare payment (less your copayment) will be accepted as payment in full. This rule prevents the provider from charging a higher amount, billing Medicare for what they will pay, and billing you for the rest (over and above the 20 percent copayment that you would normally make). Information about providers who accept Medicare assignment should be available from your local Social Security office.

✔ **Negotiate if your provider does not accept assignment from your insurance benefits.** If you ask, many providers will accept a Medicare insurance payment and your copayment as payment in full if it means keeping you as a patient. But remember that this is not always the case. Always find out up front whether the provider accepts insurance assignment.

Points to Ponder

You need to remember plenty of points when reviewing a medical insurance program for your family — certainly too many to cover in this limited space. But these few simple points can help you make a decision:

✔ **Make sure that the company selling the policy is licensed in your state.**

✔ **Check the rating of the company in one of the insurance rating services.** Best's Insurance Reports and Standard and Poor's report are two sources that can give you an idea of the company's strength and how it compares to similar companies in your state.

✓ **Take costs into account.** Consider your monthly premium (which your employer may pay in part), your deductible, and your copayment.

✓ **Think about location.** Review the listing of physicians and facilities within your area under HMO, PPO, or POS plans. If the number of physicians in your immediate area is limited, you may be unable to find a physician who meets your specific health care needs.

✓ **Make sure that you know exactly what your premiums will be and exactly what they cover.** Some coverage under a policy is available only by a special rider, which requires an extra premium. If you're paying the basic premium, you may not have the coverage you requested.

✓ **Take advantage of the "free look" provision (available in individual health policies), which is mandated by law.** If you find out that your coverage isn't what you thought you were buying, cancel it with no obligation.

✓ **Choose a policy with a stop-loss provision.** This provision limits your out-of-pocket expenses in the case of excessive medical charges within a calendar year. If the policy does not come with a stop-loss provision, check with the agent to determine whether one can be added as a rider for an additional fee.

✓ **Be sure that the policy covers prescription drugs.** Medications are very expensive and, if required for long-term treatment, can have a significant impact on your health care costs.

✓ **Check to see how preexisting conditions are covered under the policy.** If the policy excludes preexisting conditions for a period longer than six months, the coverage is of little benefit to you because any ailments you have now probably will still be with you after six months.

✓ **Check to see whether the policy duplicates coverage that you may already have under another plan.** Although most people have only one insurance plan, with both partners working these days, many people have duplicate medical coverage through both employers, each with the spouse listed as a dependent. If the plans provide for different coverage, having both may be beneficial. Otherwise, see whether either plan allows for coordination of benefits.

✓ **Don't replace your current coverage without carefully reviewing all aspects of the plan.** For example, if you have an ongoing medical problem, preexisting-condition exemptions may leave you without coverage for anywhere from six months to a year for the very reason you need the protection.

✓ *Most important:* **If you don't understand any provision of your health coverage, whether it is individual or group coverage through your employer, ask questions.** You are the most important person the health plan will ever insure. You need to understand what you're paying for and what is covered.

Chapter 9

The Where of Care: Choosing Medical Settings

● ●

In This Chapter

▶ Selecting a hospital

▶ Using outpatient and emergency services

▶ Evaluating nursing homes

▶ Considering home care as an option

● ●

*W*hen you and your family take a vacation, you shop wisely. You pick up brochures, call your travel agent several times a day, and take advantage of those rental car coupons in the Yellow Pages. You're spending a lot of money, and you want to make sure that everything goes smoothly — that you won't, for example, end up staying at a run-down motel on the wrong side of town when you expected deluxe accommodations at the Four Seasons.

Although visiting a medical facility isn't exactly a cruise, you want to take the same sorts of precautions for your family when you need the services of a hospital, health clinic, emergency room, or nursing home. Most people take for granted the choices they have in medical settings, and they head wherever their doctor recommends. But many types of facilities exist, each with its own strengths and weaknesses. To make sure that you don't end up in the medical equivalent of that run-down motel, you need to know more about your options and how they can make a difference in your family's health.

Knowing Your Hospitals

Hospitals are classified into two major categories: specialty hospitals and general medical-surgical hospitals (commonly known as general hospitals). Within these two categories, several variations exist, including community hospitals or medical centers, and teaching or nonteaching hospitals.

No one type of hospital is better than any other in the overall scheme of things. Your choice depends on your personal needs — your condition, where you live, and which doctor you visit. What may be the perfect medical setting for one person may be all wrong for you.

Specialty or general?

Specialty hospitals do just that: They specialize. A specialty hospital either treats one specific type of illness or medical condition or deals exclusively with a specific category of patients — for example, cancer, psychiatric disorders, eye problems, children, women, or the elderly.

General hospitals are what most people commonly associate with the word *hospital.* These broad-based institutions are equipped to deal with a much wider variety of medical conditions than specialty hospitals. They are, in essence, a conglomerate of smaller hospitals within a hospital, capable of treating everything from appendicitis and heart transplants to broken bones and kidney disease.

Both types of hospitals have their advantages and disadvantages. Be aware of these pros and cons when deciding which kind of hospital best suits your family's specific health care needs:

- ✔ Specialty hospitals are expert in treating certain conditions.
- ✔ Specialty hospitals have greater access to the latest technology and treatment techniques in their areas.
- ✔ General hospitals are better equipped to handle unexpected medical situations, particularly unrelated medical emergencies. For example, if you are hospitalized in an orthopedic hospital and develop cardiac complications during back surgery, a specialty hospital may not be equipped to handle this unexpected, potentially life-threatening situation. You may be stabilized and then transferred to a general hospital that is capable of treating the crisis.
- ✔ General hospitals are more common than specialty hospitals, which aren't found in every community.

Community hospital or medical center?

Community hospitals serve a particular local community with general medical and surgical services. Most community hospitals cultivate the image that they're a friendly neighbor, sending out newsletters with slogans like "We care" and being active in the community. Community hospitals possess a multitude of departments, facilities, and expensive technology, making them capable of treating a wide variety of medical conditions.

Medical centers are large institutions with various in-depth, highly sophisticated departments and expert personnel capable of handling the most serious illnesses and the widest array of medical conditions. Among the many high-tech facilities in a medical center are state-of-the-art intensive-care, coronary-care, and trauma units.

So what are the advantages and disadvantages?

- ✔ Community hospitals are large enough to handle a vast array of medical-surgical conditions yet still provide the patient-centered atmosphere that a vast medical center may lack.

- ✔ Medical centers are massive, and they continually see a wide cross-section of diverse patients and illnesses.

- ✔ Medical centers are often affiliated with universities, which brings access to the latest drugs, machines, medical-surgical techniques, and ideas.

- ✔ Medical centers usually attract top talent, young and old, who want to pioneer the next level of medical miracles.

Remember that we're generalizing here. Hospital size and preeminent staff are not necessarily indicators of the medical treatment or patient care you'll receive.

Teaching or nonteaching?

Teaching hospitals are affiliated with a medical school and provide teaching programs to their medical students, interns, and residents. Teaching hospitals may also have a school of nursing and train various other health-related professionals, including physical therapists, occupational therapists, and speech-language pathologists, to name a few.

The pros and cons of teaching hospitals center around the fact that these institutions are essentially schools.

- ✔ As educational facilities, teaching hospitals boast access to cutting-edge technology, renowned expertise, and the latest medical knowledge. However, if you don't need specialized care, a nonteaching hospital does the trick just as well.

- ✔ In teaching hospitals, students are there to learn . . . on you! These institutions exist as much to educate the next generation of medical personnel as they do to treat patients. Therefore, be prepared to deal with groups of medical students, interns, and residents regularly convening at your bedside during rounds, often discussing your case in the third person as if you weren't in the room. A teaching hospital may not be the ideal place for a relaxing, personalized hospital stay. Of course, one thing you won't be at a teaching hospital is lonely.

Also keep in mind that students in teaching hospitals, because they lack experience, may need to order plenty of tests to figure out a diagnosis. And all tests have risks. If you find yourself being poked and prodded more than seems necessary, put a stop to it.

✔ Teaching hospitals are generally more expensive than nonteaching hospitals. Because they need to provide funds for research, salaries, and top-of-the-line equipment, teaching hospitals must raise prices to cover their costs.

Selecting a Hospital

Many factors come into play when you're selecting a hospital. Of course, you want to consider the various types of hospitals discussed in the preceding section and their unique advantages and disadvantages as they pertain to your family's specific medical situation. Most important, you should base your decision on both the quality of medical care available and a patient-focused approach to care.

Choosing the best hospital for your family is a very important decision, and one that should not be taken lightly. However, don't feel overwhelmed by the variety of diverse options available. Keep the following key points in mind when evaluating prospective hospitals, and the decision becomes much easier.

Analyze accreditation

Choose a hospital that is *accredited,* which means that the institution demonstrates a certain level of quality, cleanliness, and safety, and that it has undergone an inspection by an outside body to prove it. Accreditation is a voluntary pursuit, and 75 to 80 percent of U.S. hospitals are accredited. Allopathic hospitals are accredited by the Joint Commission on Accreditation of Healthcare Organizations (JCAHO). Osteopathic hospitals are accredited by the American Osteopathic Association.

Accreditation doesn't necessarily ensure a high-quality facility, but it is a sign that a hospital has met an established national standard. Because a hospital must renew its accreditation every one to two years, you should also find out when the institution was last accredited.

Check the staff

Check out the staff's credentials and the hospital's organizational structure. (Top hospital administration officials should know this information.) Physicians should be board certified by their specialty's professional society. Be certain to determine both the doctor's and the hospital's ability to treat a specific illness or condition. How often have the parties treated this illness, and what success rates have they had?

Nurses play an extremely significant role in the delivery of your health care, so ensuring that the nursing staff is properly credentialed and not under-staffed is very important. You want a hospital that has a high ratio of registered nurses (R.N.s) to licensed practical nurses (L.P.N.s). R.N.s usually have baccalaureate degrees from a four-year college nursing program and sometimes master's degrees, whereas L.P.N.s may have just a year of nursing school. The national average is four R.N.s to every one L.P.N. A higher ratio signifies a higher level of nursing expertise. Additionally, standards suggest one nurse for every three to six patients. If the patient load is higher, ask why. You can obtain information about a hospital's nursing staff directly from the hospital, your state affiliate to the American Nurses Association, or the American Hospital Association.

Look at patient focus and special services

Patient-focused care is critical to your recovery. Determine beforehand whether the hospital has appropriate support services, including case management, counseling and social workers, patient/family educators, and a referral network for more specialized care should you need it.

Some hospitals offer the services of *patient advocates,* individuals who listen to patient complaints and problems and act as go-betweens to hospital administration. If you encounter any difficulties — from not receiving an answer to your call-button summons to billing problems — take advantage of these services if they're offered.

Hospitals and your doctor's choice

If your doctor recommends a certain hospital, ask why. Practitioners may select a certain hospital for purely selfish reasons, such as the convenience of having all their patients at a single location or the desire to meet a patient admissions quota at a specific facility in order to maintain privileges there. Sometimes a physician may tell you that a certain hospital is simply "the best."

These reasons are unacceptable. Your physician should select the best institution for *your* particular medical situation. Find out about all other hospitals that your physician could send you to and ask why he or she did not recommend them instead. If you're not satisfied with the hospitals available to you, talk to your physician about arranging possible alternatives or find a physician or health plan that meets your preferences.

Using Outpatient Clinics

Many medical services and procedures can be performed on an outpatient basis. Rather than stay overnight in a hospital as an inpatient, a patient can have a procedure performed on an outpatient basis during the day and then go home that same evening. Outpatient services and procedures are performed in a number of facilities:

- ✔ **Hospitals:** Services may be provided within the actual hospital (using the operating room or other procedure room) or within an outpatient clinic located inside the hospital walls.

- ✔ **Ambulatory care centers affiliated with hospitals:** Located off-site, these centers are generally in community settings that are more accessible and convenient for consumers.

- ✔ **Freestanding ambulatory clinics:** These clinics have no specific ties to any hospital.

Many nonsurgical treatments, such as chemotherapy, and a host of surgical procedures that used to require expensive, lengthy stays in a hospital even just a few years ago are performed on an outpatient basis today. Outpatient treatment can actually reduce your medical bill by half.

After you decide on an outpatient procedure, you need to decide which outpatient facility to use. Use these tips to help you choose:

- ✔ Remember that there is no such thing as minor surgery. If an emergency should arise, you need to know whether emergency facilities are nearby and readily accessible, whether or not the outpatient clinic is connected to a hospital.

- ✔ Find out ahead of time what happens if you don't recover completely during same-day surgery, as well as what kinds of after-care services and programs are available to ensure a quick and easy recovery.

- ✔ Ensure that the outpatient facility is licensed by the proper state agency and is subject to regular professional standards surveys. Ask about *accreditation* (whether the facility has met established national standards of quality). Inquire about the staff as well. Physicians should be board certified in their appropriate specialty.

- ✔ Visit potential outpatient centers beforehand to ensure that they are clean and professional-looking and have ample recovery room space. Location and accessibility are also factors to consider.

Getting Emergency Care

Emergency care departments, better known as emergency rooms, are the most common outpatient services in a hospital. You should know some important factors about the ER and how it works, and waiting until you or a family member needs immediate help is not the time.

Everybody knows that ER staff treat and manage a multitude of emergency cases where patients become seriously or critically ill or injured. By law, a hospital ER must provide care to everyone who seeks it. Staff judge who should be seen first. The ER can use all the hospital's resources, 24 hours a day, to care for emergencies.

Sometimes people seem to forget, or simply don't know, what constitutes a legitimate emergency. Don't rely on the ER for general health care needs: colds, ear infections, and so on. Going to the ER is expensive, time-consuming, and inefficient for nonemergencies and routine care — and it interferes with treatment for those with life-and-death problems. Plus, the ER staff do not know your medical history. You should use your primary care physician because he or she knows your background and can more readily and efficiently diagnose and treat problems.

Routine and nonemergency medical cases are best served by visiting one of a growing number of after-hours and urgent-care health care centers. These facilities are less costly and more convenient than traditional ERs, and many insurance companies promote their use. Often located in the suburbs and even in shopping malls, urgent-care centers are very accessible, with office hours generally ranging from 12 to 24 hours a day.

When a true emergency does arise, however, an ER can literally be a life-saver. Make sure that you know where the closest ER is and whom to contact for an ambulance. Most areas use the standard 911 emergency telephone number, but in some communities, you may have to call the police or fire department to obtain an ambulance. Know the quickest route to the ER, too.

Looking at Long-Term Care

Long-term care has become a large, lucrative, and growing segment within the health care industry, due in part to tremendous growth in the older population. Until recently, very little regulation existed over the long-term-care industry, resulting in neglect and abuse, untrained staff, and oftentimes unscrupulous owner-administrators. However, quality in long-term care has improved drastically since the mid-1980s due to reforms mandated by the public.

The diverse needs of the elderly have begun to be addressed. Years ago, the traditional nursing home was the only option for long-term care, even if an individual had only limited impairments. Today, however, many options exist.

Exploring your long-term options

Long-term care comes in many forms. The level of care varies according to the patient's physical and mental health. At one end of the spectrum are *nursing facilities,* which care for the most frail of patients. At the other end are *continuing care communities,* which serve a relatively healthy population. In between lie *assisted-living residences.*

Before beginning a search for a long-term-care facility, make sure that the loved one who needs the care gets a complete physical and evaluation from a primary care physician. Your choice of a facility must be based on the level of care required. You should determine whether the person needs round-the-clock care and whether dressing, bathing, eating, and other "activities of daily living" — known in medi-speak as *ADLs* — can be performed without help.

The key to selecting the appropriate nursing facility for yourself or your loved one is to match specific physical and mental needs and capabilities with the appropriate level of care. This ensures that you don't pay for services you don't need and that you receive the services you do require.

Nursing facilities

Nursing facilities, commonly known as *nursing homes* or *convalescent homes,* are generally geared toward people age 65 and over who cannot live independently because of a chronic illness or debilitating injury. However, nursing facilities exist for patients of all ages who are recovering or living with physical or mental impairments, either on a temporary or a permanent basis. Many residents of nursing facilities require 24-hour supervision and nursing and rehabilitative care.

According to the Health Care Financing Administration, the federal agency that runs the Medicare insurance program, 44 different categories of care are available in nursing facilities. Most fall into two broad levels of care:

> ✔ **Skilled nursing care facilities:** In a skilled nursing care facility, at least one registered nurse is on duty at all times. Nursing care, such as maintaining feeding tubes, inserting IVs, and applying sterile dressings, is available 24 hours a day from a registered nurse or licensed practical nurse under the guidance of an attending physician.
>
> Skilled nursing care is particularly useful for individuals who require a skilled nursing care plan, such as bedridden individuals and post-surgery patients who already have complicated chronic medical conditions, such as diabetes or heart disease.

✔ **Intermediate nursing care facilities:** These facilities provide 24-hour supervision and basic nursing care, such as dispensing medications and treating wounds. Residents are cared for by registered nurses and various therapists who help patients regain as much function and independence as possible.

People in this category are generally not bedridden and are more mobile than those who require skilled nursing care. This form of long-term care is especially useful for people with limited chronic conditions who can't live completely on their own, yet can use the social, recreational, and medical support services that intermediate nursing care facilities provide.

Skilled and intermediate care facilities used to be separate entities. Now, they are often housed together so that as individuals gain greater independence, they can transfer to the other type of facility with ease.

Continuing care communities

Also known as *life care communities,* continuing care communities include a combination of independent housing, assisted-living quarters, and skilled nursing facilities within one complex. Such communities represent a lifelong home for residents because of an inherent promise of continuing care at varying levels when and if the person needs it.

Most residents are single or widowed, are in their mid-70s, and exhibit relatively good health and high activity levels. Residents who thrive in this environment are typically those who have adapted well in the past to large settings, are outgoing, and can accept the somewhat-restrictive group lifestyle inherent in continuing care.

But what exactly is a continuing care community, and how does it differ from other forms of long-term care? The American Association of Homes and Services for the Aging, which represents the long-term-care industry, describes continuing care communities as "part housing complex, part activity center, and part health care system." Housing quarters vary widely from one community to another. Typical settings include high-rises, mid-level complexes, and spacious campus-style grounds. Individual units range from small apartments to multi-bedroom homes. Many activities and support services are available to residents, including meals, transportation, laundry/housekeeping/lawn service, security, counseling, and various social, recreational, and cultural activities.

The key factor that distinguishes continuing care communities from other long-term-care alternatives is the wide variety of health care services available. This is largely because continuing care serves such a diverse range of people for the remainder of their lives. As a resident gets older and perhaps develops more physical and mental impairments, an array of medical treatment becomes available. Health care services include less-intensive in-home care, on-site clinics, assisted-living units for bathing, meals, and other needs, a skilled nursing unit within the community or at a nearby off-site, and a variety of health, wellness, and emergency response services.

Continuing care communities can be rather costly, including a large, nonrefundable entry fee. Potential residents also must have insurance coverage and demonstrate the financial ability to meet their current and future expenses.

Assisted-living residences

Assisted-living residences are referred to by a host of different names, including *board-and-care homes, retirement homes, group homes,* and *personal-care homes.* Look beyond the name to ensure that the proposed facility contains the three components that constitute a legitimate assisted-living residence: housing, meals, and personal-care services.

Assisted living includes private housing in a single complex, meals, support services such as housekeeping, 24-hour staff monitoring, and assistance with one or more activities of daily living, including dressing and bathing. The goal of assisted living is to maintain and promote an individual's independence.

Although some assisted-living residences are affiliated with a skilled nursing facility, remember that they are not skilled nursing facilities. The most significant difference between the two is the level of medical services available. Assisted-living staff are prohibited by state law from providing medical care. Several assisted-living models exist, however, to satisfy the health care needs of its predominately elderly population:

- ✓ **Assisted-living residences as part of a continuing care community or nursing facility:** In this model, a registered nurse is often on the premises and/or on 24-hour call, as are various health care therapists.

- ✓ **Assisted-living facilities with an on-site service coordinator:** The coordinator arranges medical services from outside sources for the residents.

- ✓ **Assisted-living residences that do not provide medical care:** These communities consider medical care to be the sole responsibility of the individual and therefore do not provide health care or coordination. This model of assisted living is declining in popularity.

Assessing your alternatives

With so many long-term-care alternatives available today, how do you evaluate and choose the best option for yourself or your loved one? The key is to relax, take a deep breath, and analyze some key factors.

A word about abuse

In the 1980s, the long-term-care industry was the subject of a whirlwind of federal reforms. In the past, cases of abuse in nursing homes were rampant. In too many cases, residents were restrained or beaten, personal belongings were stolen, or patients were simply neglected, left to lie in their own filth.

Needless to say, the situation has improved. However, when no one looks out for older patients — especially those patients who depend on others for their daily needs — the possibility of abuse still looms. What can you do to prevent it?

✔ Get referrals to good facilities from others who have friends or family living there.

✔ Visit the facility and talk to residents. Ask them whether they've experienced any problems with the staff or whether they're in any way uncomfortable with their surroundings.

✔ Visit loved ones in long-term-care facilities frequently. Your presence can help deter mistreatment.

Evaluate services and personnel

Start by identifying several facilities that interest you. Ask your friends and neighbors for advice, and ask your doctor, too. Read brochures and make a list of what seem to be the best options.

Then visit the residences on your list. Evaluate the location, cost, services, facilities, residents, and management of each facility. Pay special attention to quality-of-life issues: Is the food decent? Are the rooms livable and pleasant? What sorts of activities are planned? Do residents seem well treated and respected by the staff? Also keep an eye out for safety issues: wheelchair ramps, handrails in the hallways and bathrooms, smoke detectors, emergency exits, and the like.

Verify licensing, certification, and accreditation

Long-term-care facilities can be licensed, certified, and accredited. Here's what those terms mean to you:

✔ **Licensed:** A long-term-care facility must be licensed by the state and sometimes the city and county in which it operates, according to law. A license is contingent upon an inspection by the state. The process is designed to protect residents from poor conditions and abuse.

✔ **Certified:** Long-term-care facilities have the option of becoming certified by the federal Health Care Financing Administration (HCFA). However, a facility cannot participate in the federal Medicare and Medicaid insurance programs without certification. Often, licensure and certification are intertwined in one process.

✔ **Accredited:** Long-term-care facilities can voluntarily apply for accreditation from various organizations. To receive accreditation, a facility must meet established national standards and undergo a rigorous review process.

Nursing facilities must be licensed, and certification is voluntary. Accreditation is available from the Joint Commission on Accreditation of Healthcare Organizations (JCAHO), the same group that accredits hospitals.

For continuing care communities, mandatory licenses are granted by various state agencies, such as the Department of Consumer Affairs and the Department of Health. No federal regulations exist, but facilities may voluntarily apply for accreditation from the Continuing Care Accreditation Commission of the American Association of Homes and Services for the Aging every five years. Currently, only 10 percent of continuing care communities have such accreditation. You may want to inquire as to a facility's plans to seek accreditation in the future or whether accreditation was denied.

Mandatory licensing for assisted living residences is granted by various state departments, such as the Department of Community Affairs, the Department of Health Services, and the Department of Housing, among others. Certification is optional, but, again, only certified facilities may qualify for Medicare and Medicaid reimbursement. Because assisted living doesn't provide direct medical care, few residences are certified.

Disclose costs, contracts, and taxes

Have an expert such as an attorney, accountant, or financial planner review all financial and legal matters surrounding long-term care. The contracts can be lengthy, and you want to make sure that you're not going to be held accountable for any hidden costs or troublesome requirements.

Financing long-term care

Seeking long-term care is a complex and costly endeavor. Obviously, you should seek out the best long-term-care alternative for your money, along with the best financing options.

✔ **Medicare:** You may be surprised to learn that reimbursement by Medicare is quite limited. Medicare is health insurance and doesn't cover nonmedical (though much-needed) support services such as transportation and housekeeping. Medicare coverage is also tied to acute illnesses and injuries, not to ongoing chronic conditions. If your health stabilizes, coverage ends. Additionally, Medicare does not cover continuing care or assisted-living facilities.

✔ **Medicaid:** Medicaid is the largest government payer for long-term-care services. Under Medicaid's regular program, individuals are covered indefinitely for all levels of care in certified facilities, including nursing facilities and assisted living.

The catch is that Medicaid kicks in only after personal assets dwindle to nearly nothing. This means that an individual must spend essentially all his or her money on health care before qualifying for the insurance.

✔ **Long-term-care insurance:** This is private insurance purchased specifically to finance long-term-care needs. This form of financing is controversial because many policies written in the early 1980s (when long-term-care insurance first began) contained restrictions that prevented policyholders from receiving the coverage they paid for. State reforms have changed this policy today, but it's still imperative to have experts review any insurance policy that you're considering.

✔ **Reverse mortgages:** Another form of private funding specifically for long-term-care needs, reverse mortgages allow borrowers to take out a loan against the value of their home (if they own a house or condo with little or no mortgage). The availability and types of reverse mortgages vary by state. You can find a list of lenders through the U.S. Department of Housing and Urban Development, the Area Agency on Aging, and your county property tax office, to name a few. Consult with a financial planner to determine the pros and cons.

Handling Home Health Care

People of all ages naturally prefer to remain at home rather than enter a long-term-care facility. The health care industry prefers to keep costs down. Home health care satisfies these two needs and generally results in beneficial outcomes for both patients and society. It's a growing and popular option among long-term-care alternatives.

Home health care provides medical and personal services to partially or fully dependent individuals in the home. The intent is to restore or maintain health and/or to promote independence, while minimizing the effects of physical and mental impairments.

Services are typically categorized into three levels of care:

✔ **Intensive:** The patient's needs are similar to those in a hospital or skilled nursing facility.

✔ **Intermediate:** The patient doesn't require intensive care but needs monitoring and limited medical assistance.

✔ **Maintenance:** The patient requires personal and support care.

These are some of the common home health services that are available:

- ✔ Skilled nursing care, such as intravenous feeding, oxygen therapy, blood tests, X-rays, and chemotherapy
- ✔ Personal care, such as bathing, meals, transportation, and housekeeping
- ✔ Rehabilitative therapies
- ✔ Dialysis and other "high-tech" treatments
- ✔ Delivery and setup of medical equipment and supplies

Ideal candidates for home health care are patients recently discharged from a hospital or skilled nursing facility who require rehabilitative and follow-up care. Also ideal are individuals with a chronic condition that requires frequent monitoring, as well as relatively healthy persons who have difficulty meeting basic needs, such as meals and bathing.

At first glance, home health care may appear to be the ideal solution for your loved one's long-term-care needs. The individual remains at home while still receiving the medical and personal care that he or she needs. This is particularly ideal for families agonizing over how to care for a dependent elderly parent.

Despite the obvious benefits, home health care is not always the best alternative. For example, if you have an unaccommodating home in terms of wheelchair accessibility and other limitations, home care can be difficult. The same goes for faraway family members; if you don't have enough personal support, home care may be hard to handle. Think about the needs of the patient as well. If a number of different services are required, coordinating the various agencies involved may be difficult.

What's more, highly technical or skilled services may actually be more costly with home health care than in a skilled nursing facility. Quality is hard to assess as well, especially if more than one person or organization provides home care. Discuss with your medical practitioner whether home care is a good option for you or your loved one.

Chapter 10

Undergoing Tests and Surgeries

. . . .

In This Chapter

▶ The ins and outs of medical testing

▶ Understanding the risks of common surgeries

▶ Protecting yourself from infection

▶ Finding out all about anesthesia

▶ Getting a second opinion

. . . .

*W*hen you head to a clinic for a routine blood test, you're going to undergo a medical procedure, just like a person headed for the operating room. Medical procedures come in many shapes and sizes, from diagnostic tests to complicated surgeries, and almost all have risks associated with them. It's in your best interest to find out the details of the procedure and how it can affect you and your health. That means knowing about the benefits and pitfalls of medical procedures, knowing the right questions to ask, and getting the answers you need before you proceed.

Testing the Waters of Medical Testing

Practitioners use medical testing to find valuable information about what's ailing you. Most doctors rely on medical tests, which can range from simple blood tests or X-rays to more complicated, risky procedures such as *cardiac catheterization.* (In that procedure, a thin, flexible tube is inserted through an artery into the heart to gather information about how well the heart is working. Sounds fun, huh?)

Medical tests are generally divided into four categories:

> ✔ **Screening tests:** People who appear healthy undergo screening tests to determine whether a particular problem, perhaps one they are at risk for, is present. For example, a woman with a family history of breast cancer may undergo regular mammograms as screening tests even if she doesn't have any symptoms of the disease.

- ✔ **Diagnostic tests:** Doctors use diagnostic tests to confirm or deny their impressions of what may be wrong. A sore throat, for example, may warrant a diagnostic test for streptococci, the bacteria that cause strep throat.

- ✔ **Prognostic tests:** In this case, a diagnosis has already been made, and a prognostic test is used to gather more information. A surgeon may perform a prognostic test to see how far a cancer has spread, for example.

- ✔ **Monitoring tests:** These tests are used to evaluate the effects of a medical treatment done on a patient. A person in the hospital may undergo routine blood tests after surgery to make sure that all is well.

Medical tests can be either *invasive* or *noninvasive* Invasive tests involve penetration of the body and normally pose greater risks (such as infection or doctor error) than noninvasive tests, which do not penetrate the body. An *endoscopy,* a test in which a flexible fiber-optic tube is inserted into the body (ouch!) for a look around, is an example of an invasive test. A common noninvasive test is an X-ray, which doesn't involve any too-personal poking or prodding.

Keep in mind that just because a test is noninvasive does not necessarily mean that it is risk-free. Take the X-ray example. Though noninvasive, X-rays carry some risks because of the short wavelengths they use to create images of bones and teeth. These wavelengths can damage individual cells, which may lead to cancer and also can cause birth defects. For this reason, you need to think about how necessary a test is before agreeing to have it done.

Even if the risks of a test are nil, you still want to double-check on necessity. The more tests doctors do, the more likely it is that they'll find something unusual that they want to treat (whether it needs it or not). In this way, unnecessary tests clear the way for unnecessary treatments and surgeries and the risks they carry.

Avoiding Unnecessary Testing

Whatever the problem, you want to keep testing to a minimum. The fewer tests you undergo, the less chance that something will go wrong — remember that almost every test has its downside. Of course, cost is also a factor here. You don't want to end up shelling out hundreds of dollars if you can avoid it.

A key part of avoiding tests you don't need is to ask your doctor plenty of questions about the test, why it's recommended, how it works, and what it's expected to show. Using your doctor's answers, you can evaluate for yourself whether the test is justified. Try asking these questions:

✔ **Why does this test need to be done?** A simple enough question, but an important one. If you're facing a retest, ask why it's necessary again. Was the first test flawed or inconclusive? Or will something new and important be done?

✔ **What will you be looking for in the test results?** This question requires the doctor to let you in on the process, diagnosis, and prognosis.

✔ **Will the procedure be painful, and is it dangerous?** Don't hesitate to ask this question — you won't look like a wimp. After all, if the test might lead to complications or cause more pain than the condition itself, you may want to think twice about having it done.

✔ **How much will it cost?** To get the most for your medical dollar, you can shop around for the best doctor who will perform the test at the best price. Also find out whether your insurance covers the test before consenting to have it done.

✔ **How much time will it take?** This is not a selfish or trivial question. In today's world, time is money. Certainly, you don't want to forgo essential medical care because of a tight schedule, but if a procedure's value is questionable and it means lost work time and pay, you want to take that information into consideration.

✔ **Do the potential advantages of the test outweigh the risks?** The test itself might be dangerous or cause serious problems as a side effect. Have the doctor give you a rundown of the possibilities.

✔ **Is this the most appropriate test?** A host of tests are available to diagnose or rule out a condition. Because of this, many doctors fall victim to "testitis" — they use all the tests available instead of the most comprehensive one. Watch out for the doctor who wants you to climb the test ladder. Ask your doctor which test is the most comprehensive, and find out why it wasn't recommended in the first place. Remember that one comprehensive test may be a lot cheaper than three less-comprehensive ones.

✔ **What will happen if I don't have this test done?** You must ask this question every time a procedure is recommended. What could you possibly lose by asking? And you could gain a great deal.

Before going into the hospital, see if you can get any of your preadmission testing done in advance. After you're in the hospital, they take X-rays, draw blood, and perform a whole host of tests to see what shape you're in. If you know which tests are going to be done, you can have them done quickly and less expensively before you even check yourself into the hospital.

Dealing with Common Surgeries

If medical testing is the frying pan, surgery is the fire. The last thing you want to hear when you're sitting on that cold examining table is the doctor saying, "Well, I think we'd better get you to the hospital to take care of this."

Although thoughts of surgery may lead you to ponder your own mortality, the better thing to do is to start pondering the procedure at hand. Surgery is a serious proposition — even minor surgery has its risks. You owe it to yourself and your family to get all the facts, from the credentials and qualifications of the surgeon to a list of possible complications and outcomes.

Signing on a surgeon

In Chapter 6, we go over all the information you need to know about choosing a practitioner and a specialist. A surgeon is simply a form of a specialist, so you want to ask all the appropriate questions:

- ✔ **What is your education?**

- ✔ **Are you board certified?**

- ✔ **How often have you performed the procedure required?** The more frequently a surgeon performs a procedure, the better the chances it will be a success.

- ✔ **What are the most common complications associated with this surgery?** Stay away from surgeons who hem and haw or say that no risks are involved. A good surgeon will go over all the possibilities and answer all the questions you have about them.

- ✔ **What is your success rate for this procedure?** The success rate means more than simply surviving. Ask the surgeon what your chances are of 100 percent success — that is, regaining full function. If less than 100 percent, ask how fully the doctor expects you to recover.

- ✔ **What will happen if I don't have surgery?** If you aren't keen on surgery, aren't sure how helpful it will be, and aren't in dire straits at the moment, you may want to postpone or decide against the procedure. And many conditions can be treated through means other than surgery — for example, medications or less-invasive procedures.

- ✔ **Where will I have this surgery?** It's important to get solid reasons for the choice of facility. Make sure that your doctor has your best interests — and not his or her own interests — at heart.

- ✔ **What are your fees, and how can I pay?** Even if you have insurance, be aware of the cost of your surgery. Today, most people end up paying some portion of the cost out of pocket. If you are expected to pay for a procedure yourself or are responsible for a copayment, ask whether you can pay in installments or work out some other payment plan.

> ✔ **Will you treat me yourself and personally perform any procedures we discuss, or are you in a group practice in which another doctor may provide my care?** You don't want to end up with a partner you've never met before. Make sure to get your doctor's guarantee that he or she will be at your surgery.

Signing informed consent forms

Informed consent is, simply, the idea that you have the right to available information about your condition and about the benefits and risks of any procedures the doctors want to perform on you. The information should include side effects, possible complications, likely outcomes, alternative procedures, and information about what will happen if you decide against a procedure. Then you can make an informed decision about what is done to your body and your life before you give the go-ahead or refusal.

Some doctors believe that medicine is too complicated for unschooled nonphysicians to understand, but medical consumers think that doctors ought to try to simplify medical information to make it accessible to the general public. And because doctors get paid not to talk but to perform procedures, some may consider taking time to discuss potential risks and options a loss of time and money. Also, more than a few doctors believe that if they explain things accurately, a patient may decide not to have the test, procedure, or operation.

When you enter a hospital or health care facility for a procedure, you give your informed consent by signing a consent form. This form may be a "blanket" consent form that gives the facility permission to treat your condition and applies to any and all procedures provided during your stay. Some forms may apply only to a specific procedure. Some facilities ask you to sign a consent form that includes a release against negligence on the part of the hospital or clinic or that requires you to waive your right to litigation in the event of malpractice. However, because the hospital is considered to have such a great advantage over the patient, these forms are not legally binding.

If you have not been informed to your satisfaction and/or are more than a bit unsure about giving your consent to your doctor's game plan, don't sign any form. Ask for more information. Ask about survival rates and statistical proofs of the effectiveness and safety of the procedure. (A lot of this territory should have already been covered during office visits and previous discussions.) If you are really doubtful, ask for printed materials that provide support for the route your doctor wants to take.

Also, make sure that the procedure described in the form is the same one that your doctor described to you. If it seems that the form grants permission for other procedures that you weren't aware of, don't sign the form until the point is clarified.

If you don't sign the consent form, chances are that you won't be admitted to the hospital. However, you should also know that these forms aren't set in stone, and you can revise them before signing them in order to protect your rights. A hospital consent form is not the law. The form is a contract that's subject to revision, and you have the right to revise it. You also have the right to say no to anything proposed. Although some hospital administrators may balk at your revisions, most will let you sign an amended form. This is because administrators usually realize that consent forms deny patients their rights and that refusing to amend such a form could lead to complaints or lawsuits.

Understanding mortality rates and complications

Part of informed consent, which we discussed in the preceding section, is understanding the statistics and rates that are thrown at you by doctors and hospitals before surgery. Knowing how to interpret what you hear gives you more information about the procedures — and you need as much information as you can get if you're going to make an informed decision about the surgery.

The percentage of people who die during or as a direct result of an operation is termed the *mortality rate.* The way mortality rates are determined is complicated — they're based on the total number of procedures performed over a period of time. The percentage gives you perspective on what the chances are. For example, the procedure to surgically repair a broken leg has a 3.7 percent mortality rate, which means that you have a 96.3 percent of surviving such a procedure.

The percentage of people who develop conditions as a result of a procedure is called the *morbidity rate.* Morbidity rates are even more complicated because no standards exist for what counts as a complication. One study that takes into account even minor problems may report a very high complication rate, while another that counts only really bad outcomes may report a very low one. Wide variations in these rates are commonplace.

Of course, such rates are only statistics — they may or may not apply to your personal condition. Take this into account. Your age, another medical condition, or some other factor may affect your outcome — for better or worse.

Preparing your child for surgery

Parents have twice as much to worry about when a child goes into the hospital — they not only have to think about preparing themselves for the procedures and taking care of the details, but they also need to prepare the child. Child development experts have identified issues that may arise, depending on a child's age:

✔ **2 to 4 years:** Time is pretty meaningless to most preschoolers, so don't waste yours by trying to explain how long they will be in the hospital. Instead, talk to your child a few days before surgery. Use simple explanations or drawings or use a favorite doll to show what's going to happen. Answer questions if you know the answers — never lie or make up an answer that may not be true. Even at this young age, children often have vivid fantasies: "Will the doctor cut off my arm while I'm asleep?" "Will I die like Grandma when she went to the hospital?" Encourage your child to talk and play out fantasies and work through the child's anxieties.

✔ **4 to 6 years:** Because older children may be familiar with the names of body parts and simple medical devices, you can use a little more detail here. Books can be helpful in explanations. Also at this age, children have newly developed consciences, and some begin to believe that hospitalization is punishment for a real or imagined trespass. Be especially careful to avoid equating behavior, good or bad, with the outcome of the stay.

✔ **6 to 10 years:** School-age children tend to be concerned about looking like everyone else, so many of their fears revolve around scarring and permanent damage. Asking your physician to arrange a meeting for your child with someone who has successfully undergone the procedure may help. Fears about anesthesia are also common, especially the idea of waking up before surgery is over. Beware of telling a child that anesthesia will lead to sleep — sleep disorders may develop when children associate the sleep they know with the sleep they don't know. Instead, refer to a special kind of sleep, during which no pain is felt, and that will end once the operation is over.

✔ **Teenagers:** Teens can be special problems to parents and hospital staff. They tend to fear losing control, appearing dependent, and losing privacy. Your teenager's response to a pending hospitalization may be irrational or erratic. Acknowledge the concern, but, if possible, ignore this behavior. Involve your teen as much as possible in the preparations and decisions regarding the hospitalization. If the surgery is scheduled in advance, make sure that your teen knows about it far enough in advance to become prepared.

Nose-Oh-What Infections?

Nosocomial (pronounced "nohs-oh-KOH-me-ul") doesn't quite roll off the tongue, but it's a word you should know if you're going into the hospital. By definition, nosocomial infections are infections acquired during hospitalization.

These infections are a manifestation of — here's another mouthful — *iatrogenic disease* (pronounced "eye-at-roh-JE-nick"), which comes from the Greek meaning "doctor-produced" or "doctor-caused." Iatrogenic diseases are those conditions that you end up with even though you didn't have them until a doctor did something to you — for example, accidentally cut into adjacent tissue with a scalpel or failed to remove a surgical sponge.

The ways nosocomial infections spread are numerous. Organisms can be transmitted by direct contact, in food and water, in transfused blood and intravenous fluids, in pharmaceuticals, through the air, on towels and sheets, and via the housekeeping crew, to name but a few.

Because microbes can multiply quickly in an open wound, nosocomial infections are quite risky for surgical patients. It is estimated that the recovery time necessary to combat a nosocomial infection is about four extra days in the hospital, at an average additional cost of $1,000 per day. Expensive as that is, a nosocomial infection can also be deadly: Some estimates of infection-related deaths run as high as 100,000 a year.

Studies indicate that between 5 to 10 percent of all patients (about 2 million people) develop nosocomial infections. Why are these infections so widespread? Well, for one thing, patients in modern hospitals tend to be highly susceptible to infections. And, of course, microorganisms and pathogens arrive with new patients from the community at large. Add to that the increase in invasive procedures, which often employ drugs that further weaken the immune system and leave the door open to infection. Antibiotics, ironically, also contribute to the growing numbers of nosocomial infections. Not only do some patients have bad reactions to antibiotics, but some strains of bacteria are rapidly becoming resistant to them as well.

So how can you protect yourself? You have no surefire defense if the rest of the hospital is a vast and bubbling breeding ground. So the first step in infection protection is to try to gain admission to a hospital that has a good nosocomial infection record. Ask your doctor about it. Contact your local Department of Health. Ask the hospital directly — all hospitals keep track of this statistic, though not all are eager to tell you what it is. Ideally, the rate for nosocomial infections should be zero, but rates tend to run between 5 and 10 percent. Decide against hospitals with rates that are any higher.

On guard

Hospitalization is a stressful event in any person's life — adult or child. That's why we give this advice: Don't let your child stay alone in the hospital.

Depending on the laws in your state, a preteen child cannot refuse a test or question a doctor; as a parent, you must do so if necessary. A child won't know whether a nurse is administering the wrong medication; you must double-check. Busy staff may not explain what is happening to a child; this is your job. Be your child's voice!

SAVVY CONSUMER

Hand demands

Protect yourself from nosocomial infections by demanding that all medical and nonmedical personnel wash their hands before touching you. This means everyone from Uncle Mac dropping off a bouquet of flowers to your renowned specialist. Make no exceptions!

What else can you do?

If your roommate becomes infected, you may be afraid that you'll catch an infection via the air or through the use of a common bathroom. Change your room at once if there's any chance that you might become infected, because once you are infected, it is too late. You may need to be put into isolation with your roommate.

If you are undergoing a surgery that requires the removal of hair, refuse to be shaved the night before surgery. Studies have found that chemical depilatories reduce the risk of nosocomial infections. Using barber clippers to remove hair the morning of surgery yields a low infection rate, too. Of course, you should ask whether shaving or clipping of hair is necessary at all. Removing hair before vaginal delivery or surgery in that area, for example, is probably uncalled for because clinical studies do not substantiate the old idea that hair creates a climate for infection.

Finally, have nurses regularly check the drainage of *catheters* (tubes that drain body cavities or the bladder) to help you maintain cleanliness.

All about Anesthesia

If you're going to have an invasive test or surgery done, you may have to consider *anesthesia,* a process that allows a procedure to be performed without your feeling the pain. The three different types of anesthesia are

- ✔ **Local anesthesia:** This anesthesia is used for procedures in which only a small part of the body needs to be anesthetized for a short time. Think of your dentist giving you Novocain before drilling.

- ✔ **Regional anesthesia:** With regional anesthesia, areas of the body can be numbed for up to three hours at a time.

- ✔ **General anesthesia:** If you need to be out completely for a long period of time, this is the anesthesia for you.

The type of anesthesia that you receive depends, of course, on what procedure is to be done, your condition, and your and your doctor's preferences.

As with any drug (and that's what anesthesia is, in essence), anesthesia has its side effects. For regional and general anesthesia, you may experience breathing difficulties, headaches, lightheadedness, nausea, vomiting, and pain. More serious complications of anesthesia can affect major organ systems and bring about heart attack, kidney failure, stroke, and death. However, these effects are extremely rare.

With all that in mind, you may be surprised to find out that anesthesia is relatively safe. Anesthesia itself is quite low on the list of what can go wrong during an operation. Still, the fact remains that an estimated 10,000 Americans die each year from anesthesia-related mishaps, and hundreds of thousands are injured. These injuries can range from relatively mild but prolonged numbness to conditions that handicap an individual for life.

The problem is that human errors can be made in the administration of anesthesia. Despite the safeguards that most hospitals take to prevent these tragic mistakes from occurring, they still happen. And that means it's important for you to be alert to potential problems.

Knowing who you're dealing with

An *anesthesiologist* is the specialist who's responsible for maintaining the state of sleep you're in during your surgery. Although the anesthesiologist may seem to be a minor member of your surgical team, this specialist plays a vital role.

In a hospital setting, anesthesia is usually administered by a physician who is board certified in anesthesiology. It can also be given by a certified nurse-anesthetist (a nurse with advanced training) who works under the supervision of an anesthesiologist. Both professionals are highly skilled with specialized training in their field.

Before the procedure, make sure that you speak with your anesthesiologist. Most consumers see their anesthesiologists only the night before the operation. The specialist may slip into your room, make brief introductions, and begin asking you questions about your health history. The idea is to find anything in your physical makeup that could cause trouble when you're put under, such as an allergy, heart problems, or high or low blood pressure. That really is not enough. To be fair to both you and the anesthesiologist, make an appointment to talk ahead of time. Ask the following questions:

- ✔ What type of anesthesia will you use? Why that one and not another? What dangers are there?

- ✔ What is the fee? Anesthesiologists charge separately for their services.

- ✔ What will happen just before and just after surgery?

- ✔ Will you be giving the anesthesia? Many anesthesiologists have such large practices that they can't personally be at every operation for which they are responsible. They hire help. An entirely different anesthesiologist, or a nurse-anesthetist, may stand in. You may want to tell your anesthesiologist to be there in person should any emergency arise. Get confirmation of the anesthesiologist's presence in writing. If your anesthesiologist won't give you a guarantee, you have the right to seek out one who will.

If something during your discussion with the anesthesiologist doesn't seem quite right, you have the prerogative to arrange with your surgeon and the hospital to have another well-trained, board-certified anesthesiologist present. Meet that person ahead of time, too!

Anesthesia and outpatient centers

Today, more procedures are performed in outpatient centers than ever before. Use of an outpatient center can often mean quicker recovery times and lower fees, but you also may be dealing with lesser-trained personnel. What happens if an emergency arises during your surgery that the center can't handle? Think about that possibility ahead of time.

If you're going to receive anesthesia in a nonhospital setting, make sure that the personnel are as trained and competent as in-hospital personnel. Also find out what type of backup the outpatient center has to handle emergencies. For example, they may have an ambulance available to move you to a hospital, and they may have a written agreement with a particular hospital should an emergency arise. Make sure that all staff members are trained in cardiopulmonary resuscitation (CPR). Many are not!

Sweet dreams: Anesthesia and your child

Parents play an important role in assuring that their children receive the pain relief they need should they need an operation. If your child is going to undergo a procedure, begin fulfilling that role as soon as you and the doctor agree that surgery is necessary.

In addition to asking the usual questions warranted when anesthesia is to be used, as a parent, you want to find out the following:

✔ **Are any preanesthesia sedatives used with children to lessen their anxiety?** Some centers use lollipops containing a

mild sedative, and research has found that children who receive these lollipops are more quickly anesthetized and require less postoperative pain medication than children who receive either no premedication or another oral sedative.

✔ **Can I be present during anesthesia induction?** Some hospitals encourage parents to be present while their child is being "put to sleep" and to be in the recovery room when the child awakes.

The key here is to question, question, question. Do not allow anesthesia to be administered to you in any outpatient setting unless you are completely comfortable with the competence of the practitioners involved and the emergency procedures in place.

Getting a Second Opinion

Getting another practitioner's opinion on your condition before committing to surgery is more than just a good idea — in today's world, second opinions are becoming a necessity.

Although at one time, doctors tended to frown upon second opinions (they felt as if they were being second-guessed), second opinions are widely accepted today as just another part of the process of doing all that you can to ensure that your surgery goes well. Many insurers now insist on a second opinion before they will cover some procedures, and doctors themselves often initiate second opinions by referring patients to other practitioners and specialists.Second opinions are important because not all doctors agree on medical problems — what they are, how to diagnose them, and how (or even whether) to treat them. Too often, people just go along with what their doctors recommend, whether they like it or not. In the worst case, that can lead to pain, complications, financial hardships, and perhaps even doctor-caused mishaps.

If a trip to the hospital is looming in the near future, getting a second opinion is vital. Even good doctors, convinced that the benefits of surgery outweigh less expensive and more conservative treatments, may rush patients into the operating room. A second opinion may confirm the original diagnosis and perhaps the need for hospitalization, but it also could contradict the first doctor's conclusions and thus create doubt about the need for hospitalization. You may even require a third, tie-breaking opinion.

Don't limit your search for a second opinion to recommendations involving surgery. As we said earlier in this chapter, many types of medical tests can be risky or invasive, too. Ask another doctor for a recommendation for any procedure that concerns you.

Chapter 11

Managing Medications

. . . .

In This Chapter

▶ Choosing a pharmacist

▶ Buying and using over-the-counter drugs

▶ Deciphering prescriptions

. . . .

*T*he right drugs taken the right way can be essential to your family's health. The more involved you are in prescribing, dispensing, and administering drugs for yourself and your family members, the more control you and your family have over your own health.

However, studies suggest that almost half of all prescriptions filled are never fully used. People report being confused about the side effects of the medication, about how long the medication can stay in their medicine cabinets and still be effective, and even about how to read the instructions that doctors or pharmacists gave them.

This chapter gives you the information you need about pharmacists, drug safety, and over-the-counter medicines so that you can make informed choices about any drug treatment you may require.

Enlisting a Pharmacist

Even though your family doctor may have prescribed a medication, he or she is probably not the best source for complete information about the medication. A doctor's training does not include extensive courses on drugs and their effects, and a doctor's view of a drug may be colored by the sales pitches that the doctor hears every day from drug company representatives. As a result, a pharmacist who knows your family may be a better person to answer your questions about medication.

A *pharmacist* is a professional who formulates and dispenses drugs or medications. A pharmacist also knows about drugs and their properties — their compositions, side effects, interactions, risks, and benefits. This knowledge makes pharmacists your allies in your quest for family health.

Evaluating a pharmacy

Asking plenty of questions and calling around to different pharmacies to find out their policies can be a pain in the neck. But think of it this way: If you take the time now to find the right place, with the right professional behind the counter, you can look forward to getting all your future medications hassle-free, with a family health safety net to boot.

When choosing a pharmacy, ask these questions:

- ✔ What personalized services are offered?

- ✔ Do you offer free home delivery?

- ✔ Do you have evening and weekend hours?

- ✔ Does the pharmacy accept my prescription drug insurance?

- ✔ Can refills be called in?

- ✔ What's the procedure if medication is needed when the pharmacy is closed or the pharmacist is away?

- ✔ Do you keep patient medication profiles on all customers?

- ✔ Do you offer patient counseling on drug interactions, side effects, and so on? Are consumer education materials available?

- ✔ Can you provide information about over-the-counter medications and medical equipment?

- ✔ Do you provide an area for private conversations with the pharmacist?

- ✔ Are pharmacy personnel willing to contact my family physicians if necessary?

- ✔ Does the pharmacy offer a senior-citizen discount?

Remember that the partnership your family establishes with your pharmacist has a direct bearing on your family's health and health care. Choose a pharmacist carefully. And don't hesitate to ask questions.

Working with your pharmacist

Perhaps the most important service that a pharmacist can offer your family is to monitor all the drugs you're taking in order to prevent medication errors. Doctors often do not do this monitoring, and many patients cannot accurately describe their drug treatments without their medications in hand, according to various studies.

A pharmacist uses a system called *patient medication profiles* (or simply *patient profiles*) to quickly see which previous medications worked or didn't work for your family and which caused allergic reactions or side effects. If a

You are your best defense

Pharmacists are crucial in preventing drug errors instigated by doctors. But what about errors made by pharmacists themselves?

Today, more than 46,000 Americans will walk out of their local pharmacies with either the wrong prescription medication or the wrong dosage. And over the course of the next year, 17 million people will be given the wrong prescription by pharmacists.

The consequences of these mistakes can be devastating. At least 20 percent of people admitted to hospitals are there because of a mistake made at the pharmacy, an improper drug ordered by a doctor, or an unexpected reaction to a medication. Many of those people would be home and well if a prescription error had not been made. Other victims may never enter a hospital, but they don't get better, either.

If doctors don't suspect a prescription error, they're apt to misdiagnose, which leads to more mistakes.

What we're trying to say is that you need to be vigilant against drug errors — even if you have the best pharmacist in the world.

Each time you have a prescription filled, check the label for the name of the drug and the dosage to make sure that it's correct. If the pills are different (a different shape or color, than you expected for example), double-check to make sure that you got the right prescription. If you're having a prescription filled for the first time, make sure that you get information about the drug and its side effects, and ask any questions you may have about how to use it.

possibility of a dangerous drug interaction exists, the pharmacist can alert your family and your doctor. Before your family chooses a pharmacist, find out if he or she keeps such a record for each customer and ask what information is included.

Remember, though, that a patient profile can be useful only if your family buys all your medicine from the same pharmacy. If you do go elsewhere for a prescription, make sure to tell your regular pharmacist so that your profile is up-to-date.

The American Pharmaceutical Association recommends that a patient medication profile contain the following information:

- ✔ Name, address, and phone number
- ✔ Birthdate (so that the pharmacist can check to see whether the dosage is appropriate to the age of the user)
- ✔ Any allergies, reactions, or tendencies toward adverse effects
- ✔ Any drugs that have proved ineffective

- ✔ A concise health history, including any conditions or diseases that would preclude the use of certain drugs (for example, diabetes, hypertension, or an ulcer)

- ✔ Nonprescription, or over-the-counter, medicines used (including vitamins, minerals, and alternative treatments such as herbs and other compounds)

- ✔ The date and number of each prescription filled, the name of the drug, its dosage and strength, quantity, directions for use, and price, as well as the prescriber and dispenser of each medication

Using Over-the-Counter Drugs

Studies show that more than 80 percent of all the medical care your family receives is self-care. In other words, most of the time, you are your own doctor.

The vast majority of products used in self-care are called over-the-counter (OTC) medicines and equipment, and as many as 300,000 OTC products are available in a variety of sizes, dosage forms, and strengths. Your family can buy these products at drugstores, supermarkets, and department/discount stores without a doctor's prescription.

The U.S. Food and Drug Administration (FDA) closely watches OTC products to be sure that they are safe if used according to the instructions on the label. Unlike prescription drugs, OTCs must carry labels that contain all the information needed for safe and effective use of the product. Because safety under all circumstances of use is a high priority for over-the-counter products, these products generally consist of ingredients that have a long and established safety record.

OTC products cannot do everything, though. Some conditions, such as bacterial infections or severe cuts, may need stronger products, available only by prescription. The important thing to remember is this: When in doubt, seek professional medical attention. And if you've been treating a problem yourself with OTC products and the condition either worsens or fails to improve, seek professional assistance. And be sure to tell your medical practitioner what OTC drugs you're taking.

Safety and OTC medicines

Because OTC products can be purchased by anyone, almost anywhere, without a prescription, they must have a *higher* standard of safety than prescription products. In fact, like prescription products, OTCs are regulated very closely by the U. S. Food and Drug Administration. This is to assure the consumer that the product can be used safely, following label directions.

Not only are OTC products reviewed carefully by the FDA, but they are also subject to the industry's own self-regulation for safety and effectiveness. And FDA review is not limited to new products proposed for the market. The FDA reviews, and in some cases removes, medications from over-the-counter status if evidence of a significant safety problem with a product or ingredient surfaces.

Putting an end to product tampering

Because of the publicity surrounding product tampering cases in the 1980s, manufacturers have made extensive changes in the way OTC medications are packaged and labeled. Inner and outer safety seals have been added to virtually every product to make it easier for everyone — from the store clerk to the consumer — to detect product tampering. In addition, a written warning advises against purchasing or using the product if the safety seal is broken.

Even though manufacturers have added these safety features, it's still your responsibility to examine the package, preferably before purchasing the product but definitely before using it. Look for these things when purchasing packaged medications:

- ✔ Check to see whether the container has been tampered with in any way. If the seal appears to have been disturbed, don't purchase the product. Holes, outer and inner linings that are open, or seals that are disturbed or cracked could indicate product tampering. Products with disturbed caps, cotton plugs, and wrapping also should be avoided.

- ✔ Check that pills, capsules, and tablets are not discolored, colored differently from one another, crumbly, in different sizes or shapes, or deformed. they should not give off an unusual odor.

- ✔ Check liquid medications for uniformity in color, thickness, and texture, and any unusual odors or foreign particles.

- ✔ Check creams and ointments for color and texture. Signs of discoloration or a sandy feeling could indicate a problem.

If you suspect that something may be wrong, don't purchase the product. If you have already purchased a product, return it to the store where you purchased it or contact the manufacturer. Some manufacturers have a toll-free telephone number where consumers may report problems with product packaging.

Using Prescription Drugs

With prescription drugs, safety starts even before the prescription is written. Prescription medications are powerful substances that work to alter the function of the body. But different people, even in the same family, react differently to drugs, and the medications themselves may react with other drugs or even with food or vitamins and minerals to create harmful side effects. To help determine which drug is the best for you or one of your family members, a heath practitioner should find out your health history. The questions that the health practitioner should ask include the following:

- ✔ Have you ever had an allergic reaction to a drug?

- ✔ Are you currently taking any other prescription or over-the-counter medications? Any vitamin or mineral supplements? Any alternative treatments?

- ✔ Do you have any medical conditions (such as heart disease or diabetes)?

- ✔ Are you on a special diet?

- ✔ How much alcohol do you consume?

Volunteer the information if your health practitioner doesn't ask.

To further ensure the safety and effectiveness of the drug that the health practitioner wants to prescribe, ask these questions:

- ✔ What is the name of the drug? Get the generic name as well as the brand name. (A generic drug that has the same active ingredients as the brand-name drug.) Write down both names for future reference.

- ✔ What is the drug supposed to do? How will I know that it's working?

- ✔ Has the drug been proven safe for children? Has the dosage been adjusted for my child's age and weight?

- ✔ How long has the drug been on the market? Newer drugs may be more effective than older ones, but long-term side effects will not be known.

- ✔ What are the side effects? How common are they? What should I do if these effects occur?

- ✔ Does this drug react with any foods? The effects of taking medication with certain foods can range from nausea to decreased drug effectiveness.

  Avoid giving a child any medication with fruit juices, carbonated beverages, or caffeinated drinks. Use water and give the child a tea-spoonful of jam afterward to mask the medicine's flavor if necessary.

- ✔ Does this drug interact with other medications being taken? Review with the doctor your family's prescription record and any over-the-counter or prescription drugs currently being taken. Remind the doctor of any known drug allergies as well.

✔ How should the medicine be taken? If the drug is to be given every six hours, for example, should the person taking the drug be woken during the night to receive the medication? Does "with meals" mean before or after eating? For children, can a pill be crushed and mixed with applesauce or jam to make taking the pill easier?

✔ How long does the medicine need to be taken? Antibiotics, for example, must be taken for the full prescribed course, even if you're feeling better after only a few days.

✔ Is a nondrug alternative available? Ask if the doctor can recommend nondrug therapies, such as saltwater gargle for a sore throat, that may prove equally effective.

Your family doctor may be able to give you printed materials about the drug to answer many of these questions. Or you can contact the National Council on Patient Information and Education, 666 11th St. NW, Suite 810, Washington, DC 20001-4542; 202-347-6711.

Reading a prescription

A standard prescription, written by a health professional and subsequently filled by a pharmacist, contains several basic facts: the practitioner's name and address; the patient's name and address; the name of the drug, its strength, and its dosage; special instructions that the patient must be aware of (for example, whether the drug should be taken with food or at bedtime); the practitioner's signature; and authorization for (or against) generic substitutions for a brand-name drug.

The information on most prescriptions, however, is usually coded and may be puzzling to the untrained eye. Appendix B lists phrases and terms that are frequently noted on prescription sheets.

Generic and Brand-Name Drugs: What's What?

A *generic* drug is one whose active ingredients duplicate those of the brand-name product. The name of the generic drug is designated by drug experts and approved by governmental agencies.

When a new drug is approved, the pharmaceutical company that developed the drug is granted a patent for the drug. That patent, which lasts for 17 years, gives the company the right to name the drug and to have a monopoly on the sale, marketing, and advertisement of the drug. However, when the drug comes off patent, any company may manufacture generic versions of the drug.

Generic drugs are on average 30 percent cheaper than their brand-name equivalents — and in some cases, as much as 70 percent cheaper — because their manufacturers do not go to the expense of advertising them, nor do those manufacturers spend money for research on new products.

Generic drugs need not go through all the safety and effectiveness testing done by the original manufacturer. The generic-drug manufacturer has to prove only that the generic version is *bioequivalent* to the brand-name drug. That means that the active ingredient of the generic drug is absorbed into the bloodstream at the same rate and at the same extent as is the active ingredient of the brand-name drug. The generic-drug manufacturer can then include in the drug various components known as *excipients,* such as inert fillers, preservatives, coloring agents, and binders, in order to further distinguish the generic from the brand-name version.

Keep in mind that it is not always known what kinds of side effects and allergic reactions are possible due to the inclusion of these fillers. And because the FDA allows a certain small variance rate in bioequivalency testing, the potency of various generic drugs may differ. This variance could lead to problems if one of your family members switched brands of the generic drug.

Therapeutic substitution

Therapeutic substitution allows a pharmacist to switch an entirely different drug for the drug prescribed by the physician if the pharmacist believes that the substituted drug is therapeutically similar to the prescribed drug. (Pharmacists prefer to call this practice *therapeutic interchange.*) This practice is very different from generic substitution (see the following section) because the drug dispensed is not a generic version of the pre-scribed drug, but one with an entirely different chemical composition.

The medical profession, opposed to therapeutic substitution, maintains that physicians' decisions are based on a complex body of medical information relevant to a specific patient. Make sure that that is indeed the case with your family. Be active participants in your own health care.

Generic substitution

Most states have repealed their antisubstitution laws for generic drugs. Under those laws, if a doctor prescribed a certain brand of a drug, the pharmacist could not substitute the generic version, even if the generic cost less and was the chemical twin of the prescribed brand. Now, pharmacists nearly everywhere can fill a prescription with a generic version of the prescribed drug, but the process varies depending on the state's laws. Find out your state's law concerning the substitution of generic drugs.

Medications on the Home Front

Drugs — even over-the-counter drugs — can be pretty powerful, and too often, people don't give them the respect they deserve. What do we mean by that? Well, take a look in your medicine cabinet. If you're like most people, you've got quite a mess in there — half a box of cold medicine from last winter's bout of flu, three or four heavy-duty painkillers (you took most of them when you threw your back out, but you're keeping these "just in case"), and some sort of salve that expired in 1989, all mixed in with a smattering of bandages and dental floss. But medication is serious stuff, and not something that can be mixed or matched depending on your family's needs.

Keeping drugs up-to-date

The FDA requires that drug manufacturers add an expiration date — the date beyond which a product should not be used — to the labels of most prescription and nonprescription drugs. This date is determined by appropriate stability testing. The expiration date assures you that the product you're buying has met the applicable standards of identity (that the product is, in fact, what the label says it is), strength, quality, and purity. Selling a medication that does not meet these standards is illegal.

Always check the expiration date on the medications in your home medicine cabinet. Look for a statement such as "Exp6/99," ExMay00," or "Expires 3/99" on the product's label.

Expiration dates vary somewhat. The expiration date does not mean that the product automatically loses its potency on that date. After that date, though, the product could begin to deteriorate and lose its effectiveness. (Table 11-1 lists the shelf lives of common medications.)

Table 11-1	Saving a Shelf Life
Product	*Usual Shelf Life*
Cold tablets	1 to 2 years
Laxatives	2 to 3 years
Minerals	6 years or more
Nonprescription painkiller tablets	1 to 4 years
Prescription antibiotics	2 to 3 years
Prescription antihypertension tablets	2 to 4 years
Travel sickness tablets	2 years
Vitamins	6 years or more

Potency aside, some medicines actually become harmful as the drug deteriorates with time. If you have any doubt about the expiration date of a particular medication, contact the manufacturer or discard the medicine. Always replace any medications that are old, appear strange or discolored, or give off an unusual odor.

Storing drugs properly

Always store family medications in a cool, dry place, in a locked cabinet, and out of the reach of children. Unfortunately, most medicine cabinets aren't the right place for drugs. Storing capsules or tablets in the bathroom, near the kitchen sink, or in any other damp place isn't a good idea because moisture can cause damage. If at all possible, locate your home medicine cabinet elsewhere.

Don't store medicines in the refrigerator unless you're directed to do so. Exposing medications to extremes of temperature and moisture can change the chemical makeup of the drug and lessen its effectiveness. If you then take such medicine, you may also expose yourself to the potential effects of an accidental poisoning.

Store your family's medications in the original containers, including any outside packaging material, especially if the packaging contains dosage information. The original containers are designed to protect medication from moisture and exposure to air.

And even though it may seem convenient, don't store different medications in the same bottle. This is an accident waiting to happen. And don't think that you'll be able to tell one pill from another just by size or color. Some pills and capsules look very much alike.

Medications and kids

Children learn to use drugs wisely, safely, and with a measure of skepticism from the actions of their parents and doctors. These suggestions should ensure your child's present and future safety with drugs.

- ✔ Store all medicines out of the reach of children.
- ✔ Use child-resistant safety caps, but do not rely solely on them to keep children from harm. Make sure that medications are stored where kids can't get to them.
- ✔ Never call medicine "candy." Refer to prescriptions and over-the-counter medications as "medicines," not "drugs," to distinguish between legitimate and illegal drugs.
- ✔ Make sure that your child knows why taking the medicine is necessary.

SENIOR STUFF

Hard to handle?

Child-resistant caps on medicine containers have decreased greatly the number of accidental poisonings that occur each year. Use of these caps is required by law. However, if you (or a family member) — perhaps because of arthritis or carpal tunnel syndrome — find it hard to open such caps, you may ask your pharmacist for a regular, easier-to-open cap. Of course, take extra precautions to make sure that the medications don't fall into kids' hands.

✔ Involve your child in taking medicine. Allow the child to get the spoon or glass of water. Make sure that he or she knows when to take it.

✔ Don't give a child medicine left over from an earlier illness or prescribed for someone else without first discussing it with your doctor.

✔ Keep those who care for your child informed about current medications and allergies.

Many experts emphasize that you should resist reaching for medication every time your child complains of an ache, which may teach children to see drugs as answers to life's problems. When parents see their child feeling miserable because of an illness, they too often want to demonstrate concern and boost the child's morale by rushing to the drugstore to buy an over-the-counter medication. When the illness eventually passes, the child naturally believes that the drug made it go away. That fosters a dependent attitude toward drugs that can have tragic consequences.

WARNING!

Caution with aspirin

Aspirin, which contains a salt called salicylate, has been linked to the rare but dangerous illness Reye's syndrome (also known as Reye syndrome). If your child has a viral illness, or you even suspect that he or she does, avoid giving any medication containing salicylate. (Aspirin is not the only medicine that contains this salt. Various forms of salicylate are found in over-the-counter products for relieving stomach upset and diarrhea. Read the package label to find out whether salicylate is an ingredient in the product.)

Salicylate poisoning from aspirin use is common in older people, even if they don't take excessive doses. That's because liver and kidney function decreases in old age, thus slowing the body's excretion of salicylates. Elderly people often take several drugs, many of which may contain aspirin, and are therefore more likely to develop salicylate poisoning. Report any unusual symptoms in older people to a doctor, and tell the doctor about all the medications the older person is taking.

Caution with antibiotics

Whenever possible, avoid taking antibiotics for the treatment of viral infections (most infections are viral). When you must take an antibiotic, take lactobacillus acidophilus and oral powdered nystatin along with the antibiotic — after consulting your pharmacist and practitioner, of course.

Administering medicines properly

When all is said and done, a large part of the responsibility for the safe use of medicines rests in the hands of the one taking the medicine or giving the medicine to someone else. How you actually administer the drug — in tablet, spray, or other form — is critical. The following important recommendations are from the United States Pharmacopeial Convention:

✔ When you're taking a long-acting form of a medicine, each dose should be swallowed whole. If someone in your family has difficulty swallowing an entire pill, check with your family doctor to see whether the dose can be broken, crushed, or chewed before swallowing. For children, you may be able to crush the pill and mix it with applesauce or jam to make taking the pill easier. But ask the doctor first!

✔ If someone in your family is taking a liquid medicine, consider using a specially marked measuring spoon or other device to measure each dose accurately. The average household teaspoon may not hold the right amount of liquid.

✔ If you're treating an infant or small child, seek the advice of a medical practitioner. Doing so is especially important if the child is unable to tell you exactly what his or her symptoms are. And if you're caring for a frail, elderly person or another at-risk person, seek medical advice before using OTC products.

Chapter 12

Understanding Your Medical Rights

In This Chapter

▶ Knowing your medical rights

▶ Acknowledging parents' and children's rights

▶ Establishing advance directives

*T*aking the kids to the doctor, making sure that your prescriptions are filled, finding the right health insurance for your family — isn't getting the best medical care for your family difficult enough without worrying about health care rights? But it's all too true that controversies are constantly brewing all around you. We're talking about issues such as the right to die and assisted suicide, the chasm that can exist between parents' and children's rights, and the dismal horror of a medical malpractice case.

We hear about these controversies on the news (Dr. Kevorkian, for example), daytime talk shows, and even medical dramas such as *ER* and *Chicago Hope.* What happens when a grandmother doesn't want to be put on life support? What happens when a parent doesn't want a child put on life support? What happens to the medical victim who mistakenly has the wrong foot removed in a surgical amputation, or the family of the patient who is fatally overdosed during a chemotherapy treatment?

Matters of medical malpractice and patient rights are far from cut-and-dried, but knowing a little bit about some of the issues can help you protect your family from problems — and make sure that they get what they need should a problem arise.

Testing Your Medical Rights Knowledge

We're always talking about demanding our rights — but do we really know what our rights are? Do you know for sure which legal actions are under your control and which are beyond it? Do you know what you're empowered to do when it comes to your medical care, especially the care when you are critically ill and perhaps even too ill to make decisions?

Take this quiz to test your knowledge of such issues and see what your RQ — your Rights Quotient — really is. It could mean the difference between first-class and low-class treatment, and it could help avoid family disruptions and heartbreak.

The questions and answers are based on current law, advice from People's Medical Society's legal advisers, and in part on information from a source sponsored by the American Civil Liberties Union: *The Rights of Hospital Patients* by George J. Annas (Carbondale: Southern Illinois University Press, 1989).

The questions

T   F   1. You have a legal right to health care in the United States.

T   F   2. A doctor can lie to you about the seriousness of your illness if the doctor thinks that he will spare you anxiety and grief.

T   F   3. You can override family objections and can demand to be told the nature of your illness.

T   F   4. You have the legal right to keep your illness a secret from your family.

T   F   5. Your family has the legal right to stop treatment of a competent, critically ill family member, even if the family member wants it continued.

T   F   6. As a cancer patient, you have the right to have your doctor prescribe or administer drugs, such as laetrile, that are not approved by the FDA.

T   F   7. As a competent adult, you can refuse medical care that could keep you alive.

T   F   8. You can sue a doctor if the doctor treats you against your will in order to keep you alive.

T	F	9.	You can be thrown out of a hospital if you can't pay.
T	F	10.	A doctor can (a) refuse to treat you if you can't pay or (b) stop treating you if you can't pay.
T	F	11.	If, in an emergency situation, you are brought to a hospital that does not have an emergency room, the hospital has the obligation to take you in and care for you anyway.
T	F	12.	A hospital can prevent a patient from leaving.
T	F	13.	A doctor must refer you to a specialist or seek a consultation if you request it.
T	F	14.	A doctor can refuse to continue to see you as a patient without first obtaining the services of another doctor for you.
T	F	15.	As a hospital patient, you have the right to refuse to be examined by medical students, interns, or residents.

The answers

Check your answers against the ones below:

1. F. Neither the Constitution nor the Declaration of Independence guarantees this right. The only legal right Americans have to medical care is the right to be treated in an emergency department of a hospital if they are experiencing a medical emergency.

2. F. A doctor is obligated, under all circumstances, to tell you your diagnosis and prognosis. If the doctor fails to do so, the doctor can be sued for deceit. If you have specifically expressed a desire to know your diagnosis and prognosis and the doctor does not tell you, it can be construed as a breach of fiduciary duty. And if the doctor withholds information that ultimately obstructs crucial medical, financial, or personal decisions on your part, then the doctor could be held liable for the damages that result for failure to obtain your informed consent to treatment or nontreatment.

In two instances, the doctor is off the legal hook: if you have specifically expressed a desire not to know, and if the doctor reasonably believes that bad news could be so upsetting that you would not be able to make a meaningful decision about treatment. This is known as *therapeutic privilege,* which means that the physician must seek consent from your next of kin or health care proxy.

3. T. If you are competent, your family has no right to have information relevant to your medical condition withheld from you. *You* have the right to have information withheld from your family.

4. T. You can ask that your condition be kept secret, and the doctor has to go along. Your diagnosis is confidential medical information that can be disclosed to those not involved in your treatment only with your express authorization.

5. F. If the ill person is competent (can understand the information needed to give or withhold informed consent), your family has no legal power to stop reasonable medical care. The doctor's duty is to the ill person, not to family members.

6. F. Even in states where laetrile is legal, doctors cannot prescribe it or any other drug not approved by the FDA, except in the context of an IRB-approved research protocol.

7. T. Competent adults have a constitutional and a common law right to refuse any treatment, including life-saving or life-sustaining treatment.

8. T. Despite a doctor's seemingly good intentions or ethical concerns, he or she can be sued for battery, false imprisonment, or lack of informed consent. The doctor could even end up being responsible for the cost of the care. You can also get a court order, if necessary, to force a doctor to stop treatment on penalty of contempt of court.

9. F. If you need continued care after you have been admitted, the hospital probably can't discharge you. The hospital could have you transferred to another hospital, but only if you were in stable enough condition to be moved and the new facility was better equipped to care for you. If you are discharged because you can't pay and then get worse or incur further damage, you could sue, claiming abandonment.

10. (a) T. **(b)** F. Unless there is an existing doctor-patient relationship — or the patient is a member of an HMO that has agreed to treat the patient — a doctor-patient relationship requires the consent of both parties. Once treatment has commenced, however, the physician must continue to treat the patient until treatment is no longer needed or the patient is voluntarily transferred to another physician.

11. F. Although this is technically false because only hospitals with emergency departments have a legal obligation to treat in emergency situations, the hospital should do the best it can to stabilize the patient's condition and arrange transport to the nearest emergency department.

12. F. If you are of sound mind, you can leave at any time, and the hospital can't do a thing about it — or risk a suit for false imprisonment. This applies even if you haven't paid your bill or the bill of your child. You may be asked to sign a "discharge against medical advice" form, but you have no legal obligation to do so in order to leave the hospital.

13. T. This is not a law, but good practice. It is also a portion of the American Medical Association's Principles of Medical Ethics. And if the doctor refuses your request for a referral or consultation, and it turns out that the doctor's reassurance of proper treatment was wrong, a negligence suit is probably your next (and successful) step.

14. F. The only way a doctor-patient relationship ends is if (a) both parties agree to its end, (b) it is ended by the patient, (c) the doctor is no longer needed, or (d) the doctor withdraws from the case after having given reasonable notice. Otherwise, you can make a case for abandonment.

15. T. Writes Annas: "All patients have a right to refuse to be examined by anyone in the hospital setting." In addition, fraud can be claimed if consent for an examination was given when a medical student was introduced as "doctor" to the patient, and the patient believed him or her to be a doctor.

Parents' Rights, Children's Rights

When seeking care for your kids, you may run into differences of opinion. You and your child view the tests, procedures, and therapies from your own perspectives. Your doctor provides yet another viewpoint. All of you have rights and expectations; balancing them is not always easy, but the goal of your child's good health makes the effort worthwhile.

Taking care: Parents' rights

With rare exceptions, courts have upheld parents' rights to make decisions about their young children's care, under the presumption that parents are acting in the best interests of their children, unless their actions demonstrate otherwise.

What follow are some of the basic guidelines that govern parents' rights. However, as with everything legal, gray areas exist, and depending on circumstances, these guidelines may or may not apply. For advice on these and all legal matters, consult an attorney.

✔ A physician, or any medical practitioner, is not legally permitted to care for a child without parental consent. There are two exceptions: bona fide emergencies; and several specific diseases or conditions, such as sexually transmitted diseases, where state or federal law permits a child to seek or approve treatment without necessarily requiring parental knowledge or consent.

✔ An almost absolute right of parents requires that medical practitioners provide them with all the information they need to give *informed consent* for their child's treatment. The policy of informed consent dictates that the proposed treatment or procedure must be explained thoroughly and that all questions must be answered before an individual can make a medical decision.

✔ Parents have the legal right to be with their minor child at all times — in the doctor's office or hospital — and nothing can be done for or to that child without a parent's specific permission. This right to be with your child is essential for fully informed consent. Other than in an emergency, or if you have an older child who is receiving highly personal medical care, a doctor cannot separate you from your child.

Remember that you are your child's legal and medical advocate. Don't allow yourself to be intimidated by incomprehensible medical terms, overbearing doctors, or nonphysician medical personnel who seem to have little time for your questions or concerns. You are obligated to protect the interests of your child just as you would your own.

Growing up: Children's rights

A parent's rights are not total or absolute, and they become less so as a child grows older. State law and case law have defined a number of circumstances in which children under the age of majority can make medical decisions for themselves.

✔ **Emancipated minors:** Young people become *emancipated* — that is, they are considered self-reliant for legal purposes — either by reaching a defined age or through marriage or military service. In some states, other circumstances may apply. For example, teenagers may be considered emancipated if they are self-supporting, pregnant, responsible for their own finances, or own property. Emancipated minors can consent to medical care as adults.

✔ **Mature minors:** Courts also have come to realize that teenagers who do not meet the criteria for emancipation may nevertheless be capable of informed consent for medical care. Generally, these "mature minors" are 14 to 18 years old, depending on state law or court decisions, and the following conditions apply:

- The young person understands the risks and benefits of the proposed treatment well enough to give informed consent.

- The care is for the patient's benefit, not someone else's (as it is when a child is asked to donate a kidney to a relative).

- The care is necessary based on conservative medical judgment.

- The treatment is not a high-risk procedure.

✔ **Medically emancipated minors:** States also recognize that good public health policy calls for giving adolescents the right to consent to medical care in the case of certain sensitive illnesses or conditions. Thus all states allow minors to seek treatment for sexually transmitted diseases, and most have similar statutes in the cases of alcohol and drug abuse treatment, pregnancy-related services, and outpatient mental health counseling.

When a child's and parents' rights conflict

Conflicts do arise occasionally between the rights of parents and those of their children. The possibility for conflict seems to rise as children grow older, but even infants and parents can face legal and ethical dilemmas based on differing rights. In this section, we review some of the more prominent issues where child and parental rights often conflict.

The right to refuse treatment

In competent adults, the right to refuse treatment, even life-saving therapy, is generally upheld. The legal concept of *informed consent* requires that a doctor give a patient sufficient information to make an informed decision to accept or reject the recommended therapy.

A child's age, condition, proposed treatment, and the life-and-death nature of the decision affect parents' choices about the right to refuse treatment for their children. In general, in recent years, courts have frequently been willing to intervene on a child's behalf against the parents' traditional rights in cases where parents do not appear to have the child's best interests in mind. These cases focus primarily on infants and very small children but also extend to older children whose parents have refused certain treatments on religious or philosophical grounds.

Mandatory immunizations

Parents' rights to make decisions about the health care of their young children are further restricted by the laws governing immunization. All 50 states mandate at least some vaccinations for a child by the time that child enters school. They make provisions for medical exemptions and, in some cases, philosophical or religious ones, but courts and lawmakers generally agree that the benefits to society outweigh a parent's right to refuse the shots and the risks to the child from the relatively uncommon serious side effects. (See Chapter 13 for more on the immunization controversy.)

Emergencies

In an emergency, any child can be treated without parental consent, no matter how young the child. One medical-legal expert points out that under the law, an emergency is not restricted to a condition that may cause death or disability, but simply requires prompt treatment. Court definitions of an emergency have ranged from an immediate life-threatening event to situations in which pain and suffering were eliminated.

Confidentiality

Whether you have a right to be notified that your teenager is seeking health care or to know what is in his or her medical records varies considerably from state to state and with the reason for care. Simply because a law allows a teen to seek care does not mean that it guarantees confidentiality of that care. Most laws regarding therapy for sexually transmitted diseases and for drug and alcohol abuse forbid informing parents against the child's wishes. If the child qualifies as an emancipated minor, he or she is dealt with as an adult with regard to the confidentiality of the patient-doctor relationship.

Each state tends to see parents' and children's rights a bit differently from the other states, so the details relating to age, parental notification, and such vary widely. Find out exactly how a particular issue of possible dispute is dealt with in your own state laws or how courts in your state have interpreted the laws.

Can my child . . . ?

The specific questions in this section are often asked by parents relating to their rights versus their children's rights. Please note that some of the answers differ depending on the state in which you reside.

- **Can my child get contraceptives without my permission?** Yes. In 1977, the U.S. Supreme Court ruled that minors have a right to privacy that extends to access to contraception. Federally funded family planning agencies are required by law to provide services regardless of age or marital status. Your family physician can refuse to provide contraceptives but may be obligated to refer your child to Planned Parenthood or a public clinic.

- **Can my child be treated for a sexually transmitted disease without my knowing it?** Yes. A number of states allow doctors to notify parents when their children require treatment for a sexually transmitted disease, but no state requires it.

✔ **Will my doctor perform a drug test on my child without the child's knowledge if I request it?** Probably not. The American Academy of Pediatrics issued a policy statement in 1989 recommending to doctors that older adolescents should give informed consent to any such tests.

✔ **Can my daughter get an abortion without my consent?** Yes, in many cases. In 1976, the U.S. Supreme Court ruled that parents or guardians cannot prevent an abortion in a consenting minor. Three years later, the court again ruled on the issue, this time agreeing that states can require parental consent, but only if the child has an alternative. Known as *judicial bypass,* these proceedings allow a child to apply to the court instead of her parents; if the judge declares her "mature" and thus competent to decide, she may do so without her parents' consent. If the judge does not think that she is legally mature, the court must decide whether an abortion is in her best interests. However, pro- and anti-abortion groups continually lobby state legislatures, so laws in this area undergo constant change.

✔ **Can I require my pregnant teenager to have an abortion?** No. Although fewer court cases are involving parents trying to force their daughters to have an abortion, youth law experts agree that a teenager's right to privacy extends to her right to give birth if she chooses. Doctors rarely agree to perform an abortion on someone who does not want one.

✔ **Am I responsible for paying for medical care that my child consents to without my involvement?** No, unless it is emergency care. Many of the laws enabling minors to consent to care specify that the minors are legally responsible for the care. If the condition is one for which confidentiality is guaranteed, which is often the case with sexually transmitted diseases, then neither the parents nor their insurance company can be told, even for billing purposes, without the minor's consent.

Resolving conflicts

Communication is the key among you, your child, and health care professionals. Keep your child involved in his or her care from the very beginning. Encourage your child to express feelings, ask questions, and learn as much as possible about a condition or proposed procedure.

If you and your teenager disagree over his or her therapy in a nonemergency situation, we offer these suggestions:

✔ **Make sure that both of you have enough accurate information to make an informed decision.** For example, a teen may believe that scarring from the recommended surgery will be disfiguring, when in fact it will not; perhaps you could arrange for your child to talk with another young person who has undergone the therapy. Invite a nurse, another doctor, or another professional whom you and your teen trust to answer your questions and discuss the options.

✔ **Look for areas of agreement or steps that may lead either of you to change your mind.** Will your teen agree to a different test that could clarify the prospects for recovery? Will you both agree to medical therapy, rather than surgery, even though the outcome is less certain? Aim for consensus rather than confrontation.

As your child matures, conflicts in areas large and small, including health care, are inevitable. If you have encouraged your child to be an informed consumer, not a victim, of health care professionals, then you, as well as the doctor, must respect your teen's decisions. Take comfort in the knowledge that you have armed your child well to face off against those who control medical care.

Death and Dying Issues

Death used to be simple. If you stopped breathing, your heart stopped, and your pupils dilated, you were dead. Not so today. No longer is the traditional heart-and-lungs concept of death applicable in every case. So if you are concerned about the issue known as *dying with dignity,* you need to understand how the medical and legal worlds are redefining death.

Over the years, advances in technology have made it possible to prolong lives and maintain heartbeat and breathing functions even in the face of serious illnesses. As a result, the definition of death has come under scrutiny, making it sometimes difficult to determine your rights concerning the end of life.

Advance directives: A patient's right to decide

All adult individuals in hospitals, nursing homes, and other health care settings have certain rights. For example, you have a right to confidentiality of your personal and medical records and a right to know what treatment you will receive.

You also have another right: to fill out a paper known as an *advance directive.* The paper says in advance what kind of treatment you want or do not want under special, serious medical conditions — conditions that would prevent you from telling your doctor how you want to be treated. For example, if you were taken to a hospital in a coma, would you want the hospital's medical staff to know your specific wishes about decisions affecting your treatment?

The two most common types of advance directives are the living will and the durable power of attorney for health care.

No state agency presides over advance directives. So, in most instances, the federally funded health care institution will be able to fully explain your state's provision for advance directives. You should be aware of one notable exception, according to the organization Choice in Dying: Institutions with their own ethical or moral codes (for example, a hospital with religious affiliations) may impose their own restrictions on your treatment. Usually, these institutions will inform you of their policies when you are admitted.

Living wills

A *living will* is a document that lists an individual's preferences concerning life support, other life-sustaining procedures or "heroic" measures, and instructions about therapies that one wishes to have or not have.

It's generally agreed that an individual has the right to decide whether he or she wants to be subjected to futile measures that may prolong an otherwise inevitable outcome. The individual can decide whether to be put on a respirator or dialysis machine, be resuscitated, or be nourished intravenously. Specifically, a person can refuse to receive CPR (cardiopulmonary resuscitation) by placing a *DNR (Do Not Resuscitate)* order in his or her advance directive.

Assisted suicide, euthanasia, and the terminally ill

Growing numbers of people believe that ending life with dignity and on their own terms is a basic human right. For some people who are terminally ill, death with dignity is especially crucial. However, controversy surrounds *euthanasia,* the practice of painlessly killing or permitting the death of someone who is terminally ill, and *assisted suicide,* in which the dying person requests that another help end his or her life. Laws vary from state to state, but nearly everywhere, a person who assists in the suicide of a dying family member or friend risks prosecution as an accessory to a crime.

Even when a patient and the patient's family believe that a person has the right to control his or her own death, the difficulties of such a decision can be great. If you or someone you know is suffering from a terminal illness and is considering suicide, you may want to contact Choice in Dying, Inc. (1035 30th Street, Washington, DC 20007; 202-338-9790) or the Hemlock Society (P. O. Box 101810, Denver, Colorado 80250; 800-247-7421). These organizations provide information about euthanasia and assisted suicide and the current laws on an individual's rights regarding death and dying.

In hospitals and nursing homes across the country, DNR means that, should respiration or heartbeat fail, CPR will not be started or carried out. A DNR order means that the patient will not be given brief emergency CPR, nor will the patient be placed on long-term mechanical life-support equipment.

Knowing about DNR orders — when, how, and by whom they're issued, and how they work — is an important step in gaining more control over the circumstances of your death. A few questions then arise: Upon admission to the hospital, should you routinely discuss your wishes for resuscitation? At what point in the course of your illness/hospitalization can the decision about resuscitation best be made? What can you do if your decision about resuscitation changes over time?

The important thing is to avoid the potential complications that can arise — between family members and between your family and the hospital and doctors, and the need for determination by outside parties such as the hospital ethics committee or legal counsel. Follow these suggestions to avoid problems:

- ✔ Talk to your physician about the appropriateness of a Do Not Resuscitate order — before it's needed, and even before admission to the hospital, if possible.

- ✔ Discuss the matter with your family so that they'll know your wishes and will be able to act confidently in your behalf if necessary.

- ✔ Document your wishes concerning emergency resuscitation, and have your physician make this a part of your medical record.

- ✔ Remember, too, that a DNR order is not an irrevocable decision. If the outcome of another day in the hospital or another hospital stay causes you to have second thoughts, just speak up — and document your decision, of course. Any major improvement in your condition also would nullify the DNR order.

A living will, which can be revoked at any time, can be drafted by the individual or can be obtained from state agencies or Choice in Dying. If you decide to write or sign a living will, notify your lawyer, physician, and family and make sure that they understand your wishes. Also, you should check the living will legislation of your particular state because laws and stipulations vary from state to state. All states — except Massachusetts, Michigan, and New York — and the District of Columbia have living will legislation.

Durable Power of Attorney for Health Care

A *Durable Power of Attorney* (DPA) is a document that names a legal agent who will carry out your desired method of treatment or who will make those decisions for you at the time of death or when you become incompetent.

Even though you can spell out your desired methods of treatment in a Durable Power of Attorney, having both a living will and a Durable Power of Attorney or a Durable Power of Attorney for Health Care (a limited form of Durable Power of Attorney) is a good idea. The document must be signed, dated, and witnessed and can be canceled (in writing) at any time.

The most critical issue is deciding who is the appropriate decision-maker. Most experts recommend that you consider these factors: Whom would you trust with life-and-death decisions? Who knows you best — your attitudes and values? Who would respect your wishes? Most people appoint spouses or close family members — good choices because they know you well — but if they are beneficiaries of your estate, they may have a conflict of interest.

As with any advance directive, you should keep the directive in a safe place. The family, physician, designated proxy, and lawyer should be notified of your instructions and directions and should hold a copy of the document. Because states differ in advance directive legislation in terms of definition and limitations, make sure that you know your state's policy concerning advance directives.

For further information about advance directives, the specific laws of your state, legal advice concerning death, or the registration of living wills, contact Choice in Dying (1035 30th Street, Washington, DC 20007; 202-338-9790).

Hospice care

Hospices are facilities that exist solely to assist dying patients — typically, cancer patients who have exhausted the various forms of curative treatment — and to help them live their remaining weeks or months as free from symptoms and as much in control as possible.

Deliberately created as alternatives to traditional long-term institutions, hospices provide *palliative care* (care intended to comfort and ease pain) to patients and their families, and also provide bereavement counseling to families following a patient's death. In short, a hospice is an alternative to a hospital and nursing home that can offer the patient personalized care, attention, emotional support, and relief from pain.

Hospice care can be performed in a hospice facility (a freestanding facility or one associated with a hospital or nursing home) or at home, where a primary caregiver (usually a family member) works with the hospice team to tend to the patient. Unlike hospital care, the active contributions and support of family members are welcomed and, in fact, are an integral part of the hospice care system.

Part IV
Different Strokes: Kids, Teens, Moms, and Dads

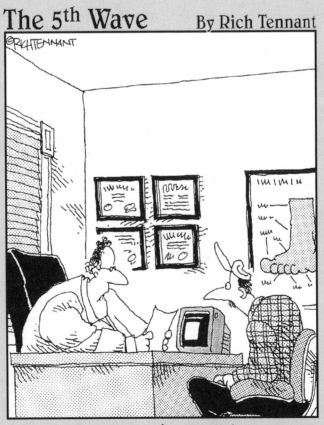

The 5th Wave   By Rich Tennant

"Please, Mr. Dugan, I'm a podiatrist. I can't be expected to advise you on why your car stalls at stoplights. You'd need to talk to an internist for that."

In this part . . .

Each person in your family has his or her own special needs, and this part addresses those needs. These "family matters" can be serious stuff — no sitcoms on this channel. Stay tuned to find out about children's and adolescents' issues, as well as men's and women's special issues.

Chapter 13

Tending Tots: Children's Health

. . . .

In This Chapter

▶ Monitoring your child's health and development

▶ Knowing when to call the doctor

▶ Understanding symptoms

▶ Coping with common childhood conditions

. . . .

*Y*ou can't talk about family health without talking about kids. In fact, kids tend to monopolize the conversation. From the moment of birth (and even before), parents worry about their children's well-being. And it's a lifetime of worry — one filled with skinned knees, chicken pox, ear infections, and much more.

We can't turn you into a pediatrician in a single chapter. But we *can* present you with the basics on what's normal, what's not, how to tell when something's wrong, and what to do about it. We cover immunizations, development, emotional health, and a host of childhood conditions and symptoms that you're pretty sure to face as your son or daughter grows up.

Everyone's always saying that kids are tougher than you think — that they bounce back quickly. That's true enough, but don't make the mistake of trying to treat your kids without a doctor's advice and diagnosis. And don't rely on this book as a substitute for medical care. We believe that parents are the best advocates and, in most cases, the best caretakers for their children — but they need professional advice and support to do it right.

Choosing a Pediatrician

Pediatricians provide primary medical care to children. In many ways, searching for a pediatrician is like looking for any other specialist. (See Chapter 6 for more on choosing a practitioner.) However, you should know what you want in a doctor when making your choice. For example, do you want a doctor who will serve as a resource at all times, or one who will just care for your child during illness? Do you want a doctor who explains the pros and cons of each procedure and lets you decide, or one who makes decisions for you and your family?

Also ask yourself these questions:

- ✔ Does my lifestyle demand certain features — for example, office hours at nights and on weekends?
- ✔ Is cost a factor?
- ✔ Does my managed care plan allow for freedom of choice?
- ✔ Does my child have special health care needs?
- ✔ Do I prefer male or female, young or old, solo or group practitioner?
- ✔ How important is a "big-name" doctor — one with the best reputation in town?
- ✔ Why did I change pediatricians in the past? What do I want my new doctor to do differently?

Knowing When to Call the Doctor

All parents sometimes hesitate about whether to call the doctor. Sure, in an emergency situation, you're on the phone in a minute, but what about those "gray areas" — especially if it's a weekend or 2:00 in the morning? Can it wait until morning? Are you overreacting? Are you risking your child's health?

In his classic child care book, *Dr. Spock's Baby and Child Care* (New York: Pocket Books, 1998), pediatrician Benjamin Spock, M.D., offers this basic rule: Call your doctor "if a baby or child *looks different* (in general appearance) or *acts differently*." Your physician may provide general guidelines.

Call a doctor if a newborn or infant

- ✔ Does not pass the meconium (the first, dark, bowel movement) within 36 hours of birth
- ✔ Appears to be jaundiced (the whites of the eyes are yellowish)
- ✔ Vomits forcefully or more frequently than usual
- ✔ Refuses food for more than six to eight hours
- ✔ Has a fever of 100.5 degrees Farenheit or higher
- ✔ Has a persistent cough
- ✔ Cries louder or more persistently, sleeps more or less than usual, or is unusually cranky or passive
- ✔ Turns very pale or flushed

> ✔ Has serious diarrhea or other changes in the pattern or color of bowel movements

> ✔ Appears dehydrated (produces less urine and saliva or has a drowsy, lethargic attitude)

Call a doctor if your toddler or school-age child shows the following symptoms:

> ✔ Temperature over 104 degrees Fahrenheit without other symptoms, or fever without other symptoms lasting more than 24 hours, or fever in a child with a serious underlying disease

> ✔ Serious diarrhea

> ✔ Blood in the urine or stool

> ✔ Sudden loss of appetite lasting 2 to 3 days or more

> ✔ Hoarseness, unusual crying, or difficulty breathing

> ✔ Unusual vomiting

> ✔ Off-color appearance

> ✔ Listlessness or behavior change

> ✔ Convulsions or fits (seizures)

> ✔ Eye or ear injuries or infections

> ✔ Blows to the head causing unconsciousness (even briefly), or with effects lasting longer than 15 minutes

> ✔ Burns with blisters or unusual rashes

> ✔ Indications of pain, such as limping

> ✔ Suspected poisoning

> ✔ Stress or anxiety

> ✔ Swallowing of a foreign object

If you can't decide whether to contact your doctor, err on the side of safety and make the call. *Any* pediatrician would rather deal with an overanxious parent than risk a child's health.

When you call the doctor, be prepared to answer basic questions about the situation. Don't expect that the doctor has your child's medical history memorized; provide details about relevant recent care. Relate main symptoms and their duration, any medications that you've given your child, and any circumstances that you suspect may be causing the problem.

Before you hang up the phone, make sure that you know what changes to expect if the condition worsens, what you should do at home, when you should seek help again, and how long the condition usually lasts.

Nurturing Healthy Emotions

The quality of your child's emotional health depends on two things: his or her biological makeup (nature) and your approach to parenting (nurture). One of the most important gifts you can give your child is a healthy sense of self-esteem.

Nurturing of emotional health begins the first time your child lies in your arms. Throughout childhood, a child turns to parents for approval and guidance. They need to learn how to make decisions, and they will make mistakes. The process requires your careful input. Your job is to help them understand what the consequences are, how to make amends, and how to show sympathy for others, all the while providing a gentle, guiding hand. Doing so takes thought and time on your part, but the outcome is worth it.

Reaching Developmental Milestones

Parents anxiously watch their babies develop new skills and wonder whether they are progressing and growing "normally." The human body develops in a predictable sequence, which is described in terms of developmental milestones. You needn't assess your child yourself. At each doctor's visit, your pediatrician should do so for you, asking a series of questions to be sure that your child is within the normal range.

If you suspect that your child is not developing properly, talk with your doctor as soon as possible. Don't take a wait-and-see attitude. With a thorough examination, a doctor can determine whether your child has a medical condition, such as a hearing loss or a vision problem, and can prescribe treatment to prevent further developmental problems.

What to expect from a newborn

A quick rundown of the typical sequence of events follows, although you should remember that all children are different:

- ✔ Just after birth, a newborn can suck; that's called the *rooting reflex*.
- ✔ By 2 months, an infant can move the arms and legs smoothly, hold the head at a 45-degree angle for a few minutes, and hold an object for a brief time.
- ✔ By 3 months, a child can sit supported, although the head still bobs.
- ✔ By 4 months, an infant can sit for 10 minutes or so and maintain good control over the head.

- By 5 months, an infant can put the feet in the mouth and suck on the toes.

- By 6 months, an infant can roll from the stomach to the back.

- By 7 months, an infant can sit easily with a little support or alone. He or she can also bang two objects together.

- By 8 months, an infant can crawl and maybe even stand with support. He or she can also attempt to pick up objects.

- By 9 months, an infant can master picking up objects with the thumb and pointer finger and can crawl while grasping one toy.

- By 10 months, an infant can walk if both the hands are held, or can even walk alone while holding on to the furniture. Walking alone can begin anytime between 10 and 14 months.

- By 11 months, an infant can wave, climb, squat, stoop, and stand alone and may be able to grasp a spoon and bring it to the mouth.

- By 12 months, an infant can walk but still prefers crawling to get around. He or she can point with the index finger and take the covers off containers.

Infants usually begin to babble around the seventh month and may begin forming short words by the first birthday.

What to expect from a 1-year-old

Between the ages of 1 and 2, a child discovers the outside world and begins to take the first steps toward independence. Between 10 and 14 months, most babies pull themselves up into a standing position, walk with the aid of a walker, parents, or the furniture (called *cruising*), and finally take their first solo steps across the room. By this age, they have also graduated to solid foods and are learning how to feed themselves.

Most babies say their first words by 12 to 14 months. Some, however, put it off as they master walking. By 18 months, a baby should speak at least 15 words and enjoy verbal games. By the age of 2, a child should be speaking in two-word sentences, although pronunciation may not be clear.

What to expect from toddlers and preschool-age children

From their second birthday until they start school (at 4 or 5 years of age), children develop into social beings with physical coordination, strong verbal skills, and the ability to work with other children in a concentrated effort.

Between the ages of 2 and 3, a child develops greater coordination, enough to safely climb up and down stairs and even stand on one foot. By the age of 3, a child should be able to climb well, walk up and down stairs alternating feet, kick a ball, run easily, pedal a tricycle, and bend over without falling. A child should also have developed certain fine motor skills, such as making vertical, horizontal, and circular strokes with a pencil or crayon and turning a book's pages one at a time.

After birthday number two, most children can tell you their names and the names of common objects. Their vocabulary should be about 50 words or more. They can speak in three- or four-word sentences and even hold a brief conversation. At 3 years of age, many children can recognize several numbers and letters, use pronouns, and understand plurals. By the time they are 4 years old, they can speak clearly enough for a stranger to understand them and are capable of telling a story. Some children are also able to write letters of the alphabet at this age.

By age 5, a child can dress and undress. A 5-year-old can stand on one foot for ten seconds or longer, hop, do a somersault, swing, climb, and perhaps skip. The child's abilities to use the hands are also fully developed. A 5-year-old can also recall part of a story, speak in sentences that are longer than five words, use future tense, tell longer stories, and say his or her name and address.

Immunizing

Immunization is the process of making individuals resistant to certain viruses and bacteria. Immunizations are just as much a part of growing up as developmental milestones are. A baby born this year will receive 20 shots before the age of 2. That's a lot of vaccinations! But the process is worth it. Today, the risk of contracting the childhood diseases that were once common and sometimes life-altering or deadly is practically nil, thanks to immunizations.

Understanding how vaccines work

A *vaccine* is a substance that contains the germ of the specific disease. Some vaccines are called "live" because they contain a weakened germ of the disease. Other vaccines contain a dead disease germ. When these vaccinations enter your child's body, the immune system goes to work making antibodies that fight the germs.

Vaccinations give the body the chance to practice fighting the weak germs so that when the real, strong disease germs invade the child's body, the antibodies know how to destroy them and the child does not become ill. Protective antibodies remain in the child's system even after the disease is gone, and they safeguard the child from the real disease germ. If left to chance, the child's first exposure to the disease may be from a germ that is too strong for the immune system to fight.

Putting vaccinations into action

As diseases such as measles are virtually wiped out in the United States, it's tempting to think that vaccines are unnecessary. But germs that cause these illnesses are still circulating in the environment and are a very real threat to you and your children. Immunization protects not only the individual but the community as well, because these diseases are highly contagious.

 Ask your doctor about which immunizations are necessary for your child and when. Some doctors even provide charts that you can use as part of your medical record to help you keep track of vaccinations. And even if you're pretty sure that your child's immunizations are up-to-date, double-check with your doctor to be certain that you are following the most current guidelines.

At each office visit with your child's doctor, you should receive information about the vaccinations that will be required at the next visit. Read the material in its entirety and call your doctor if you have any questions. Federal law dictates that your doctor provide you with material that out-lines the risks and benefits of vaccinations. Generally, doctors give parents the material distributed by the Centers for Disease Control and Prevention.

If you have any questions or concerns about immunizations, you can contact the Centers for Disease Control and Prevention's National Immunization Hotline at 800-232-2522 (English) or 800-232-0233 (Spanish) and talk to an information specialist, or visit their Web site at www.cdc.gov/nip.

What's preventable through immunization?

Many childhood diseases are potentially dangerous and life-threatening, but they are preventable through immunization. But one problem does exist: Some immunizations have side effects, ranging from soreness where the shot was administered to fever, allergic reactions, and more. As with any test or procedure, ask your doctor about the risks and benefits of immunization and how often they occur. Brief discussions of the diseases prevented by immunizations, along with information about possible side effects, follow:

> ✔ **Hepatitis B:** A viral illness that is most commonly spread by blood or through sexual contact. It can lead to cirrhosis and liver cancer. Doc-tors call the vaccine that protects against this disease Hep B. Side effects from the Hep B injection occur in 1 to 3 percent of those who get the shot; they include fever and swelling at the site of the injection.

✔ **Polio:** A virus that causes muscle pain, difficulty breathing, and, occasionally, paralysis. Through immunization, the disease is virtually nonexistent in the United States. The recommended vaccination is now the inactivated poliovirus vaccine (IPV), instead of the oral polio vaccine (OPV) provided in past years. Polio vaccines are generally not known to cause side effects, but the IPV can cause some soreness at the site of the injection and a low-grade fever.

✔ **Measles, mumps, and rubella:** Three mild childhood diseases that become life-threatening in rare cases. These diseases are spread when viruses pass from an infected person to the nose or throat of others. Measles causes a rash, cough, and fever, but it can lead to ear infection, pneumonia, diarrhea, seizures, brain damage, and even death. Mumps causes fever, headache, and swollen glands under the jaw. It can also lead to hearing loss and meningitis, and males can have painful, swollen testicles. Rubella (or German measles) can cause rash, mild fever, swollen glands, and arthritis. Pregnant women and their infants can suffer greatly from being exposed to rubella; babies can be born deaf and/or blind, or suffer from heart disease, brain damage, and other serious problems.

Immunizations for measles, mumps, and rubella are combined in one vaccine called MMR. Possible side effects from the vaccination include soreness, redness, or swelling at the site of the injection; rash; fever; swelling of the glands in the cheeks, neck, or under the jaw; seizure; and joint stiffness or swelling.

✔ **Diphtheria, tetanus (or lockjaw), and pertussis (or whooping cough):** Bacterial infections. Diphtheria and pertussis spread when germs pass from an infected person to the nose or throat of others. Tetanus is caused by a germ that enters the body through a cut or wound. Diphtheria causes a thick coating in the nose, throat, or airway and can lead to breathing problems, heart failure, paralysis, and even death. Tetanus causes serious, painful spasms of all muscles and can lead to "locking" of the jaw so that the patient cannot open the mouth or even swallow. It can be fatal. Pertussis causes coughing and choking for several weeks, making it hard for infants to eat, drink, or breathe. The disease can lead to pneumonia, seizures, brain damage, and death.

Immunizations for these diseases are combined in one vaccine called DTP. Rarely, DTP is associated with neurological reactions. In 1991, the FDA approved a version known as acellular pertussis vaccine, which uses only purified portions of the bacteria cell. This vaccine reportedly causes fewer side effects.

✔ *Haemophilus influenzae* **type B:** A highly contagious bacterium that causes several life-threatening diseases, including meningitis and *epiglottitis* (swelling of the windpipe). Doctors call the vaccine that protects against this disease Hib. About 25 percent of children experience side effects from the injections, including tenderness at the site of injection and fever.

Immunizations: Marking your calendar

The American Academy of Pediatrics' Committee on Infectious Diseases, the Advisory Committee on Immunization Practices of the Centers for Disease Control and Prevention, and the American Academy of Family Physicians issue recommendations for scheduling immunizations. These recommendations are based on research into the best timing for greatest effectiveness and are timed to coincide with commonly scheduled visits to the doctor. The guidelines change as new vaccines are developed or more information about effectiveness or side effects becomes known. At present, most doctors follow this schedule.

Recommended Age	*Immunization*
Birth to 2 months	Hepatitis B (Hep B) #1
1 month to 4 months	Hepatitis B #2
2 months	Diphtheria, tetanus, pertussis (DTP) #1
	Inactivated poliovirus vaccine (IPV) #1 or oral polio vaccine (OPV) #1
	Haemophilus influenzae type B (Hib) #1
4 months	DTP #2
	IPV or OPV #2
	Hib #2
6 months	DTP #3
	Hib #3
6 months to 18 months	Hep B #3
	IPV or OPV #3
12 months to 15 months	Hib #4
	Measles, mumps, rubella (MMR) #1
12 months to 18 months	Varicella
15 months to 18 months	DTP #4
4 to 6 years	DTP #5
	IPV or OPV #4
	MMR #2
11 to 12 years or 14 to 16 years	Tetanus and diphtheria (Td)

The American Academy of Pediatrics cites numerous exceptions, cautions, and alternatives to this basic schedule. Ask your pediatrician for more information regarding your child's particular situation, or consult the AAP's Web site (www.aap.org) for more information about any special risks or circumstances surrounding immunization.

✔ **Varicella (or chicken pox):** A common childhood viral illness that is highly contagious and causes an itchy, blistery rash. It is usually not dangerous, but it can lead to pneumonia, encephalitis, and infection of open sores. The chicken pox vaccination is new. Side effects include a mild rash with only a few blisters in 7 percent of the cases, and pain at the site of injection and fever in 20 percent of the cases. If a rash does develop, contact your child's doctor.

Very rarely, a child has a serious reaction to a vaccine. In this case, contact your doctor immediately. Write down what happened and the date and time it happened. Ask your doctor, nurse, or department to file a Vaccine Adverse Event Report form. The National Vaccine Injury Compensation Program gives compensation for persons thought to be injured by vaccines. You can reach the program at 800-338-2382.

Dealing with Common Symptoms

If you know a little about symptoms, what causes them, and how to treat them, you become better equipped to handle related conditions. Understanding symptoms becomes especially important when you're dealing with conditions that can't be treated directly. For example, viral infections are impervious to antibiotics and must be allowed to run their course. In such cases, you need to focus on fighting the symptoms to make your child more comfortable.

Constipation

Constipation is rarely a problem in breast-fed infants. It can, however, occur in bottle-fed babies and older children who are eating solid foods. In general, it occurs when the muscles at the end of the large intestine tighten and prevent the stool from passing through normally. The longer the stool remains there, the firmer and drier it becomes.

Parents who are familiar with their child's bowel habits are in the best position to know when constipation occurs. In general, in newborns, the signs of constipation include passing firm stools less than once a day. In older children, the stools are hard and compact, with three or four days between them. A child may also experience abdominal pain, which disappears after the bowel movement, and the outside of the stools may be streaked with blood.

Changes in diet are the main means of treating constipation. If it appears that your child is constipated, try adding extra water to his or her diet and decrease amounts of constipating foods such as rice, bananas, and low-fiber cereal. If your child has just graduated from formula to milk, try returning to the usual formula. Infant formula can be less constipating than unmodified cow's milk.

If your child is eating solid food and has problems with constipation, you may need to add high-fiber foods to the diet. Such foods include prunes, apricots, plums, raisins, peas, beans, broccoli, and whole-grain cereals and bread products. Keep in mind that fat produces harder stools and that fiber softens stools, making them easier to pass through the muscles of the large intestine.

In more severe cases, your child's doctor may prescribe a laxative or perhaps even an enema. Do not, however, try either without the consent of your child's doctor.

Dehydration

Dehydration — a serious symptom in children — occurs when the body loses more fluid than it is able to take in. It is caused by excessive perspiration from fever, vomiting, diarrhea, or refusal to drink fluids. Children have higher metabolic rates than adults and need more fluids, so they are especially prone to dehydration when they are ill.

Signs of dehydration include a dry or sticky mouth, lack of tears when crying, a decrease in urinating (for infants, fewer than six wet diapers a day), and lethargy. Another symptom is skin that is less elastic than usual; for example, when the skin is pinched and let go, it doesn't return to its normal appearance.

If your child is severely dehydrated, additional symptoms may be fussiness; excessive sleepiness; sunken eyes; cool, discolored hands and feet; and wrinkled skin. A severely dehydrated child may go 8 to 12 hours without urinating.

Severe dehydration can develop quickly, and it can be life-threatening. For this reason, never try to treat your child without advice from your doctor. If you suspect dehydration, contact your doctor immediately for help. For mild to moderate dehydration, you may be advised to give your child a commercially prepared electrolyte solution. Breast-fed babies should continue feeding in addition to receiving an electrolyte solution in a bottle. If you think that your child is severely dehydrated, go to the emergency room immediately. In this case, your child may need to be hospitalized and rehydrated intravenously.

Diarrhea

As a parent, you become all too familiar with your child's toilet habits. An occasional loose stool is no cause for alarm, but if you notice that the bowel pattern suddenly changes to frequent, loose, watery stools, your child has diarrhea. Diarrhea occurs when the inner lining of the intestine is injured and the intestine cannot properly digest or absorb the nutrients that your child eats and drinks. A viral or bacterial infection may be the cause.

Your doctor is the best source of advice about diarrhea and can help diagnose and treat its cause. Prompt treatment is best because one common complication of diarrhea is dehydration — a potentially serious condition. If your child is exhibiting the signs of dehydration, call your doctor immediately. (See "Dehydration," earlier in this chapter, for more information.)

You can probably handle a mild case of diarrhea yourself. If your child doesn't have a fever, is active and hungry, and isn't suffering from dehydration, continue to feed your child the same diet, although you may want to increase fluids. Do not give a "clear liquid diet" that contains sweetened beverages, such as juices, Jell-O, or soda, because the high sugar content will make the diarrhea worse. In infants, diarrhea usually lasts about 72 hours; in older children, it may last up to a week.

Over-the-counter medications should not be given to children under 2, and they should be used with caution with older children. Consult your child's doctor before using one of these treatments.

Earache

If your child is experiencing pain in the ear, contact your doctor as soon as possible, especially if the pain is accompanied by other symptoms such as fever, cough, and discharge from the ear canal — signs of infection. Only a doctor can determine how to treat the infection appropriately. (See "Ear infections," later in this chapter, for more information.)

In the meantime, you can help reduce the discomfort of the earache with acetaminophen, along with a heating pad on a low setting or a hot-water bottle placed around the ear. Never give a child who is 2 years old or younger any medication without your doctor's advice.

Under no circumstances should you insert a cotton swab, tissue, or anything else in the ear canal to remove discharge or relieve an itch. Doing so can only damage the delicate skin and remove the thin layer of earwax that serves as a protective barrier against germs. Removing the earwax or adding tiny scratches to the canal's skin only provides a place for microbes to reside and thrive.

Fever

The body normally reacts to an infection with fever; an increased temperature indicates that the body is attempting to fight off invading microorganisms. The normal average temperature is 98.6 degrees Fahrenheit, although a child's normal temperature may be a bit higher or lower. A child's temperature may also be lower in the morning and higher in the afternoon. Temperature may be elevated after physical exercise, in hot weather, after warm food or drink, or when a child is dressed too warmly.

A high temperature may indicate an infection. Report your child's fever to your doctor if any of the following conditions apply:

- ✔ Your child is 3 months old or younger and has a rectal temperature of 100 degrees Fahrenheit or higher.

- ✔ Your child is 3 to 6 months old and has a temperature of 101 degrees Fahrenheit or higher.

- ✔ Your child is 6 to 12 months old and has a temperature of 103 degrees Fahrenheit or higher.

- ✔ Your child is older than 1 year and has a temperature of 104 degrees Fahrenheit or higher.

- ✔ Your child's fever persists for more than 24 hours.

- ✔ Your child becomes delirious.

- ✔ Your child has a febrile convulsion, or seizure.

- ✔ Your child is lethargic or extremely irritable.

- ✔ Your child hasn't urinated in 8 to 12 hours.

- ✔ Your child has other symptoms, such as a stiff and sore neck, sore throat, earache, or body rash.

Temperatures under 101 degrees Fahrenheit do not need to be treated unless your child has a history of febrile convulsions or is uncomfortable. Even higher temperatures are not in themselves dangerous, but an examination rules out any possible infection or disease. If your child is eating and sleeping well and has periods of playfulness, treatment probably isn't needed.

Take the following steps to make your child more comfortable during a fever:

- ✔ Give acetaminophen, which blocks the mechanisms that cause a fever. Never give aspirin to children under the age of 19. Aspirin is directly linked to a rare but serious and life-threatening condition called Reye's syndrome.

✔ Give your child a sponge bath. Seat your child in 1 to 2 inches of tepid water (85 to 90 degrees Fahrenheit) and use a clean washcloth or sponge to spread a film of water over his or her trunk, arms, and legs. The water evaporates and cools the body. This method usually brings the temperature down in 30 to 45 minutes. If your child cannot sit still for this long, don't force the issue. Let your child play quietly in the water or end the bath — whatever keeps your child calm. Sponging is ideal if your child is allergic to, or is unable to tolerate, fever-reducing drugs.

✔ Keep your child's room cool and dress your child lightly so that excess body heat can escape.

✔ Encourage your child to drink plenty of fluids. The body loses fluids through the excess perspiration that a fever produces.

✔ Avoid fatty foods and foods that are difficult to digest. Fever reduces the activity and effectiveness of the stomach. However, don't stop giving your child milk or formula.

✔ Avoid strenuous activity, although your child doesn't need to stay in bed. Quiet play is safe.

Sore throat

Children commonly awake in the morning with a dry throat that needs soothing. If your child's sore throat does not go away with the first cup of juice or milk, however, contact a doctor. If your child is also experiencing a stomachache, fever, headache, stiff neck, or fatigue, call a doctor immediately. A sore throat can be a sign of any number of conditions, including strep throat, tonsillitis, and even measles.

To help soothe a sore throat and make swallowing less painful, try adding soft foods and more liquids to your child's diet. Ice cream, Popsicles, soothing teas, and warm soups are good choices. Also encourage your child to drink plenty of fluids to prevent dehydration. If your child is old enough, offer a gargle of double-strength tea or warm, salty water. Make sure that your child spits out the salty water, though, and doesn't swallow it, because it can upset the stomach. Dry air can aggravate a sore throat, too, especially at night. Add moisture to the air with a cool-mist humidifier.

Stomachache

Even as you read this, we bet that millions of kids across the country are pulling on their parents' shirtsleeves, complaining, "I have a tummyache!" — a testament to the wide range of illnesses that can trigger this common childhood symptom. Indigestion, gas, overeating, constipation, pulled muscles, and emotional distress are only a few of the reasons behind stomachaches.

Many times, the discomfort of a stomachache can be relieved by sitting in a warm bath or by placing a warm towel on the abdomen. Encourage your child to take frequent sips of clear liquids. Don't limit your child's diet to only water for more than a day. If your child has a stomachache, don't use medications without your doctor's instructions, particularly with infants and toddlers. Some medications may contain ingredients that are dangerous to small children.

If your child is experiencing constant stomachache or severe cramping that causes crying or doubling over, or if your child is running a fever, contact a doctor immediately. These symptoms could mean appendicitis, particularly if pain occurs in the lower-right abdomen.

Vomiting

Vomiting is the body's way of removing harmful substances. Vomiting has many causes, including a viral or bacterial infection, intestinal obstruction, poisoning, severe coughing, and motion sickness. In infants, vomiting should not be confused with spitting up. Vomiting is forceful and often described as projectile, bringing up a large amount of fluid at one time.

Contact your doctor if your child is vomiting. The treatment prescribed is greatly affected by your child's age, medical history, and other symptoms, such as fever. Dehydration is a common complication of vomiting. Contact your doctor immediately if your child shows any sign of dehydration. (See "Dehydration," earlier in this chapter, for more information.) Seek immediate medical attention if your child has severe abdominal pain or a stiff neck, has suffered a recent head injury, or is throwing up blood.

If you suspect that your child is vomiting because of exposure to something poisonous, call the poison control hotline in your local area immediately and follow the instructions provided. See Chapter 5 for details on poison emergencies.

Giving your child acetaminophen or ibuprofen

Don't give a baby younger than 3 months acetaminophen or any other medication without the advice of your pediatrician. For older babies and children, the dose should be based on weight, not age.

Although ibuprofen is now approved for use with infants and children, it is still relatively new. According to the American Academy of Pediatrics, not much is known about its side effects. Contact your child's doctor before using ibuprofen.

Taking your child's temperature

One patented skill of parenthood is to simply lay your hand on your child's feverish forehead and magically know the temperature. For those of us who want to be more precise, many types of thermometers are on the market today. The American Medical Association recommends a glass or digital thermometer for exact readings, but you may want to experiment to find one that is accurate and easy for you to use.

You can use three different methods — rectal, *axillary* (under the arm), and oral — to take your child's temperature. Reset a digital thermometer or shake down a rectal thermometer (which has a shorter bulb than an oral thermometer) so that it reads below 96 degrees Fahrenheit and then follow these instructions:

✔ **To take a rectal temperature:** Lubricate the tip of the thermometer with a water-soluble jelly, not petroleum jelly. Place your baby belly-down across your lap and support the head with your hand. Have an older child lie down on a flat surface, preferably the floor. Hold your child with your hand at the middle of the lower back and gently insert the thermometer into the rectum. Insert only the bulb, and nothing more, and hold onto it while it is in your child. Remove a glass thermometer after two minutes. For a digital type, wait for the beep. Rectal readings are usually 1 degree higher than oral readings.

✔ **To take an axillary temperature:** Insert the thermometer in your child's armpit and fold the arm across the chest. Hold the oral thermometer in place for four to five minutes; a digital one beeps when it's ready. Be sure that the thermometer is not sticking out the other side of the armpit, and also try to avoid placing it in an air pocket — make sure that it is surrounded by skin. Many doctors prefer that parents take a rectal temperature on a young child and a baby because it is more accurate than an axillary temperature, which can be about 3 degrees lower than a rectal temperature. However, the axillary temperature can be useful in screening your child for a fever. Do not take an axillary temperature soon after physical activity or after a bath.

✔ **To take an oral temperature:** Make sure that your child's mouth is clear of candy, gum, or food, and then place the thermometer's tip under your child's tongue. The child should close his or her lips around it and should not bite the thermometer or talk while it's in his or her mouth. Remove a glass thermometer after three to five minutes. A digital thermometer beeps when it's ready. Wait 20 to 30 minutes after your child has finished drinking or eating to take an oral temperature.

Handling Childhood Conditions

Germs, the harbingers of disease, are a natural part of the environment. And as your child becomes more active and social — perhaps attending day care or preschool — it's only a matter of time before germs move in to do their dirty work.

Preventing the spread of all germs is impossible, but you can help reduce the risks by taking simple precautions. The best and easiest is to wash your hands often and encourage your child to do the same, particularly before meals and at bedtime. Our hands are the quickest route that germs can take to our noses and mouths, where they find the perfect environment to grow. Also remember to keep a sick person's utensils and drinking cups separate from the rest of the family's, and keep older children who are sick away from younger ones. Wash children's toys regularly, especially if your children are teething or they often put things in their mouths.

These precautions can help prevent illness much of the time, but every child gets sick now and then. The following sections describe the most common childhood illnesses, along with their symptoms, the usual treatments, and what you can do to help your child recover at home. With the proper treatment, you can greatly reduce the risk of complications, and your child can return to a normal, active life in no time.

Chicken pox

Chicken pox is a condition that parents get to know all too well. Also called *varicella,* chicken pox is a mild but contagious childhood disease best known by the itchy rash that it causes. More than 90 percent of chicken pox cases, which are triggered by a herpes virus, occur in children younger than 12. The disease is spread through contact with airborne droplets carrying the virus (launched by a cough or a sneeze) or through contact with the rash.

Most children with chicken pox recover without complications. However, some 9,000 people are hospitalized with the condition each year, and, in rare cases, it results in death. In adults — and even older children, who can get this condition — the same virus causes a painful nerve condition called shingles.

Recognizing the signs

The symptoms of chicken pox include a low-grade fever, runny nose, slight cough, decrease in appetite, and fatigue and weakness. Anywhere between 24 and 48 hours later, a rash develops on the body, starting on the chest, back, or face. The rash may also appear in the mouth as white ulcers, or as ulcers in the ears and eyes.

Children are contagious from two days before the rash develops until all the lesions have crusted over, usually five to ten days after the rash breaks out.

Making it better

With viral infections, time is the greatest healer; they must be allowed to run their course. At times, antihistamines may be prescribed to help relieve itching. In serious cases (for example, when a person has a depressed immune system), the drug acyclovir may be recommended.

To make your child more comfortable and to avoid minor complications, try the following:

- ✔ Have your child drink plenty of fluids.

- ✔ Apply calamine lotion to itchy areas.

- ✔ Trim your child's nails or have the child wear mittens to discourage scratching open the rash, which can cause a skin infection.

- ✔ Soothe the rash with a bath. Add $1/2$ cup of uncooked oatmeal or $1/2$ cup of baking soda to a warm bath, and let your child soak for 15 minutes. Do not rinse the skin, but do pat dry gently. (To avoid plugging the drain, put oatmeal in a nylon stocking, or use a powdered infant oatmeal cereal.)

- ✔ Use acetaminophen to treat a fever. Never give aspirin or salicylates to a child under the age of 19. Aspirin has been directly linked to a rare but serious and life-threatening condition called Reye's syndrome.

Contact a doctor immediately if your child

- ✔ Finds that the itching is uncontrollable

- ✔ Is vomiting

- ✔ Experiences a painful and stiff neck

- ✔ Is very sleepy or has trouble walking

- ✔ Has a temperature higher than 102 degrees Fahrenheit, or has a fever after the fourth day of illness

- ✔ Has a serious illness, or is on steroids and comes down with this illness

The best way to prevent chicken pox is with the varicella vaccine, a relatively new vaccine that protects against chicken pox. (See "Immunizing," earlier in this chapter.)

Colds and flu

The common cold is a viral infection that attacks the upper respiratory tract: the nose, throat, sinuses, ears, eustachian tubes, trachea, larynx, and bronchial tubes. In an age of day-care centers, play dates, and preschool, it's not uncommon for kids to get one cold after another. Young children commonly experience 5 to 12 colds per year.

A common misconception is that colds are caused by exposure to cold or wet weather. Although these conditions can depress the body's immune system, making you more vulnerable to illness, colds are caused by germs, plain and simple.

Recognizing the signs

Children who are otherwise healthy suffer from a cold for 7 to 14 days. The contagious phase is the first two to four days after symptoms appear. These symptoms can be so minor, such as a tickle in the throat, that the cold can go undetected during the contagious phase, giving it a chance to spread easily to others.

As the cold progresses, the symptoms become more pronounced and uncomfortable. The most common symptoms are sneezing, stuffy or runny nose, watery eyes, cough, earache, sore throat, and fever.

Making it better

As with any viral infection, time is the best healer because the virus must run its course. To reduce the effects of a cold and make your child more comfortable, you can take several steps:

- ✔ Make sure that your child gets plenty of bed rest.

- ✔ Encourage your child to drink plenty of fluids.

- ✔ Increase the humidity in the air by using a cool-mist humidifier. Make sure to rinse it out daily. Bleach it at least once a week to prevent sending germs into the air. Also, consider filling it with distilled water.

- ✔ For infants and very young children who cannot blow their noses, use a nasal syringe to remove mucus. Bear in mind, though, that overuse can increase nasal secretions.

- ✔ Treat a fever with acetaminophen. Never give aspirin to children under the age of 19. Aspirin is directly linked to a rare but serious and life-threatening disease called Reye's syndrome.

- ✔ Apply petroleum jelly on the skin under the nose to soothe rawness.

- ✔ Give older children sugarless hard candy or cough drops to suck on to relieve sore throats.

- ✔ Check with your doctor before giving your child any cold remedy. Over-the-counter medications can dry out the nasal passages and cause side effects.

Contact a doctor immediately if your child

- ✔ Is under 6 months of age (a time during which a small infant can quickly develop a more serious condition such as pneumonia)

- ✔ Widens the nostrils with each breath or has difficulty breathing

✔ Has symptoms that interfere with sleeping, eating, and drinking

✔ Does not urinate for more than 8 to 12 hours (a sign of dehydration)

✔ Has blue lips or nails

✔ Complains of increased throat pain or difficulty swallowing

✔ Has thick, green mucus instead of clear mucus

✔ Has a cough that lasts longer than two weeks, or a cough so strong that it causes choking or vomiting

✔ Complains of chest pain or shortness of breath

✔ Has pain in the ear

✔ Shivers and has chills

✔ Has a temperature higher than 102 degrees Fahrenheit, or has a temperature higher than 101 degrees Fahrenheit that lasts several days, or develops another fever after the initial fever subsides (a sign of a secondary bacterial infection)

✔ Is excessively sleepy or cranky

To prevent spreading the cold to others, be sure that your child covers his or her mouth when sneezing or coughing and washes hands after blowing his or her nose. Discard used tissues immediately. These simple tasks can be difficult for a small child, so it's important to take the time to teach kids these measures. You can find more information about colds in Chapter 17.

Diaper rash

This form of dermatitis is characterized by a red, irritating rash followed by dry, scaly skin on the buttocks and genitals of an infant. It usually results from an infant sitting in a wet diaper, because the ammonia in the urine may irritate the skin. Diaper rash may last up to ten days, although most cases clear within a day.

To relieve diaper rash on your own at home, allow the baby to go without a diaper under your supervision. Use a zinc oxide ointment to soothe the rash. In serious cases, topical corticosteroids may be prescribed to stop the rash. An antifungal drug may be used to prevent yeast infections. In either case, be sure to talk with your baby's doctor first before medicating, and check product directions to find out whether use is not recommended for children.

To prevent diaper rash, change the infant's diaper — cloth or disposable — as often as possible. When you wash cloth diapers, add 1 ounce of vinegar per 1 gallon of water in the rinse cycle to match the pH of the diapers to the pH of the baby's skin.

Ear infections (Otitis media)

Ear infection, or *otitis media,* is the inflammation of the middle ear, the area located behind the eardrum. Two out of three children experience at least one bout of the infection by the time they are 3 years old.

Recognizing the signs and knowing for sure

The symptoms of an ear infection in an older child are pain in the ear, a sensation of fullness in the ear, hearing loss, and fever. In a younger child, symptoms are irritability and fussiness, difficulty in sleeping, pulling at the ear, difficulty in or painful sucking, and fever.

An unresolved ear infection can lead to complications, so a child with the symptoms discussed in the preceding section should always be seen by a physician, especially if symptoms include a fever and previous upper respiratory infection. Other conditions also lead to earaches: teething, a foreign object in the ear, an ear canal injury from a cotton swab, or hard earwax. Only a doctor can determine the exact cause of an earache and provide the best treatment.

Making it better

As many as 85 percent of otitis media cases are caused by bacteria, which can be eradicated by antibiotics. Some children do not feel relief until 48 hours after starting the antibiotics, but if your child experiences no relief at all, discuss with your doctor the possibility of a viral infection (which cannot be treated with antibiotics) or allergies. Finding the culprit of recurrent ear infections is important because they can affect a child's hearing and speech development.

Anytime your child is sick, ask your child's doctor to check for fluid in the middle ear. Even if your child is not in pain, the fluid can affect hearing, something that young children in particular cannot communicate to others.

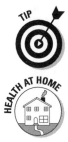

At home, make your child more comfortable. Position the child with the infected ear up; the bulging of the tympanic membrane causes pain, and with the ear up, gravity helps to reverse this process. A warm compress on the ear and acetaminophen can help reduce pain and pressure. As long as the infection is not contagious, a child with an ear infection can go outside and play with others. Swimming is not recommended, though, because water entering the ear aggravates the condition.

An ounce of prevention

In infants, the natural immunities passed on through breast-feeding can help reduce the risk of contracting ear infections. The position that a baby takes during breast-feeding also helps reduce the chance of fluid entering the middle ear. Bottle-fed babies benefit from being in an upright position during feedings, with the head kept higher than the belly. Do not lie a child flat during feedings or allow a child to take a bottle to bed.

Measles

Although measles is usually associated with a severe skin rash, it is actually a respiratory infection. Initial symptoms usually appear anywhere from 9 to 11 days after exposure to the measles virus, and illness lasts 10 to 14 days. The measles virus spreads in fluid from the nose or mouth, and in airborne droplets from sneezes and coughs. It is a highly contagious disease.

Recognizing the signs and knowing for sure

The first symptoms of measles are irritability, runny nose, eyes that are red and sensitive to light (*conjunctivitis,* or *pinkeye* as it is commonly called), hacking cough, and a fever as high as 105 degrees Fahrenheit.

Within eight days after early symptoms develop, a rash appears. After the rash begins to develop, the initial symptoms subside, except for the cough, which can continue throughout the course of the illness. The rash usually begins on the forehead and works its way down the face, neck, and body. It looks like large, flat blotches that are somewhere between red and brown in color. They often overlap each other to completely cover the skin, especially on the face and shoulders. Within three days, the rash makes its way to the feet. It lasts about six days and then starts to disappear, again beginning with the forehead and working its way down. As it sheds in a finely textured peel, the skin may look brown. This is only temporary.

One unmistakable sign of measles is *Koplik's spots,* small, red, irregularly shaped spots with blue-white centers found inside the mouth. They usually appear one to two days before the skin rash sets in, and a doctor may notice them upon examining a child who is suffering from a high fever and cough.

Making it better

As with any viral infection, antibiotics are not effective. Treatment usually involves making the child comfortable and watching for complications such as pneumonia. Someone with measles is contagious from five days after exposure to the virus until five days after the rash disappears.

Keep your child home and away from other children during this time. A child should get plenty of bed rest and avoid busy play and activity. To make your child more comfortable during recovery, try these suggestions:

- ✔ Encourage your child to drink plenty of fluids to prevent dehydration.
- ✔ Use a cool-mist humidifier to relieve the child's cough and soothe the breathing passages.
- ✔ Give acetaminophen to control a fever of 103 degrees Fahrenheit or higher. (Never give aspirin to a child younger than 19.)
- ✔ Darken your child's room. The pinkeye that sometimes accompanies the illness can make it painful for your child to be in bright sunlight.
- ✔ Take your child's temperature at least once each morning and night to monitor progress and spot complications.

Children who suffer from measles are often susceptible to bacterial infections, especially those involving the ears and the lungs. A doctor can treat this infections with antibiotics.

Contact a doctor immediately if your child

- ✔ Develops a sore throat
- ✔ Complains of an earache or heaviness in the ear
- ✔ Develops a cough that produces a colored mucus and/or lasts longer than four days
- ✔ Has difficulty breathing or breathes very fast
- ✔ Has lips or nails that turn bluish or gray
- ✔ Has a temperature above 103 degrees Fahrenheit

Mumps

Mumps is a viral infection that spreads throughout the body, but its symptoms are especially focused on the *parotid* salivary glands. When infected, the parotid glands become swollen and painful over a period of one to three days. Other glands around the face may also become involved.

Mumps infections are rare in children younger than 2 years. Children ages 10 to 19 are most likely to get mumps. Symptoms set in anywhere from 12 to 25 days after the child is exposed to the virus; the average is 18 days. Most children recover in 10 to 12 days. It usually takes a week for the swelling to disappear in each parotid salivary gland, but both glands usually don't swell at the same time.

Experts have a varied opinion of how long mumps can be contagious. Some say that the infection is contagious from two days before the symptoms begin to as long as six days after the symptoms end. Others say that it lasts from six days before the glands begin to swell to two weeks later. In any case, the virus is highly contagious because it lives in the infected child's saliva and can be spread on cups and utensils and through the droplets spread by sneezes and coughs. It can also survive in a child's urine for two to three weeks.

Recognizing the signs

Thanks to the mumps vaccine, most children will not contract the illness. But if your child is not immunized, you should know the signs and be able to distinguish them from those of other illnesses.

Symptoms include swelling of one or both glands along the sides of the cheeks, fever for three to five days, pain when the swollen area is touched or when the child opens the mouth, nausea and occasional vomiting, headache, a general feeling of weakness, loss of appetite, swelling and pain in the joints, and swelling of the testes in boys.

Making it better

No specific treatment for mumps exists. As with all viral infections, antibiotics are not effective, and the disease must run its natural course. The only measure a parent or doctor can take is to make the child as comfortable as possible and watch for complications. Try these suggestions:

- ✔ Give your child acetaminophen for fever and pain. (Never give aspirin to a child under 19.)

- ✔ Add liquids and soft, noncitrus, easy-to-swallow foods to your child's diet. Hard foods that require a lot of chewing also cause the glands to produce more saliva and cause more pain. So do acidic citrus juices and foods.

- ✔ Keep a glass of fresh water or noncitrus juice nearby and encourage your child to take sips. Although a child with mumps will find drinking and swallowing painful, fluids prevent dehydration.

- ✔ Apply a cold or warm compress over the swollen glands to give short-term relief.

- ✔ Take your child's temperature at least once each morning and again at night. If a fever goes higher than 103 degrees Fahrenheit, give your child acetaminophen.

Contact a doctor immediately if your child

- ✔ Worsens in overall condition

- ✔ Feels pain in the testes (in boys)

- ✔ Has severe abdominal pain

- ✔ Is extremely listless

- ✔ Exhibits signs of mumps and has received the vaccine

Respiratory problems

The lungs, windpipe, and other components of the respiratory system work to get the body the oxygen that it needs. However, conditions such as asthma, bronchiolitis, croup, and pneumonia may affect your child's breathing. This section provides a quick rundown of these conditions.

Asthma

Asthma is a lung disease that causes breathing problems for nearly 10 million people in the United States. Most cases of asthma develop in children — even infants — although it may also occur in adults. Asthma is a chronic disorder and can be life-threatening in some cases, but by recognizing and responding to early warning signs, you and your child can manage attacks.

An asthma attack occurs when the muscle layer of the breathing passages narrows and spasms. The delicate lining of the airways, called *mucosa,* swell, and an excessive, sticky mucus is produced. This can cause a tightness in the chest, wheezing, coughing, restlessness, or trouble breathing. Colds, flus, allergies, weather, air pollution, vigorous exercise, and, infrequently, emotional stress and excitement can trigger asthma attacks.

Contact your doctor if your child has chest, throat, or neck pain or severe trouble breathing that seems to be getting worse, especially if the child is breathing rapidly. Pulling at the chest during inhalation and forceful grunting during exhalation are also signs of asthma. Also watch for other, less obvious signs: eyes or fingertips that appear blue or skin that seems darkened. A child with asthma may act agitated, extremely lethargic, or confused.

A complete evaluation of your child's condition helps pinpoint a medication that eases the symptoms. Regular checkups, education about early warning signs, and routine monitoring of lung air capacity with a peak flow meter can help decrease your child's chance of experiencing a frightening and severe attack.

Bronchiolitis

Bronchiolitis is an infection of the small breathing tubes of the lungs, called *bronchioles.* Don't confuse this condition with *bronchitis,* an infection of the larger, more central airways. Infants are more susceptible to this infection than older children because their airways are smaller and are more easily blocked when infection and inflammation occur.

If your infant has bronchiolitis, it will start with signs of a cold: runny nose, mild cough, and sometimes fever. After a day or two, the cough becomes more pronounced, and the baby will begin to breathe more rapidly and with more difficulty. A child may also eat poorly because the effort to breathe may make sucking and swallowing difficult.

Contact your doctor immediately if your baby shows any signs of breathing difficulty, or if the fever lasts more than three days, or if a fever is present in an infant younger than 3 months. Because taking fluids can be difficult for both older children and infants, it's important to watch for signs of dehydration. The signs include dry mouth, taking less than a normal amount of fluids, shedding no tears when crying, and urinating less than normal or not wetting a diaper for 8 to 12 hours.

Because bronchiolitis is caused by a virus, antibiotics are useless against the infection itself. However, a bronchodilating drug that opens the breathing tubes may be prescribed. Hospitalization may be recommended if your child is having breathing difficulties or is suffering from dehydration. If your doctor recommends that your child should be treated at home, all you can do is try to make your child more comfortable and ease cold symptoms. See "Colds and flu," earlier in this chapter, for self-care tips.

Croup

Croup is an inflammation of the larynx and trachea that narrows the airway just below the vocal cords and makes breathing noisy and difficult. The condition can happen at any time of the year, but it is more common between October and March. Children are most susceptible between 6 months and 3 years of age. The greatest danger of croup is that the airway may continue to swell and narrow, making it first difficult and then impossible to breathe.

If your child awakens in the middle of the night with the distinctive croup bark, take him or her into the bathroom and run the shower with the hottest water possible. This creates a steam that helps reduce the swelling of the airway. (Be sure to keep your child away from the water to avoid scalding.) Close the bathroom door and sit in the steamy room for 15 to 20 minutes. Afterwards, your child will still have a croup cough but should be able to breathe more easily. Using a cool-mist humidifier in your child's room for several nights is also recommended. Put the humidifier as close to the bed as possible so that your child gets the full benefits of the moist air.

With croup, contact your child's doctor immediately, regardless of the hour, for advice on treatment. Some doctors recommend decongestants for spasmodic croup and cortisone medications to reduce swelling from viral croup. Cough syrups are not recommended because they do not affect the larynx or trachea where the infection is located, and they may interfere with your child's ability to cough up the secretions produced by the infection.

In rare cases, hospitalization may be a course of action. There, your child can benefit from an oxygen croup tent, intravenous nutrients, and aerosol medication. To bypass the swelling in the larynx and trachea, a tube may be inserted through the nose or mouth into the windpipe so that your child can regain normal breathing during recovery.

Take your child to the emergency room immediately if he or she

- Makes a whistling sound that gets louder with each breath
- Can't speak for lack of breath
- Seems to be struggling to get a breath

Pneumonia

Most pneumonia develops after a respiratory tract infection spreads to the chest. Pneumonia can also be a complication that follows other viral infections such as chicken pox, measles, herpes, infectious mononucleosis, and rubella. It can be caused by a bacterial infection as well. Although the illness was once considered extremely dangerous, today most children recover completely with proper and prompt medical treatment.

The symptoms of pneumonia include fever, sweating, chills, flushed skin, general discomfort, loss of appetite and energy, cough, fast and labored breathing, wheezing, and a bluish tint to the lips or nails. Contact your child's doctor if you notice any of these signs.

Your doctor may prescribe an antibiotic because it's difficult to determine whether the illness is caused by a virus or bacteria. If your child does have viral pneumonia, the illness should disappear in a few days, but you should still give your child all the antibiotic for as long as prescribed to ensure that all the bacteria are eradicated. At home, do not give your child cough suppressants; coughing is necessary to clear the excessive secretions caused by the infection.

Be sure to check back with your doctor if your child has a fever that lasts more than two or three days after the antibiotics are started, has difficulty breathing, or experiences red, swollen joints, bone pain, stiffness in the neck, or vomiting. These are all signs of a possible infection elsewhere in the body.

Strep throat

Group A streptococci are bacteria that cause a painful inflammation of the throat called *pharyngitis*. Commonly known as strep throat, this condition is most common during the cold winter months when people are crowded together indoors. The strep bacteria are contained in the droplets of sneezes and coughs, and it can also be spread through close contact with someone who is already infected. Of all age groups, children ages 5 to 15 are the most commonly affected.

The incubation time for strep throat is two to seven days after exposure to the bacteria. Consider your child contagious until after treatment by antibiotics for 24 hours.

Recognizing the signs and knowing for sure

In older children, symptoms of strep throat include painful throat; difficulty swallowing and eating; fever above 101 degrees Fahrenheit; chills; body aches; nausea, vomiting, and abdominal pain; red, swollen tonsils that are dotted with whitish or yellowing specks of pus; and swollen glands in the neck. In infants, the symptoms may not be focused on the throat. They may include runny nose, crusting and sores around the nostrils, a low-grade fever, and poor feedings.

If your child shows any signs of strep throat, see a doctor for diagnosis and treatment. If left untreated or treated incompletely with antibiotics, the bacteria can lead to other, more serious complications, including kidney problems, rheumatic fever, sinusitis, ear infections, pneumonia, and skin infections. At times, a rash accompanies the strep infection. The illness is then called *scarlet fever* or *scarlatina,* but it is no more serious than strep throat alone.

To diagnose strep throat, the doctor runs a rapid strep test or takes a *culture* (a test in which the throat is gently swabbed) from your child's throat with a cotton swab. The procedure is painless, but it may make your child gag, so you may want to hold your child in your lap while the sample is taken.

Making it better

The illness is typically treated with penicillin for ten days. If your child is allergic to penicillin, the doctor will prescribe another antibiotic. You can expect your child's fever to stop within three to five days, and the sore throat to subside soon afterward.

To make your child more comfortable during recovery, try the following suggestions:

- ✔ Add soft foods and more liquids to the diet, because swallowing can be painful. Try ice cream, Popsicles, soothing teas, warm soups, and milkshakes.
- ✔ Encourage your child to drink plenty of fluids to prevent dehydration.
- ✔ Let the child rest in bed and play quietly.
- ✔ Help your child gargle. Try a double-strength tea or warm, salty water. Make sure that your child spits out the salty water after gargling, because it can upset the stomach.
- ✔ Use a cool-mist humidifier to add moisture to the air.
- ✔ Place a moist, warm towel around your child's neck to help soothe swollen glands.

Finally, to prevent complications, be sure that your child takes all the antibiotics for as long as they are prescribed.

Contact the doctor immediately if your child

✔ Develops a second fever after several days of normal temperature

✔ Develops a skin rash

✔ Complains of an earache or, in a younger child, pulls at the ear

✔ Has a nasal discharge with discolored or bloody mucus

✔ Develops a cough, especially if it produces mucus

✔ Experiences chest pain, shortness of breath, or extreme tiredness

✔ Has convulsions

✔ Has painful, red, and swollen joints

✔ Is nauseated or vomiting

Tonsillitis

The tonsils are clusters of tissue that lie in two bands at the back of the throat. They contain cells that produce antibodies that fight viruses and bacteria. *Tonsillitis,* an infection and inflammation of the tonsils, can be caused by viruses or bacteria. In either case, the tonsils become enlarged and red and are often coated with a yellow, gray, or white membrane.

Whether caused by bacteria or a virus, tonsillitis is highly contagious. It usually spreads from person to person by contact with the throat or nasal fluids of someone who is already sick, perhaps by sneezing, coughing, or drinking from a cup used by the infected person. The illness can last anywhere from 2 to 12 days, depending on whether the infection is viral or bacterial. Several weeks may pass before the tonsils and swollen glands return to normal size.

Recognizing the signs and knowing for sure

In an older child, the symptoms of tonsillitis are a sudden sore throat, pain upon swallowing, stiff neck, loss of appetite, general ill feeling, chills, a fever higher than 101 degrees Fahrenheit, and swollen and tender glands under the neck. In infants, the symptoms of tonsillitis may not be as focused on the throat. Their most noticeable symptoms may be poor feedings, runny nose, and a slight fever.

A doctor diagnoses tonsillitis by examining the tonsils. A culture may also be taken to determine which virus or bacteria is causing the infection.

Making it better

In 30 percent of tonsillitis cases, the bacteria called *Group A streptococci* (also called *strep*) is responsible for the illness, and a course of antibiotics will treat the infection. In the other 70 percent of cases, the infection is viral, in which case antibiotics will not help — the illness must run its course.

In tonsillitis caused by strep bacteria, the fever and sore throat usually last three to five days. When tonsillitis is caused by a virus, its duration depends on the virus involved. Most people recover almost completely within a week.

To make your child more comfortable during recovery, take these steps:

- ✔ Because pain during swallowing can make eating difficult, try including more liquids and soft foods, such as soothing teas, warm soups, cooling soft drinks, milkshakes, and Popsicles, in your child's diet.

- ✔ Make sure that your child drinks plenty of fluids.

- ✔ Check your child's temperature at least once in the morning and once at night. Report any increase in temperature to your doctor.

- ✔ Give acetaminophen to relieve pain and reduce fever. (Never give aspirin to a child younger than 19, because it is directly linked to Reye's syndrome, a serious and life-threatening condition.)

- ✔ Encourage older children to gargle with double-strength tea or warm, salty water. Be sure that your child doesn't swallow the salty water, though, because it can upset the stomach.

- ✔ Because dry air can aggravate a sore throat, use a cool-mist humidifier to add moisture to the air, especially during the night.

- ✔ If your child is taking antibiotics, to prevent complications, be sure that he or she takes the medication as directed for as long as prescribed.

When a child suffers frequently from tonsillitis (usually seven times in one year, or five times in a year for two years in a row), doctors sometimes suggest surgical removal of the tonsils. The procedure, called a tonsillectomy, was once a common form of treatment — almost a rite of passage — but now many doctors question its effectiveness in preventing further throat infections and therefore recommend it less frequently. Research has also shown the benefit of the tonsils in the immune system response.

Contact a doctor immediately if your child

✔ Develops a second fever a few days after the initial fever disappears (possibly indicating a second infection)

✔ Develops a skin rash

✔ Complains of an earache

✔ Has convulsions

✔ Has a nasal discharge that's discolored or streaked with blood

✔ Develops a cough, especially if it produces mucus

✔ Complains of chest pain, shortness of breath, or extreme tiredness

✔ Has painful, red, or swollen joints

✔ Is nauseated or vomiting

Chapter 14

Surviving Puberty: Adolescent Health

*L*eaving childhood and heading into adulthood is a physical and emotional roller coaster, both for teens and their parents. Adolescents today have many options and opportunities available to them that their parents never did. They must also overcome some challenges and pitfalls that their parents never faced.

Growing up is difficult in terms of health as well. As a teenager, you need to understand what's going on with your body, how to handle those changes, and how to start taking responsibility for your own health.

Raging Hormones: Puberty and Sexual Development

Puberty is an ugly word. Upon pronunciation, it almost *sounds* embarrassing. But it's really nothing to be shy about. After all, everyone goes through it. And if you want to be healthy, you need to know all the details — gory as you may think they are.

What is puberty, exactly? According to *Webster's Dictionary,* puberty is the stage of physical development when secondary sex characteristics develop and sexual reproduction first becomes possible.

In the following pages, we talk about the changes that come with puberty. But before you begin comparing yourself to your friends, keep this in mind: The outward signs of puberty vary from one person to the next. One young person may begin development at 8 years of age, while another may not show development until 14 or 15. Generally, girls tend to enter puberty two years ahead of boys. Don't fret if you feel that you're not up to speed. "Normal" is relative.

Girls growing up

When a girl is between the ages of 8 and 13, her *ovaries* — the organs that produce eggs for reproduction — get the signal to begin producing more of a hormone called *estrogen,* which kicks off a chain of events that doesn't wrap up for about four to five years.

The first visible changes in a girl's body are the emergence of breasts and the growth of sparse pubic hair. About one year or so after breasts begin to develop, a girl usually experiences *menarche* (pronounced "meh-NAR-key"), her first menstrual period.

Menstruation, illustrated in Figure 14-1, is the completion of a cycle that goes on inside the body. A menstrual period may appear suddenly one day, but (thanks to estrogen) the "preparations" for this event have been going on internally for some time.

Females have two ovaries, each containing thousands of tiny eggs. Females are born with all the eggs they'll have throughout their lifetimes. Once a month, one of the ovaries releases an egg in a process called *ovulation.* Each month before ovulation, the uterus readies itself for a possible pregnancy by forming a lining composed of tissue and blood.

The released egg travels toward the uterus (or womb) through one of two fallopian tubes. Most of the time, the egg breaks up before it reaches the uterus. If, however, sperm (the male reproductive cell) meets and joins the egg on its travels, fertilization takes place. The fertilized egg then travels to its "nesting place," the uterus, where it attaches itself to the lining and develops over the course of nine months into a baby.

If fertilization does not occur, the special lining in the uterus is not needed. The tissue and blood flow out of the uterus, down through the cervix and vagina and out of the body. This is the menstrual period, which generally lasts three to seven days. Usually, 14 days elapse between ovulation and a period. However, the time from the beginning of the period to the next ovulation may vary, so not all women's cycles are the same. The whole cycle, from release of the egg to formation of the lining to the start of the menstrual period, is regulated by estrogen and other hormones.

After ovulation occurs for the first time, pregnancy is possible — even if you haven't yet had a menstrual period. If you are sexually active and are concerned about preventing pregnancy and sexually transmitted diseases (as you should be), find out about contraception and safer sex! Discussion

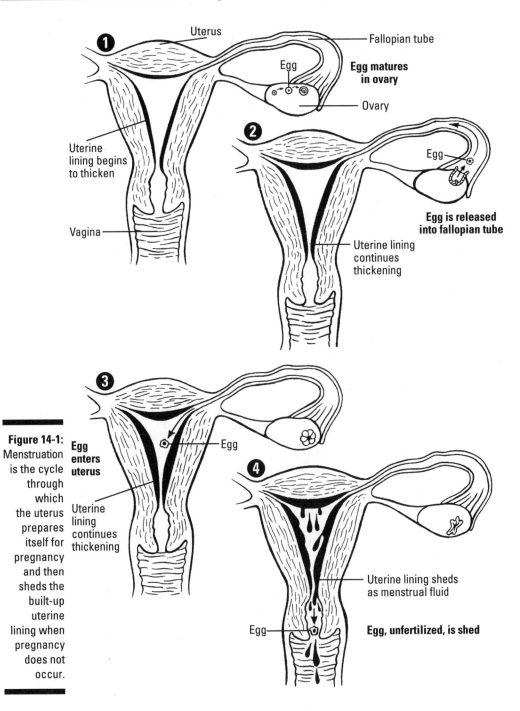

① Uterus — Fallopian tube

Egg

Egg matures in ovary

Ovary

Uterine lining begins to thicken

Vagina

②

Egg

Egg is released into fallopian tube

Uterine lining continues thickening

③

Egg enters uterus

Egg

Uterine lining continues thickening

④

Uterine lining sheds as menstrual fluid

Egg

Egg, unfertilized, is shed

Figure 14-1: Menstruation is the cycle through which the uterus prepares itself for pregnancy and then sheds the built-up uterine lining when pregnancy does not occur.

with a parent, doctor, school nurse, guidance counselor, or some other trusted adult will provide the information you need. (We talk about all these ideas, too, in Chapter 19.)

Puberty, of course, doesn't end with menstruation. Usually after menarche, girls begin to grow taller. Underarm hair begins to grow, and pubic hair becomes thicker. The breasts, of course, continue to enlarge, and the hips begin to widen. The libido, or sex drive, awakens. Girls' voices also deepen during puberty, though not as much as boys' voices do. Puberty is generally complete by age 18.

Boys becoming men

Hormones — in this case, testosterone — are responsible for puberty in boys. For guys, the first outward sign of puberty is the appearance of hair in the pubic area, under the arms, and on the face. The voice gradually deepens, sometimes "cracking" as the vocal cords thicken and adjust, and the libido, or sex drive, becomes more active.

The hormones also cause the testicles to enlarge and the scrotum to become darker. The penis gradually becomes longer and thicker. And after testosterone begins circulating, the male body begins to produce sperm, the male reproductive cells.

A boy is able to have an erection at birth, but *ejaculation* (the emission of fluid called *semen* from the penis at the height of sexual excitement) doesn't occur until puberty sets in. Around this time, spontaneous erection and ejaculation may occur during sleep — what's called a *nocturnal emission* or "wet dream." These are signs of ongoing sexual maturation.

More than 50 percent of boys develop some degree of adolescent *gynecomastia* — breast enlargement — during adolescence. The condition may be accompanied by minor lumps and some pain, but the main problem is embarrassment. However, it's not a reason to worry. Temporary hormonal imbalance is the cause, and any enlargement normally fades in 12 to 16 months.

We told the girls, and now we'll tell you: If you are sexually active, find out about contraception and safer sex in order to protect yourself against pregnancy and sexually transmitted disease! Discussion with a parent, doctor, school nurse, guidance counselor, or some other trusted adult will provide the information you need. (We talk about all these ideas in Chapter 19.)

Health Conditions and Concerns

Teens have many of the same health conditions that men, women, and children may worry about: the flu, a broken bone, allergies, and so on. But a few health concerns — such as acne and eating disorders — commonly haunt adolescents.

Reacting to acne

When it comes to your skin, you can pretty safely blame hormones for just about everything that goes wrong. In the case of acne, the hormones of puberty work to increase the oil production of glands within the skin. The boost in oil production causes clogged pores that may become inflamed and develop into pimples.

To help fight acne, wash your face regularly and keep your hair (which is covered with oils of its own) off your face and forehead. Use only oil-free products and cosmetics on your face. Most important: Don't pick at your pimples. Doing so can only make matters worse and may lead to permanent scarring.

If acne is particularly bothersome and doesn't subside, talk with a dermatologist or your medical practitioner about what you can do. A number of prescription drugs (notably Accutane) are available for treating the condition.

Fighting back against eating disorders

During adolescence, you may look at yourself in the mirror and wonder how the "finished product" will look after this period of adolescence ends. You probably never focus so much attention on your physical appearance as you do during your teens.

For some adolescents, though, this self-focus becomes an obsession with weight and appearance. The pressure to conform to what the marketing industry "mandates" leads many young people to go on diets. Although a sensible diet and an exercise program under medical supervision may be healthy, many adolescents, especially girls, go to unhealthy extremes to maintain their "ideal weights." From these extremes, eating disorders may result. The three common types of eating disorders are

> ✔ **Anorexia nervosa:** This eating disorder, characterized by an obsession with thinness, mostly affects adolescent girls. A girl may become as thin as a toothpick but still insist that she needs to lose weight. The extreme weight loss of anorexia causes serious side effects, such as loss of muscle, bone minerals, and menstrual periods. A weakened heart, anemia, and liver and kidney damage may occur as well. In some

cases, anorexia leads to death. Adolescents who have anorexia need immediate medical care and psychological counseling.

- **Bulimia nervosa:** Bulimia nervosa involves *bingeing and purging:* eating large amounts of food in a short period and then purging (emptying) the food from the body by inducing vomiting, using laxatives, or fasting. The physical results of bulimia are not as noticeable as with anorexia because those with bulimia tend to maintain normal weights. Some negative side effects may include upsetting the body's fluid and mineral balance, damage to the bowels, internal bleeding and infection, and tooth damage and lesions in the esophagus due to exposure to stomach acid during repeated vomiting. In some cases, bulimia may lead to death.

- **Binge eating disorder:** Those who binge consume food frequently and repeatedly, often in secret. This disorder usually has its roots in stress, anxiety, or depression; genetics, socioeconomic status, and culture also may play a role. Males are more likely to have binge eating disorder than anorexia or bulimia.

The first step in treatment is a physical examination to determine the extent of the disease. Mild cases are often treated with *psychotherapy,* a form of counseling that involves talking and working to restructure eating habits and behavior. In more serious cases, immediate hospitalization may be necessary to restore the health of the person with the disorder before therapy can begin.

For more information about eating disorders, contact the American Anorexia/Bulimia Association, 293 Central Park W., Suite 1R, New York, NY 10024, 212-501-8351; or visit their Web site at members.aol.com/amanbu.

Boosting emotional health

At the beginning of this chapter, we described adolescence as a type of roller coaster. During these years, emotions seesaw as you ride the wave of adolescence. Part of the ride can be attributed to hormones, which do affect mood and sex drive. The other part comes from the conflicts that come with growing up: your changing relationships with your parents and friends, pressure from peers, and perhaps the awkwardness with which the body changes.

Emotional health, of course, has much to do with physical health. You may be able to run laps around the football field and still not be truly healthy unless you have peace of mind. And we're not talking metaphorically, either: Stress weakens the immune system and makes you more likely to be sick.

Unfortunately, the combination of adolescent stress and/or family problems sometimes sets the stage for serious emotional problems. These stresses may even precipitate mental illness. Professional help is the only alternative.

We all experience short "down" periods now and then. These are even more common during adolescence. However, when depression becomes prolonged, it's time to seek help. Just as with a physical ailment, recovery is quicker if the emotional illness is addressed sooner. And depression is treatable. Some signs of depression are

✔ Chronic sadness

✔ Feelings of hopelessness

✔ Avoidance of family and friends

✔ Diminishing interest in food, school, or recreational activities

✔ Inability to focus and concentrate

✔ Physical symptoms such as fatigue, headache, or stomachache

✔ Insomnia or hypersomnia (sleeping too much)

For free information about depression, you and your parents can contact the National Institute of Mental Health's D/ART (Depression/Awareness, Recognition, Treatment) Program. Write them at D/ART, Room 10-85, 5600 Fishers Lane, National Institute of Mental Health, Rockville, MD 20857; or call 301-443-4140. For free brochures on depression, call 800-421-4211 or visit D/ART's Web page at www.nimh.nih.gov/publicat/eduprogs/ dart.htm.

Making Smart Health Choices

Choices surround you during adolescence. Your parents guided you toward choices when you were a child, but now the responsibility increasingly falls upon your shoulders. You hear warnings about outside influences from your parents, teachers, and perhaps clergy members. You may listen, but you want to be "one of the gang." Peer approval is very important to you. And this may become a real problem regarding the temptations that lure adolescents. The temptations we refer to are drugs, alcohol, tobacco, and sex. (See Chapter 19 for a discussion of sex and sexually transmitted diseases.)

True, everyone has his or her own beliefs about what is right and wrong. But the truth is that all these behaviors can pose threats to your health, and you can't argue with that. If you want to be at your best, you need to know the facts about habits that can affect your health. So here they are: the facts, according to the National Clearinghouse for Alcohol and Drug Information.

✔ **Tobacco:** In your teenage years, your body is at a very important stage of development. Cigarettes contain some 4,000 chemicals (200 of which are known poisons) that can throw off that process. The risks include poor sense of taste, weakened immune system, smoker's cough, stomach ulcers, bronchitis, increased heart rate, heightened blood pressure, premature wrinkles, emphysema, heart disease, stroke, and cancer of the mouth, larynx, pharynx, esophagus, lungs, pancreas, cervix, uterus, and bladder.

✔ **Alcohol:** Alcohol is a legal drug for those who are of age, but it's still a drug. Next time you're offered a beer at a party, think of these statistics: Alcohol contributes to more than 100,000 deaths annually, and it's the third leading cause of preventable deaths in the U.S. In the short term, alcohol distorts vision, impairs judgment, and causes bad breath and hangovers. In the long term, habitual alcohol drinkers suffer from vitamin deficiencies, skin problems, stomach ailments, impotence, liver damage, heart and nervous system damage, and memory loss. Heavy drinking can harm almost every organ and system in the body, and it carries with it an increased risk for cancer.

✔ **Marijuana:** In the short term, this drug can cause fatigue, impaired memory, increased heart rate, dry mouth, paranoia, and hallucinations. In the long term, it can mean enhanced cancer risk, decreased test-osterone levels and sperm counts for men, increase in testosterone levels for women, diminished fertility, and diminished sexual pleasure.

✔ **Cocaine:** Cocaine, a stimulant, is highly addictive and often results in the user sacrificing all else in life to obtain and use the drug. Its risks are serious and include sexual dysfunction; increased blood pressure, heart rate, breathing rate, and body temperature; heart attack; stroke; lung failure; hepatitis or AIDS through contaminated shared needles; brain seizures; weakened immune system; paranoid behavior; halluci-nations; anxiety; and loss of touch with reality.

Keeping your eyes open

Knowing whether a friend or relative is in trouble with drugs is sometimes hard. The National Clearinghouse for Alcohol and Drug Information suggests that if a loved one has one or more of the following signs, that person may have a drug or alcohol problem:

✔ Getting high or drunk regularly

✔ Lying about the amount of drugs or alcohol being used

✔ Avoiding you and others to get drunk or high

✔ Giving up activities such as sports, home-work, or hanging out with friends who don't drink or use drugs

✔ Having to use more alcohol or drugs to get the same effect (a tendency called *tolerance*)

✔ Constantly talking about drugs or alcohol

✔ Believing that drugs and alcohol have to be part of a good time

✔ Pressuring others to drink or use drugs

✔ Getting into trouble with the law

✔ Getting suspended

✔ Taking risks (unprotected sex, driving drunk, and so forth)

✔ Feeling depressed, run-down, or suicidal

✔ Performing poorly at school or work

Chapter 15

Feeling Your Best: Women's Health

• •

In This Chapter

▶ Understanding the ups and downs of pregnancy

▶ Handling common conditions: Endometriosis, fibroids, and PMS

▶ Breezing through menopause

▶ Dealing with breast cancer

• •

*I*n many ways, women's health concerns are the same as men's. After all, most of the systems of the human body are common to both genders. But you don't need to be told that major differences exist between the two — notably the aspect of, shall we say, indoor versus outdoor plumbing.

In this chapter, we share some of the concerns and conditions that are unique to women and common among them: pregnancy, of course, as well as endometriosis, fibroids, premenstrual syndrome, menopause, and breast and other cancers.

Having a Baby: Pregnancy and Childbirth

One day a fertilized egg implants itself in a woman's uterus, and her world is never the same. For the next 266 days or so, she has permission to eat for two, get a whole new wardrobe, ask for Chinese food in the middle of the night, and have all the mood swings she wants. Doesn't sound so bad!

Recognizing the signs and knowing for sure

Most women begin to suspect that they are pregnant when they experience the following symptoms:

- A missed menstrual period
- Nausea
- Tender breasts
- Frequent urination
- Fatigue
- Headache

A pregnancy test helps you find out for sure whether you're pregnant. Whether taken in a doctor's office or at home, these tests analyze blood or urine for the presence of human chorionic gonadotropin (HCG). It is present in the blood just 6 to 8 days after conception and shows up in the urine in 17 to 28 days. Blood tests are considered more accurate than urine tests and can detect a pregnancy even before a missed period is noticed.

Choosing a birth practitioner

When you're expecting a bundle of joy, you want to choose the right practitioner to help with the delivery. Several options are available for mothers-to-be:

- **Obstetrician-gynecologist (ob-gyn):** A licensed medical doctor with specialized training concerning the female reproductive system and the birth process.

- **Family practitioner:** A licensed medical doctor with generalized or specialized training that covers the birth process. Not every family practitioner will help you deliver, especially if you or your baby has health problems.

- **Midwife:** A certified practitioner (not a physician) with specialized training in the birth process. Depending on the laws in your state, midwives may practice independently or may be part of a birth center under the supervision of a physician. Most midwives specialize in natural births without medications or other interventions.

Before you choose a birth practitioner, think about the type of birth you'd like to have. Do you want to be awake during the birth, or are you comforted by the thought of having anesthetics on hand if needed? Would you feel safer in a hospital, surrounded by technology, or would you prefer the more intimate setting of a freestanding birth center? Do you have any medical conditions, such as diabetes, that may complicate your pregnancy?

If your practitioner has the same values and feelings about birth that you do, you're more likely to have the kind of birthing experience you want. Find out these things from any practitioner you're considering:

✔ How long have you been in practice? What are your credentials?

✔ What is the cost of maternity care? Are payment plans available?

✔ Do you accept my insurance coverage?

✔ Will the same practitioner who provides my prenatal care attend the birth?

✔ What method of childbirth preparation do you prefer?

✔ What prenatal tests and procedures do you recommend?

✔ Do you encourage or allow the partner's presence, both in prenatal visits and during labor and birth? What about during a cesarean section?

✔ Do you encourage women to try different birthing positions? What about birth methods such as Lamaze? What options are available?

✔ What is your cesarean-section rate? What circumstances require a cesarean?

✔ In what percentage of your patients do you induce labor? Are episiotomies routine in your practice? What about forceps delivery or vacuum extraction — in what percentage of the births in your practice do you use these procedures?

✔ Do you routinely use drugs — analgesic or anesthetic — in the management of pain during labor? If so, what are the most common ones?

✔ Is electronic fetal heart-rate monitoring a routine procedure in the childbirths you attend?

(See "Avoiding childbirth interventions," later in this chapter, for more information about these and other interventions.)

Making sure that all is well

After you become pregnant, a number of tests are available to help determine the health of your child. When all goes right, these tests can reassure you that your fetus is coming along just fine or alert you to problems that need to be addressed.

Not all tests done during pregnancy are risk-free, so speak with your practitioner about whether a test is necessary before you have it done. Blood tests and ultrasound are widely recognized as safe, but invasive procedures such as amniocentesis carry a small risk of miscarriage. You may not want to choose an invasive test unless the benefits outweigh the risks — for example, if a hereditary disease runs in your family. The most common tests that pregnant women undergo include the following:

✔ **Alpha-fetoprotein:** This blood test, conducted at 15 to 20 weeks, looks for the presence of alpha-fetoprotein (AFP), a chemical found in the baby's neural tube. If AFP levels are high, the neural tube may not be forming correctly.

- ✔ **Alpha-fetoprotein-3:** Given during the 16th week of gestation to all pregnant women, this blood test measures the amounts of three substances: AFP, estriol, and human chorionic gonadotropin (HCG). Abnormal levels of these substances may indicate a problem with the pregnancy, such as a fetus forming without a full brain or with an incomplete spine.

- ✔ **Amniocentesis:** This test may be performed at 15 weeks. Amniotic fluid is removed from the womb through a needle inserted through the woman's abdomen. The sample is then examined for chromosomal defects. Parents-to-be can also find out the baby's gender from this test.

- ✔ **Chorionic villus sampling (CVS):** Capable of being performed earlier than amnio (at 9 to 12 weeks), CVS involves threading a catheter into the womb and removing some of the fingerlike projections on the placenta. CVS carries a slightly higher risk of miscarriage than amniocentesis and, in rare cases, may damage the fetus's limbs. The test looks for chromosomal abnormalities and also can determine gender.

- ✔ **Ultrasound:** During this familiar test, a device called a *transducer* is passed over the abdomen. The device emits sound waves to create an accurate picture of the developing baby. Usually performed at 18 weeks, an ultrasound helps determine how old the fetus is, how well it is growing, and even (at times) its gender.

Boosting health before and during pregnancy

Because a fetus grows so quickly, all mothers-to-be should do all they can right from the start — even before conception — to ensure a healthy pregnancy and delivery.

Have a rubella vaccination

One of the best prepregnancy moves you can make is to have a rubella vaccination if you have not been exposed to the disease. Women who are vaccinated must wait three months before trying to conceive but no longer have to be concerned that their fetus will develop heart, eye, or ear problems if they are exposed to rubella while pregnant.

Eat right

A low-fat, high-fiber diet that provides plenty of vitamins and minerals is a good idea for any woman, but essential for one who is pregnant or thinking about becoming pregnant. In addition, researchers recently discovered that moms-to-be need to increase their intake of folate, which you can get from lentils, garbanzo beans, black beans, black-eyed peas, and dark green and bright-colored vegetables such as broccoli, bok choy, and spinach. Folate prevents *spina bifida,* a condition in which the baby's vertebrae fail to fuse completely.

Work out and shape up

Who wouldn't want to have an easy labor and get back to her prepregnancy weight fast? The quickest way to accomplish both goals is to exercise while pregnant. But some forms of exercise should be avoided — anything that requires bouncing, jerking, or twisting or that involves more than 15 continuous minutes of strenuous exercise. Walking and swimming are excellent for pregnant women. Ask your doctor about which regimen is right for you.

Live the good life

How a woman lives her life also affects her pregnancy. To avoid fetal alcohol syndrome, the leading cause of preventable retardation, women should not drink during pregnancy. Babies born with fetal alcohol syndrome may have small heads and other abnormal facial characteristics and may experience developmental delays from which they never recover.

Next to avoiding alcohol, the most important thing a pregnant woman can do for her baby is to give up smoking. Women who smoke are more likely to give birth to underweight babies and are ten times more likely to see their infants die from sudden infant death syndrome. As if that weren't bad enough, nicotine and carbon monoxide also reduce oxygen flow to the fetus's brain, speed up the fetal heartbeat, and increase the fetus's blood pressure.

Other sensible precautions include postponing dental X-rays whenever possible, avoiding prescription drugs that may harm the fetus (such as Accutane for acne), and letting your partner or children change the cat's litter box to prevent getting toxoplasmosis.

Anticipating common complications

Not every pregnancy goes smoothly. Despite the best care and intentions, some women experience a complication such as gestational diabetes, Rh factor incompatibility, miscarriage, or ectopic pregnancy.

- **Gestational diabetes:** During the second or third trimester, some women develop a temporary form of diabetes. The good news is that it rarely causes serious harm to the pregnancy and can be controlled through diet and medication. Women who have a family history of diabetes or are otherwise at risk should speak with their doctors about the possibility of gestational diabetes. Women diagnosed with diabetes should be considered to have high-risk pregnancies and should be monitored closely by their physicians.

✔ **Rh factor incompatibility:** Differences in the immune system substance known as *Rh factor* may cause complications for a mother and child. If the mother is Rh-negative and her fetus is Rh-positive, the mother's body may begin forming antibodies against the fetus. Although rarely a problem in a first pregnancy, the Rh difference can cause problems in subsequent pregnancies. Rh differences can be successfully treated, however. Women whose partners are Rh incompatible can be vaccinated with Rh immunoglobulin at 28 weeks of pregnancy and again several days before delivery. If Rh incompatibility is discovered later, after the mother's body has begun making antibodies against the baby, a blood transfusion may help the problem.

✔ **Miscarriage:** Two out of every ten pregnancies end in miscarriage, usually between the eighth and tenth weeks. The body may spontaneously end a pregnancy in which the fetus is abnormal, or the miscarriage may occur because of another problem. A pregnant woman should consult her physician immediately if she experiences bleeding, spotting, severe abdominal pain, cramps, or dizziness.

✔ **Ectopic pregnancy:** Ectopic pregnancy occurs when a fertilized egg implants itself outside the uterus. Only 2 percent of pregnancies occur outside the womb, but when they do occur, they carry the risk of rupturing the fallopian tube, bleeding, infection, and possible death. Symptoms of an ectopic pregnancy include cramps, spotting, bleeding, shoulder pain, dizziness, and severe abdominal pain. Ectopic pregnancy is an emergency situation that calls for immediate medical treatment. It always results in the loss of the pregnancy.

Other complications include *cervical incompetence* (in which the *cervix,* the opening of the uterus, isn't completely closed), *gestational hypertension* (high blood pressure during pregnancy), and *preeclampsia* and *eclampsia* (very serious conditions marked by high blood pressure, protein in the urine, and, rarely, convulsions and coma).

Pregnancy after age 35

In the last 30 years, the number of first-time mothers giving birth between the ages of 40 and 44 has doubled. Many of these pregnancies are just as uneventful as those experienced by younger women. If an older woman doesn't have diabetes or high blood pressure before pregnancy, she is likely to be treated no differently than any other pregnant woman and is just as likely to resume her shape when it's all over. However, women over 35 are five times as likely to have a premature baby, twice as likely to have uterine fibroid tumors (which can lead to cesarean sections), and three times as likely to have high blood pressure. More than 50 percent of women over 45 miscarry, and older mothers are more likely to carry a child with a chromosomal defect.

The big finale: Labor and delivery

To get through the labor process, some women use a natural childbirth method such as the Bradley method (which emphasizes relaxation, calmness, and reassurance for the mother), the Lamaze method (which utilizes different types of breathing), or the Dick-Read method (which uses physical awareness, breathing control, and relaxation techniques). These methods, which usually involve coaching from a partner or friend, help women control pain and ease labor. Medications to ease pain may be used in conjunction with these methods. Early in your pregnancy, talk with your practitioner about your preferences.

Avoiding childbirth interventions

Experts report that 90 percent of all births can occur naturally and without any assistance. However, in some cases, a doctor may use drugs or a procedure to help the process along. Such action is called an *intervention.* Possible interventions include

- **Electronic fetal monitoring:** In this procedure, a monitor is used to check contractions and the heart rate of the child during labor.

- **Induction or augmentation of labor:** This intervention involves the use of drugs or an *amniotomy* (a procedure in which the amniotic sac is pierced) to speed or stimulate labor.

- **Pain relief:** A number of drugs may be administered during labor to ease pain. An *epidural,* anesthesia injected into the spine to numb the lower part of the body, is a common childbirth intervention.

- **Forceps or vacuum extraction:** Metal blades, called *forceps,* or a special instrument that uses suction may be used to gently pull the child through the birth canal.

- **Episiotomy:** In this procedure, an incision is made in the tissue that extends from the vagina toward the anus to widen the birth canal. This incision gives the baby more room to move and prevents tearing of the tissue.

- **Cesarean section:** When a child cannot be delivered vaginally, a practitioner makes an incision in the abdomen and uterus and removes the child surgically.

Interventions often save the lives of both mothers and children, but make sure that you don't choose an intervention-happy practitioner if you want to avoid problems. Like all medical procedures, interventions have risks: An episiotomy may lead to infection; pain-relieving drugs may slow fetal breathing and heart rates; forceps and vacuum extractors can damage a child's head and brain. Although at times such procedures are necessary, some practitioners turn to them to speed labor and ease their workload. Find out before labor begins what your practitioner's philosophies on interventions are and how often he or she uses them.

Easing Endometriosis

Endometriosis — which most commonly affects women between the ages of 25 and 40 — occurs when tissue from the lining of the uterus (called the *endometrium*) finds its way into the pelvic cavity. Even outside the uterus, the monthly hormonal cycles that govern menstruation affect the errant tissue. However, in the pelvic cavity, no outlet exists for the tissue to break down and pass out of the body during menstruation, so the tissue remains there, often causing pain, the development of cysts, and the growth of scar tissue that may lead to infertility. Figure 15-1 shows what endometriosis looks like.

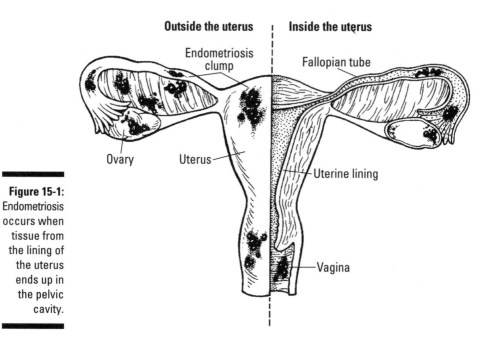

Outside the uterus   **Inside the uterus**

Endometriosis clump

Fallopian tube

Ovary   Uterus

Uterine lining

Vagina

Figure 15-1: Endometriosis occurs when tissue from the lining of the uterus ends up in the pelvic cavity.

Recognizing the signs and knowing for sure

One-third of women with endometriosis have no symptoms and are unaware that they have endometriosis. Others experience one or more of the following symptoms:

- Painful ovulation and menstruation
- Heavy, lengthy menstrual periods
- Painful intercourse
- Constipation, diarrhea, and painful bowel movements and urination
- Vomiting
- Low-grade fever
- Lower back pain

Physicians sometimes make the diagnosis by using a thin viewing scope (a *laparoscope*), which is inserted through a 1-inch incision in the abdomen during an outpatient surgical procedure called a *laparoscopy*. A *laparotomy*, which requires opening the abdomen with a longer incision, may also be used to diagnose the condition.

Magnetic resonance imaging (MRI), a noninvasive procedure that uses magnetic imaging to see the inside of the body, is increasingly being used to diagnose the condition. MRIs can detect 96 percent of cases of endometriosis without making an incision.

Making it better

Endometriosis may disappear during pregnancy or after menopause, when periods come to an end. If it is mild, it may not require treatment at all. However, treatment is recommended if endometriosis is painful or if the woman wants to have children in the future (the disease can interfere with fertility).

Some diet and exercise tips may help ease endometriosis symptoms. Regular workouts reduce the risk of developing the condition and also reduce the weight gain and depression associated with the drugs used to treat it. Also, stay away from saturated fats and hydrogenated oils, which contribute to severe menstrual cramps. You can ease some symptoms by getting enough of the vitamins C, E, and B complex and the minerals selenium, calcium, and magnesium.

Medications, commonly nonsteroidal anti-inflammatory drugs (called NSAIDs), may be prescribed to ease pain. Naproxen sodium is thought to be helpful, too.

Hormonal drug treatments work by interrupting the menstrual cycle and suppressing ovulation. The growths can also be removed through surgery, most commonly through the performance of dilation and curettage (D&C), cauterization, or laser surgery. As a last resort, a *hysterectomy* (removal of the uterus) may be performed.

For more information about endometriosis, contact the Endometriosis Association, 8585 N. 76th Pl., Milwaukee, WI 53223, 414-355-2200, 800-992-3636; or find them on the Web at www.endometriosisassn.org.

Figuring Out Fibroids

Fibroids, sometimes called *leiomyomas,* are noncancerous, solid tumors made up of irregular cells in the uterus (see Figure 15-2). Often, they produce no symptoms, and the women who have them are unaware of their existence. Whether or not you are troubled by them depends on how big they are and where they form. About 25 percent of women in their 30s and 40s suffer from fibroids. Some groups are prone to the condition: An estimated half of all African-American women in their 30s and 40s have fibroids. Asian women seem more likely to get them, too.

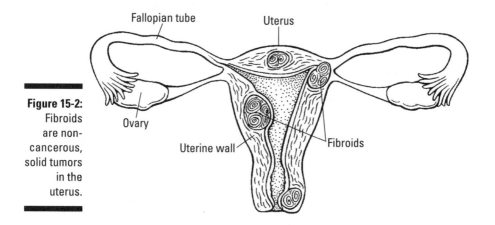

Figure 15-2: Fibroids are non-cancerous, solid tumors in the uterus.

Fallopian tube

Uterus

Ovary

Uterine wall

Fibroids

Recognizing the signs and knowing for sure

Fibroids don't always cause symptoms, but they may trigger excessive menstrual bleeding, frequent urination, constipation, or bloating.

A practitioner may be able to feel fibroids during a pelvic examination. They can also be diagnosed by using ultrasound (which uses sound waves to create an image of the uterus) or magnetic resonance imaging (which uses magnetic waves to create an image). In difficult cases, a laparoscopy may be done. In that procedure, a fiber-optic scope is inserted through a small incision in the abdomen to view the uterus.

Making it better

Fibroids usually disappear on their own after menopause. In the meantime, women can choose from a variety of treatment options.

Aspirin, ibuprofen, or another over-the-counter pain reliever may be recommended for women with occasional symptoms. If pain or pressure becomes intolerable, surgery may be an option. The procedures available include hormonal treatments (prescribed in the short-term to shrink fibroids), *myomectomy* (surgical removal of fibroids that leaves the uterus intact), *endometrial ablation* (which uses heat or electrical current to destroy the lining of the uterus), and hysterectomy (which removes the entire uterus and results in infertility).

If a hysterectomy is recommended for your fibroids, get a second opinion. More hysterectomies are performed as a result of fibroids than any other cause, but conservative practitioners argue that they're not necessary except as a last resort — for example, if pain and bleeding are severe and fibroids can't be treated in any other way.

Defining Premenstrual Syndrome

Premenstrual syndrome — or PMS — has been giving women a bad name for years. Some blame those three little letters for every bad day, and others don't think that it exists at all. Well, take heart: It's not all in your mind. Experts recognize 150 symptoms as part of PMS and now believe that it's caused by the peak progesterone levels that occur in women just before menstruation. The most likely sufferers are women over 30 and those who are approaching menopause.

Recognizing the signs and knowing for sure

A *syndrome* is a condition characterized by a collection of symptoms. The most common symptoms of PMS include bloating, breast tenderness, changes in appetite and cravings, and emotional changes such as mood swings, anxiety, and irritability.

The best way to tell whether you have PMS is to chart your symptoms for three months. If the chart shows a consistent pattern of problems that develop after you ovulate and go away a week after you finish menstruating, you probably have PMS. Be sure to get a pelvic examination from your practitioner, too, to rule out different problems (such as fibroids).

Making it better

To reduce your PMS symptoms on your own, follow these hints:

- ✔ Exercise.
- ✔ Limit the intake of alcohol and caffeine.
- ✔ Eat less salt.
- ✔ Explore complementary therapies such as herbal treatments, yoga, massage, relaxation techniques, and reflexology.

Medical treatment for PMS includes oral contraceptives (which regulate menstruation and hormones), diuretics (which remove water from the system and prevent bloating), vitamins and minerals, hormones, and tranquilizers. The tranquilizer Xanax, along with the antidepressants Prozac and Zoloft, shows promise in treating PMS symptoms.

Managing Menopause

Have you met your hypothalamus gland? Women over the age of 51, the average age when menopause begins, may become quite familiar with this little body temperature regulator because it is responsible for setting off that unpleasant harbinger of menopause: the hot flash. Your skin may turn red, your heart may pound, you may sweat and experience chills — all within a 30-second to 5-minute period. Seventy-five percent of menopausal women get hot flashes, although heavyset women are virtually immune to them.

Of course, menopause involves much more than hot flashes. It is a phase of life in which ovulation ends and the ovaries begin to produce less of the hormone estrogen. Menopause can occur in women as young as 35, and it usually lasts 2 to 3 years, although it can last as long as 12.

Recognizing the signs

Menopause can be thought of as puberty in reverse. Common signs include

- ✔ Headache
- ✔ Insomnia
- ✔ Hot flashes
- ✔ Vaginal dryness and thinning
- ✔ Reduction in or loss of sexual desire
- ✔ Night sweats

Making it better

Menopause isn't a disease and doesn't call for treatment; it's a natural phase of life. Some lucky women — about 10 to 15 percent — get through meno-pause and the decade or so leading up to it with no discomfort whatsoever. (They're probably the same people who never had a pimple in their lives.) On the other end of the spectrum, about 10 to 15 percent of women become somewhat physically or emotionally disabled by menopausal changes.

You can take some measures on your own to temper the symptoms of menopause. Hot flashes, vaginal dryness, and mood swings can be com-bated with measures such as these:

- ✔ Exercise regularly, maintain a healthy diet, and try to drink eight glasses of water daily to prevent hot flashes. Other tips include keeping rooms cool and avoiding spicy and hot foods.

- ✔ If a hot flash strikes, try taking a cool shower. Dress in layers of light, comfortable clothing that can be removed if a flash comes on.

- ✔ Try complementary medicine. Homeopathy, Chinese medicine, and biofeedback are among those therapies that are thought to ease menopausal symptoms.

- ✔ Start a tofu habit. Asian women have few problems with menopause, experts say, because they eat a diet rich in soy, which contains plant estrogens. Try drinking low-fat soy milk or mixing soy powder in your favorite juice. Eat tofu, tofu burgers, and toasted soy nuts.

✔ To fight vaginal dryness, try an over-the-counter lubricant such as Replens. Frequent intercourse also helps keep the vaginal lining flexible and promotes natural lubrication.

✔ Practice Kegel exercises, which are done by tightening and relaxing the muscles used for urination. Strengthening these muscles helps improve urinary and sexual functions as well.

Doctors can help relieve symptoms of menopause as well. Hormone replacement therapy (HRT) can be prescribed to relieve symptoms such as hot flashes and vaginal dryness. HRT also helps prevent the long-term health conditions associated with menopause: osteoporosis and heart disease.

Although most doctors recommend going with HRT, disadvantages do exist. Painful, lumpy breasts may develop. Fibroids and the lining of the uterus may thicken and grow — bad for women with endometriosis or fibroids. HRT may also exacerbate gallstones and liver conditions.

To HRT or not to HRT?

Every woman bumping up against menopause has some tough decisions to make. Will you opt for hormone replacement therapy (HRT), which can lessen your risk of heart disease and osteoporosis, seek other, natural ways to replace estrogen, or do nothing?

Whatever you choose, don't let someone else make the decision for you. Some doctors believe HRT to be the greatest thing since sliced bread and push it on all their patients, and others shun the regimen, saying that menopause is all-natural, come what may. Certainly, you need to speak with your doctor about your options, but make up your own mind based on your own circumstances.

You might consider HRT if

✔ Heart disease runs in your family.

✔ Osteoporosis runs in your family, or you have weakened bones.

✔ You faced menopause at an early age, perhaps before age 45.

You might think twice about HRT if

✔ Breast or endometrial cancer runs in your family.

✔ You have unexplained vaginal bleeding, migraines, endometriosis, fibroids, diabetes, or gallbladder disease.

Coping with Breast Cancer

A number of types of cancer target women, and we talk about cancer in a general sense in Chapter 18. However, we want to discuss breast cancer here because of its astounding emotional and physical effects on women. Although heart disease is a bigger killer of women, breast cancer is the disease that women fear most.

Recognizing the signs and knowing for sure

The earliest signs of breast cancer can be detected only with a *mammogram,* an X-ray of the breast. (Chapter 3 talks about the importance of routine mammography and some of the issues surrounding it.) Outward signs, which appear in the cancer's later stages, include

- A lump within the breast
- Thickening or distortion of the breast or nipple
- Swelling of the breast

The diagnosis of breast cancer cannot be made without a *biopsy,* the removal of breast tissue for study under a microscope. Don't panic if your doctor recommends a biopsy, though. Eighty percent of them reveal no cancer.

You may encounter two types of biopsies. In a nonsurgical *needle biopsy,* a needle is inserted into the suspicious tissue and a sample is drawn out. Needle biopsies can be done in a doctor's office, often without anesthetic. *Open biopsies* surgically remove a suspicious breast lump for analysis.

Many women are understandably upset when a biopsy is suggested, and they don't know what to expect. To get as much information as possible — and therefore empower yourself — be sure to ask these questions:

- What type of biopsy do you recommend? Why?
- Who will perform it?
- What are the possible side effects?
- When will I know the results?
- What happens if the biopsy shows cancer?
- Will my insurance cover the biopsy?
- How accurate is the biopsy? What are the chances that the results will be wrong?

Making it better

When cancer is present, treatment depends on whether the cancer is confined to the breast (in-situ) or has spread (invasive).

The two surgical options are lumpectomy and mastectomy. *Lumpectomy,* for the most part, spares the breast, taking only the cancerous lump and the surrounding tissue. A *mastectomy* is the surgical removal of the entire breast and — in the case of a radical mastectomy — lymph nodes and chest muscles, too. A ten-year study by the National Cancer Institute suggests that the combination of a lumpectomy and radiation is as effective as a mastectomy in the treatment of early-stage breast cancer.

In addition to surgery, women may also receive an *adjuvant,* or additional, therapy such as chemotherapy, radiation, hormone therapy, or immunotherapy. See Chapter 18 for the rundown on these options.

The drug tamoxifen may also be recommended. A powerful anticancer drug, tamoxifen is suitable for women with hormone-sensitive breast cancer. Some 74 percent of women using tamoxifen will not have a recurrence, compared with 54 percent who don't take the drug.

An ounce of prevention

The National Cancer Institute recently completed a federally funded study showing that tamoxifen can significantly cut a woman's chances of getting breast cancer. The study, which followed 13,000 at-risk women for five years, found that the drug cut the incidence of breast cancer across all age groups by 45 percent. But for women over 50, the drug increased the chances of developing endometrial cancer and blood clots.

Women of average risk can significantly protect themselves from breast cancer by making certain lifestyle changes:

✔ Exercise.

✔ Eat a diet rich in fish oils, soy products, green leafy vegetables, broccoli, brussels sprouts, cauliflower, and carrots.

✔ Boost your fiber intake.

For more information about breast cancer, contact the American Cancer Society, 1599 Clifton Rd., N.E., Atlanta, GA 30329-4251, 404-320-3333, 800-ACS-2345; or find them on the Web at www.cancer.org.

Other Cancers in Women

Cervical and endometrial cancers affect women exclusively. Both cancers involve the uterus. In cervical cancer, abnormal cells develop in the cervix. Endometrial cancer affects the lining of the uterus (the *endometrium*).

Cervical cancer

The number of cases of cervical cancer has dropped dramatically over the past 15 years, thanks to widespread use of the *Pap test,* a screening test that can detect the presence of abnormal cells in the cervix even before they become cancerous. When the cancer is caught in its earliest stages, it is 99 percent curable. (See Chapter 3 for more on Pap tests.)

Symptoms of cervical cancer include

- ✔ Redness, inflammation, or sores on the cervix (visible during a pelvic exam)
- ✔ Abnormal bleeding
- ✔ Heavy, lengthy menstrual periods
- ✔ Bleeding after menopause
- ✔ Increased vaginal discharge

Although a Pap test detects abnormal cells, cancer is definitively diagnosed through a *cervical biopsy,* a sampling of the cervical cells for examination.

The cancer can be removed through *cryosurgery* (freezing the lesions) or *laser surgery* (using concentrated light to cut away lesions). Electrosurgical procedures and conization (also used for biopsy) may also be used to treat the cancer. In advanced cases, a hysterectomy may be performed. After the cancer is removed, radiation therapy or chemotherapy may be employed to eradicate any remaining cells.

Endometrial cancer

Endometrial cancer attacks the lining of the uterus and most commonly affects women over 50 years of age. Symptoms of this cancer include

- ✔ Abnormal bleeding after menopause
- ✔ Irregular periods
- ✔ Bleeding between periods
- ✔ Weight loss and pain (in advanced stages)

Unlike cervical cancer, endometrial cancer cannot be detected with a Pap test because the abnormal cells are too far within the uterus. Diagnosis is done through *biopsy,* the collection of a tissue sample for microscopic examination. The sample can be collected during a pelvic exam or through *endometrial aspiration* (which uses a vacuum apparatus) or dilation and curettage (D& C).

An ultrasound, which uses sound waves to create an image of the uterus, may be used to spot cancer. A *hysteroscopy,* a procedure in which a fiber-optic viewing scope is inserted into the uterus, may also be helpful.

Endometrial cancer is usually treated by performing a hysterectomy, followed by radiation therapy or chemotherapy. Hormones that discourage cancer growth may also be recommended.

Chapter 16

What Guys Need to Know: Men's Health

· ·

In This Chapter

▶ Handling hair loss

▶ The truth about male menopause

▶ Understanding your prostate

▶ Coping with cancers

· ·

Men don't like to talk about health. Women may chat about pregnancy, PMS, and even yeast infections, but men tend to be strong, silent types — even when it comes to doctors' visits. Studies show that men make about 150 million fewer visits to the doctor than women and are less likely to seek help for problems. It often takes a health crisis such as a heart attack to send a guy to the doctor.

Breaking that silence, we present in this chapter some information about a few of the conditions that affect men: hair loss, male menopause, prostate disease, and prostate and other male cancers.

Hair Loss

For most men, hair loss is a fact of life. More than two-thirds of all men experience some degree of hair loss, or *alopecia*. Those who become bald usually have significant loss by age 35.

Hair loss can usually be attributed to male-pattern baldness, known medically as *androgenetic alopecia,* which results from an inherited sensitivity to male hormones called *androgens*. There's no stopping it. At a genetically predetermined time, hair follicles begin to convert the androgen known as *testosterone* into one called *dihydrotestosterone* (DHT), which causes the follicles to shrink. Hair produced by the shrunken follicles grows thinner until all that remains is "peach fuzz" — fine, colorless hair, technically known as *vellus hair.*

Male-pattern baldness usually progresses in this way, as shown in Figure 16-1:

✔ The hairline recedes, forming a "widow's peak."

✔ The hair on the crown thins, eventually causing a bald spot.

✔ The receding hairline and the expanding bald spot connect, leaving only a ring of hair around the sides and back of the head.

Despite the U.S. Food and Drug Administration's ban on unproven hair-loss remedies, advertisements for growing new hair are everywhere you look. Do all these things work? Nope. Couldn't there be a "secret ingredient" in any of these products that will grow hair on your head? Not likely. Just think about how long something so desirable would stay "secret."

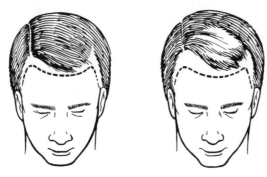

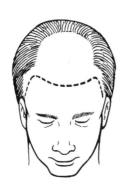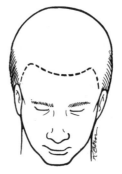

Figure 16-1:
Male-pattern baldness usually goes through these stages.

But if your resolution is firm, medical solutions do exist. First, we'll talk about medications:

- ✓ **Minoxidil (brand name Rogaine),** now available over the counter, is the first drug to be FDA-approved for the treatment of hair loss. Rubbed on the top of the head twice a day, minoxidil helps preserve follicles that may shrink, but it doesn't regrow hair that's already lost. Any hair that's preserved falls out when the use of the drug is stopped. Minor side effects include itching and dryness of the scalp.

- ✓ **Finasteride (brand name Propecia),** taken orally, works by inhibiting the enzyme that changes testosterone into dihydrotestosterone. But unwelcome side effects occur in rare cases: erection problems, loss of sex drive, and reduced sperm count. Finasteride was originally designed to treat prostate disease.

According to clinical trials, about 50 percent of those who used either minoxidil or finasteride reported an increase in hair growth. No studies comparing the two drugs have been done to date.

If medication isn't for you, surgery is another option. Surgery works best if you have mild to moderate hair loss on the front of your head. Men with thick, curly hair and blond or gray hair tend to have better results. Surgery to combat baldness is expensive, though, and is not covered by medical insurance. The four main surgical techniques are hair transplantation, scalp reduction, scalp lifts, and hair flaps:

- ✓ **Hair transplantation (also known as grafting or "plugs"):** Grafts of hair are moved from the side or back of the head to the thinning area on top or in front.

- ✓ **Scalp reduction:** In this procedure, a surgeon reduces the size of your bald spot by cutting out a piece of skin from the scalp, pulling the remaining edges together, and stitching them shut.

- ✓ **Scalp lift:** In this radical scalp reduction, a surgeon separates the scalp from the skull down to the back of the head or the neck, removes a large bald spot, and pulls the loosened scalp back over the patch. Later, hair transplants are used to create a frontal hairline.

- ✓ **Hair flap:** A hair flap is a hair-bearing strip of scalp that a surgeon transplants to the front of the head.

For more information about hair loss, contact the American Hair Loss Council, P. O. Box 809313, 401 N. Michigan Ave., 22nd Floor, Chicago, IL 60606-9319; 312-321-5128; 800-274-8717; or find them on the Web at www.ahlc.org.

Contemplating Male Menopause

In women, menopause signals the end of menstruation and is accompanied by decreased levels of the hormone estrogen that can cause fatigue, hot flashes, vaginal dryness, mood swings, and depression.

Menopause in men, usually called *andropause* or *viripause,* refers to a slow decline in levels of testosterone. Levels generally drop by only 1 percent a year. The decline may start anytime between the ages of 40 and 50. An estimated 15 percent of older men have testosterone levels low enough to be considered *hypogonadism,* a condition in which the body produces insufficient amounts of the hormone.

Recognizing the signs and knowing for sure

In most cases, the decline in testosterone is so slight that it is never noticed. However, in some men, the decrease in hormones can result in loss of libido, less-frequent erections, loss of muscle, fatigue, and bone loss contributing to osteoporosis.

Testosterone replacement is not recommended for those who have not been definitively diagnosed with hypogonadism. Testosterone levels can be checked with a blood test; however, normal testosterone levels vary widely from person to person — anywhere from 200 ng/dl to 400 ng/dl — so a blood test alone cannot be used for diagnosis. Any symptoms of sexual dysfunction should be evaluated to determine whether their cause is a low testosterone level.

Before testosterone replacement is prescribed, screening for prostate cancer — a digital rectal exam and a prostate-specific antigen test — must be done. Prostate cancer is not caused by hormones, but it can grow faster in their presence. (See "Prostate cancer," later in this chapter, for more information about these tests.)

Making it better

If a man is found to have hypogonadism, testosterone replacement therapy can be provided through injection into a muscle or via a patch that delivers a dose through the skin. Injections tend to raise hormone levels suddenly and then drop them sharply, while the patches keep testosterone levels steadier.

The therapy does have potential side effects. Because it promotes muscle growth and fluid retention, testosterone replacement may cause weight gain.

In younger men and teenagers being treated for hypogonadism, acne and *gynecomastia* (enlargement of breast tissue) may occur. *Sleep apnea,* a condition in which the airways become momentarily blocked during sleep, may develop or worsen. In rare cases, liver disorders (such as cysts in the liver) may occur. Supplemental testosterone can also interfere with fertility.

Keep in mind that hormone replacement therapy is appropriate only for a small number of men. It's not a fountain of youth or the key to staving off stiff joints, wrinkles, gray hairs, and a sluggish sex life — no matter what the media says. Nonetheless, don't hesitate to talk with your doctor about any health or sexual health problem you may be having. Too often, men keep their symptoms to themselves, ignoring problems that can be treated easily.

Getting to Know Prostate Disease

The prostate isn't a sexy organ, although it's located in the right neighborhood. The prostate is actually a gland of the male reproductive system. The secretions produced by the prostate gland make up 30 percent of the milky *semen,* the fluid that contains and nourishes sperm (the male reproductive cells).

Shaped like a walnut, the prostate weighs less than an ounce and is located in front of the rectum and at the base of the bladder (the organ that stores urine). The prostate surrounds a part of the *urethra,* the tube that carries urine from the bladder out through the penis.

Three different types of disease affect the prostate gland: *prostatitis* (inflammation of the prostate), *benign prostatic hyperplasia* (or BPH, a noncancerous enlargement of the prostate), and prostate cancer. Figure 16-2 shows both a normal and an abnormal prostate.

Figure 16-2:
The prostate gland is part of the male reproductive system and can be affected by three different types of disease.

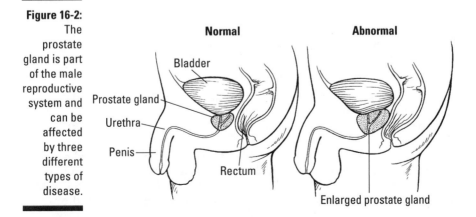

Bacterial and nonbacterial prostatitis

Prostatitis, or inflammation of the prostate, can affect you at any age, and most men visit the doctor for this condition at least once in a lifetime. The two main types of prostatitis are nonbacterial and bacterial.

Nonbacterial prostatitis, the most common form of prostatitis, describes two separate conditions: *congestive prostatitis* and *prostatodynia.*

- ✔ **Congestive prostatitis** occurs when prostatic fluid collects in the gland instead of being ejaculated out of the body. Your prostate produces prostatic fluid based on how often you ejaculate. If your ejaculation rate suddenly drops drastically, then the fluid builds up in the prostate, causing it to swell.

- ✔ **Prostatodynia** ("painful prostate") indicates a condition in which pain seems to be coming from the prostate gland, although usually the pain comes from the surrounding muscles or from inflammation in the pelvic bones. In most of these cases, the prostate is normal. Experts aren't sure what causes this condition, but evidence suggests that it is stress-related.

Bacterial prostatitis (infectious prostatitis) can be either acute or chronic. The acute form is a rare and serious disease caused by bacteria in the prostate gland. Chronic bacterial prostatitis is a recurring prostate infection that usually results when invading bacteria are not eradicated for one reason or another. Bacterial prostatitis is not contagious and cannot be sexually transmitted.

Recognizing the signs and knowing for sure

The symptoms for both nonbacterial and bacterial prostatitis are similar. They include the following:

- ✔ Discharge from the penis
- ✔ Pain or itching deep within the penis
- ✔ Discomfort during urination, or difficulty urinating
- ✔ Fever, aches, and pains
- ✔ Lower back pain (with acute bacterial prostatitis)

Many of these symptoms are also symptoms of sexually transmitted diseases (which are contagious), so make sure that you have a definitive diagnosis before you begin treatment.

Diagnosis is done through a series of tests and examinations, including a physical examination and a medical history. A laboratory analysis of your urine *(urinalysis)* may be done to check for signs of infection, which would indicate bacterial prostatitis. A *digital rectal exam* (DRE), in which the doctor inserts a gloved, lubricated finger into your rectum to feel the prostate, is also performed. An enlarged, spongy prostate may indicate nonbacterial prostatitis.

Proper diagnosis is essential in treating prostatitis because the various forms are handled differently. A diagnosis of prostatitis does not indicate any greater risk of benign prostatic hyperplasia (BPH) or prostate cancer.

Making it better

Bacterial prostatitis is treated with antibiotics. If symptoms are severe, painkillers and bed rest may be prescribed. If the urethra becomes blocked, fever leads to dehydration, or there is a risk that the bacteria may spread throughout the body, hospitalization may be necessary.

If you're taking antibiotics for bacterial prostatitis, be diligent about taking your medication as directed. Antibiotic treatment must be thorough and complete to eradicate all the bacteria.

Surgical removal of the prostate may be considered as a last resort if bacterial prostatitis is causing complications such as urinary retention (inability to urinate) or kidney problems.

Antibiotics are not effective for nonbacterial prostatitis. For congestive prostatitis, regular ejaculation (through intercourse or masturbation) is often prescribed. Prostatodynia can be treated with over-the-counter medications such as ibuprofen or aspirin. Muscle relaxants may be prescribed for prostatodynia because the condition is considered to be stress related.

Benign prostatic hyperplasia

Benign prostatic hyperplasia (BPH) is a noncancerous enlargement of the prostate gland. In BPH, the prostate slowly becomes larger, squeezing the urethra and hindering, if not obstructing, urination. BPH can lead to bladder problems, frequent urinary tract infections, and possibly urinary retention, in which you become unable to urinate.

BPH, also called enlarged prostate, affects more than 50 percent of men over the age of 50 and approximately 80 to 90 percent of men over the age of 80.

No one is sure what causes BPH, but researchers feel that its development is somehow linked to the production of testosterone, the male sex hormone. BPH does not occur in men who have had their testicles surgically removed or in men with low levels of an enzyme known as *5-alpha-reductase,* which converts the hormone testosterone into another hormone, called *dihydrotestosterone* (DHT).

Some recent studies point to a high-fat and high-cholesterol diet as a risk factor for BPH because the body converts cholesterol into male hormones. In addition, studies have shown that Asian men who eat lower-fat diets than American men have a lower rate of BPH. Obesity is also being eyed as a risk factor for prostate enlargement, although currently no conclusive evidence of a link between obesity and BPH exists.

Recognizing the signs and knowing for sure

The symptoms of BPH are often described as either irritative or obstructive:

- ✔ **Irritative symptoms,** which result from the inability to completely empty the bladder, include *urgency* (the frequent need to urinate) and numerous trips to the bathroom at night (called *nocturia*). These are generally the first symptoms of prostate problems, even though they may not be noticeable until years after the prostate has begun to grow.

- ✔ **Obstructive symptoms** relate to problems with urine flow. They include the inability to urinate (called *urinary retention*), trouble starting or stopping the flow of urine, a weak urine flow, and dribbling after urination.

Other symptoms include frequent urinary tract infections, marked by a burning feeling during urination and strong-smelling urine. Blood in the urine (or *hematuria*), which occurs when growing prostate tissue stretches and breaks blood vessels, is another symptom.

If you have any of these warning signs, consult your family physician or a *urologist,* a specialist in urinary and men's reproductive health. Although BPH isn't cancerous, kidney damage or failure may occur in advanced cases.

BPH is diagnosed through urine tests, blood tests, and imaging tests such as X-rays, *ultrasound* (a noninvasive test in which sound waves are used to create an image of the prostate), and *cystoscopy* (which allows visual examination of the urinary tract by means of a lighted viewing tube passed through the urethra and into the bladder).

Although none of these tests alone can definitively diagnose BPH, as a group the tests can confirm a diagnosis.

Making it better

Plenty of options exist for enlarged prostate. But before we get into explaining treatments for BPH, we need to mention one option that's not a treatment at all: watchful waiting. Men who choose watchful waiting are monitored carefully by their physicians, but they don't receive treatment. The idea is that the side effects and risks of medical treatment may outweigh the benefits of treatment in men with mild symptoms. Studies have shown that 30 to 50 percent of those with BPH exhibit some improvement on their own.

Medication helps control BPH but does not cure it. If you suffer from BPH and drugs are prescribed for you, you must take the drugs every day or the symptoms will return. Two major types of medication are used to treat an enlarged prostate: alpha blockers (also called *alpha-adrenergic blockers,* a type of antihypertensive) and 5-alpha-reductase inhibitors.

Alpha blockers such as terazosin (Hytrin) work by relaxing the muscles of the prostate, allowing urine to flow more freely. Alpha blockers help about 75 percent of the men who try them, according to the American Academy of Family Physicians. Potential side effects include low blood pressure and dizziness.

The 5-alpha-reductase inhibitors, such as Proscar (finasteride) and episteride, relieve symptoms by blocking the conversion of testosterone into the hormone dihydrotestosterone (DHT), which is thought to contribute to the enlargement of the prostate. Although these drugs take three to six months to produce results, they have been shown to reduce prostate size by up to 30 percent. Studies say that Proscar provides some relief for 60 percent of the men who have used it, but side effects such as erection problems and a decreased interest in sex may result.

Evidence shows that finasteride reduces *prostate-specific antigen* (PSA) levels in the bloodstream by about one-half. PSA testing is used in screening for prostate cancer; therefore, if you're taking finasteride, you should know that it may interfere with the test's ability to detect the cancer. (See "Prostate cancer," later in this chapter, for more information about the PSA.)

Surgical procedures center around removing or reducing prostate tissue in a procedure known as a *prostatectomy* (or partial prostatectomy because only part of the prostate is removed). Open and closed prostatectomies (the latter does not involve an abdominal incision) are the two varieties of this procedure.

But prostatectomy isn't your only option. In balloon urethroplasty, a balloon is inserted into the urethra and then inflated in the area where the prostrate is restricting the flow of urine. Expanding the balloon enlarges the area within the urethra, allowing a stronger flow of urine. The results are usually temporary.

Recently, several new surgical methods were developed. Microwave thermotherapy (or *hyperthermia*) uses heat to destroy some of the obstructive prostate tissue. *Intraurethral stents* (small, tubelike structures) are inserted into the urethra to enlarge it. And *transurethral needle ablation* (TUNA) employs lasers to cut away excess prostate tissue. The long-term effects of these procedures are not yet known.

The treatment option you choose depends on a variety of factors: your age, the severity of your symptoms, your overall health, and your personal preferences, just to name a few. You also want to take into account statistics such as mortality rates and complication rates. Talk with your doctor about your options and also do some research on your own before making a choice.

To complicate matters, studies show that surgery for BPH can safely be delayed for years — if not indefinitely — if the symptoms do not become intolerable. But don't decide on your own to postpone surgery; see your practitioner. If surgery is recommended, seek a second opinion, as you should with every invasive procedure.

For more information about prostate problems, contact the National Kidney and Urological Diseases Information Clearinghouse, Box NKUDIC, 3 Information Way, Bethesda, MD 20892-3580; or find them on the Web at www.niddk.nih.gov.

Prostate cancer

Prostate cancer is defined as the slow growth of abnormal cells in the prostate gland. Approximately 184,500 men are diagnosed with the disease each year in the United States, and 39,200 men die from prostate cancer annually, making it the second-leading cancer killer of men (after lung cancer) — although admittedly it's a very distant second.

Prostate cancer usually grows very slowly. In fact, in some men it may grow so slowly that no treatment is required. Because of its slow growth, prostate cancer is easy to treat and cure. (For more information about cancer in general, see Chapter 18.)

Most of what is known about prostate cancer risk factors pertains to personal characteristics — your age, your family medical history, and so on — that are likely to be only indirectly associated with what actually causes this disease. Your risk may be increased if you identify with any of the following statements:

- ✔ **I'm African-American.** The incidence of prostate cancer is nearly two times higher in African-American men than in Caucasian men. However, black men living in Africa have among the lowest rates of prostate cancer in the world. When they emigrate to the United States, their risk of developing prostate cancer increases tenfold. Similar findings are associated with Asians who emigrate to this country and abandon their traditional low-fat diet. So race may not be as critical a factor as diet.

- ✔ **I'm getting older.** Besides gender, age is the single most important risk factor for the development of prostate cancer. Around 80 percent of those diagnosed with prostate cancer are over 65.

✔ **I have a family history of prostate cancer.** Some studies have shown that the risk of prostate cancer increases two to three times in men with a positive family history of the disease. The number of affected family relatives and a younger age at diagnosis appear to be influential familial factors.

✔ **I eat a high-fat diet.** A diet high in animal fat may approximately double your risk of developing prostate cancer.

Recognizing the signs and knowing for sure

In the early stages, prostate cancer has no outward symptoms. As the disease progresses, the major symptoms include

✔ Difficulty in starting and stopping the flow of urine

✔ Frequent nighttime visits to the bathroom

✔ Weak urine flow

✔ Blood in the urine

✔ Painful ejaculation

✔ Lower back, pelvis, or thigh pain

Some of these symptoms are similar to those for enlarged prostate (benign prostatic enlargement, or BPH), which we talked about earlier in this chapter.

Often prostate cancer goes undetected for a long time because it grows so slowly. Many times it is discovered by accident during a screening for another condition. The two most common tests used to screen for prostate cancer are the digital rectal exam (DRE) and the prostate-specific antigen (PSA) test.

Digital rectal exams

The DRE, in which a doctor examines the prostate for lumps or other abnormalities by inserting a gloved, lubricated finger into the rectum, does not diagnose cancer but locates abnormalities that may be cancerous.

Although the DRE is the standard test for prostate cancer, studies show that this test may not be effective in catching cancer before it spreads. Tumors in their early stages are often too small to be felt or are located in the back of the gland, where a physician cannot feel them. Nonetheless, the American Cancer Society recommends that men over the age of 50 have a DRE as part of their yearly physical. Men with risk factors for prostate cancer may want to be tested earlier.

Prostate-specific antigen (PSA) testing

The prostate-specific antigen (PSA) test is a simple blood test that measures levels of *prostate-specific antigen,* a protein generated by the prostate gland. PSA is produced by both normal prostate cells and cancerous prostate cells, but cancerous cells produce more of it. Therefore, higher PSA levels may indicate cancer.

But an enlarged prostate, because it contains more tissue than a normal prostate, also produces more PSA. Like the DRE, the PSA can indicate that cancer may be present. Neither test definitively diagnoses prostate cancer. Only a *biopsy,* a procedure that collects tissue for examination, can confirm or rule out cancer.

Making it better

The type of treatment received depends on the severity of the cancer, as well as on other factors such as age, risk of the treatments, quality of life issues, and present health. Be sure to talk with your practitioner about all possible treatments if you are diagnosed with prostate cancer.

TIP

Sorting out the PSA controversy

Questions abound about the accuracy — and the value — of the PSA test. Although experts agree that the PSA test is more accurate than the DRE, the PSA test is very sensitive and often gives incorrect results. Many factors other than cancer are thought to affect PSA levels — so many, in fact, that the test loses much of its reliability.

Experts also question the value of the PSA test even when it's correct. Some fear that an early detection of prostate cancer leads men to choose unnecessary treatment that may do more harm than good.

As a result of the controversy, recommendations on when and how often to have the PSA vary:

✔ The American Cancer Society and the American Urological Association recommend that all men over age 50 have a PSA test each year and that men at risk for the disease have the test annually after age 40.

✔ The U.S. Preventive Services Task Force, the American Academy of Family Practitioners, and the American College of Physicians do not recommend the test but suggest that you talk with your doctor about its risks and benefits.

✔ The National Cancer Institute is waiting for more evidence and currently makes no recommendation about the test.

The choice whether to have the test is up to you. If you fall into one of the groups at high risk of prostate cancer, screening may be to your advantage. Be sure that the test is accompanied by a DRE to help avoid a diagnosis of no cancer based solely on the PSA test. And if you do have high PSA levels, remember that they do not necessarily mean cancer. Seek a second opinion before you go ahead with either an invasive diagnostic procedure or a cancer treatment.

Watchful waiting

The watchful waiting approach uses careful observation with no action to treat the cancer. Because prostate cancer tends to grow slowly and treatment often has serious side effects, the best course may be simply to monitor the disease. Although 30 to 40 percent of men over the age of 50 have prostate cancer, evidence suggests that only 4 to 8 percent have cancer that is significant or requires treatment.

Hormonal therapy

In some cases, hormonal therapy may be used either to block the activity of testosterone, the male sex hormone that feeds the cancer, or to prohibit the production of testosterone. Surgery to remove the testicles is another, more drastic technique to reduce hormone levels. Hormonal therapy is used in men with advanced cancers who can't have surgery or radiation. The possible side effects from the hormonal changes include erection problems, tender breasts, and hot flashes.

Surgery

When the cancer is confined to the prostate gland, the surgical procedure known as the *radical prostatectomy* is done to remove the prostate gland and seminal vesicles (two structures underneath the bladder that contribute to the production of semen) in order to wipe out the cancer. This surgery is considered very successful in treating cancer.

Because the prostatectomy is serious surgery, it's risky. Possible complications include infection, injury to the bladder (which may result in urinary incontinence), and erection problems. However, refinements in surgical methods have limited the chance of such problems. This surgery is usually not recommended for men over age 70 because it has not been proven to add any years to life and because of the possibility of serious side effects.

Another surgical procedure is the transurethral resection (also used for an enlarged prostate). In this procedure, the cancerous section of the prostate gland is removed through the urethra. This surgery is often performed in men who cannot have a radical prostatectomy due to age or other illnesses.

Radiation therapy and chemotherapy

Radiation therapy (using high-energy X-rays) may be used by itself to treat small cancers or cancers that have spread beyond the prostate. It may also be used to supplement radical prostatectomy, killing any cells that have been left behind. Radiation may be administered from machines outside the body *(external beam radiation)* or through *brachytherapy* (implanting radioactive pellets in the prostate gland). Side effects such as rectal problems and urinary troubles, as well as impotence, are possible with either form of radiation treatment. Chemotherapy is sometimes used for cancer that recurs after other treatment.

An ounce of prevention

Follow these guidelines to help prevent prostate cancer:

- Eat more vegetables.
- Fill up on tomatoes.
- Maintain a healthy weight.
- Eat less saturated fat.
- Get enough vitamin E.

Other Cancers in Men

Testicular and penile cancers are relatively rare. Testicular cancer involves the growth of abnormal cells within the *testes,* the male sex glands. In the United States, about 7,600 cases are diagnosed each year, and about 400 men die annually from the disease. Penile cancer affects the skin and tissues of the penis. About 1,500 cases are diagnosed annually, with 200 deaths each year. (For more information about cancer in general, see Chapter 18.)

Testicular cancer

The two main types of testicular cancer are *seminomas* and *nonseminomas.* Seminomas are slow-growing and usually don't spread beyond the testicle. Nonseminomas grow rapidly and often spread before they are discovered.

Symptoms of testicular cancer include

- A lump in a testicle, enlargement of a testicle, or pain or discomfort in a testicle
- A dull ache in the groin
- Enlargement or tenderness of the breasts

Diagnosis of testicular cancer is done through a physical examination, X-rays, and blood and urine tests. If these tests do not show an infection or another disorder, a biopsy should be done to see whether cancer is present.

The problem with a biopsy is that it involves surgically removing the entire affected testicle. If cancer is present, cutting into the testicle may cause the cancer to spread. Also, prompt removal halts growth if cancer is present. Removal of one testicle has no effect on fertility or the ability to have an erection. Only a 1 percent chance exists of cancer developing in the remaining testicle at a later time.

If cancer is present, chemotherapy and radiation may be used after the testicle has been removed to kill any remaining cancer cells that have spread to the lymph nodes and surrounding areas. If these therapies are not successful, lymph nodes can be surgically removed.

Testicular cancer is more often a disease of young men. Self-examination (discussed in Chapter 3) is recommended and could save your life.

Penile cancer

Cancer of the penis is rare in the United States, but one-fourth of all men diagnosed with the condition die from it. Despite its high mortality rate, penile cancer is quite curable in early stages because it grows slowly. However, embarrassment and fear often keep men from seeking treatment for the condition.

Symptoms of penile cancer include

✔ A red spot, wart, crusted area, or sore on the penis

✔ Discharge from the penis

✔ Pain in the penis

✔ A lump in the groin

✔ Bleeding during erection or intercourse

Keep in mind that these symptoms are similar to those of sexually transmitted diseases, so it's important to see a doctor for a diagnosis.

Diagnosis involves examination of the penis and a biopsy of tissue from the affected area. If cancer is detected, samples of fluid may be taken from nearby lymph nodes to determine whether the cancer has spread to other parts of the body.

Penile cancer is usually treated by removing the affected tissue. This may involve only a small area, or it can mean partial or total amputation of the penis. Despite this radical treatment, some men are still able to have erections and orgasms when the remaining genital tissue is stimulated.

Radiation and chemotherapy may be employed after surgical treatment to destroy any remaining cancer cells, or it may be used alone in cases where the cancer has not yet spread.

Part V
Managing Medical Conditions

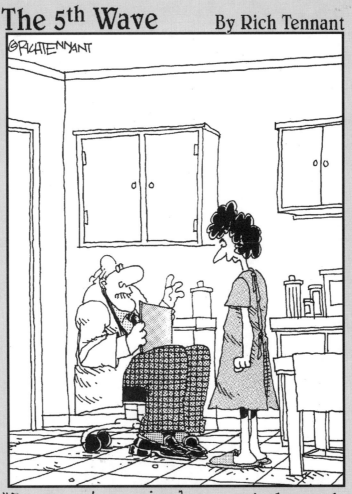

The 5th Wave   By Rich Tennant

"I was just surprised you put the word 'Marriage' next to the question asking if you suffered from a chronic condition."

In this part . . .

"I just dropped in to see what condition my condition was in. . . ." If that describes you, then you've come to the right part. This section tells you about acute and chronic conditions, and it also discusses sexual health.

Chapter 17

Passing Pains: Dealing with Acute Conditions

*I*f you or a family member has a medical condition, the more you know about that condition, the better — for several reasons:

✔ You know what you're up against.

✔ You're better able to wisely choose among your treatment options.

✔ You can take care of yourself more effectively.

In this chapter, we talk about *acute* conditions: those illnesses that come on suddenly and usually stick around only a short while. For each condition, we describe what it is, what the symptoms are, how it's diagnosed, and your treatment options (at home and at the doctor's office), plus how to prevent it, if possible.

For information about *chronic* conditions — those that linger for months or even years — see Chapter 18. There, we discuss problems such as cancer, diabetes, and arthritis. In Chapter 19, we touch on some of the conditions that may affect your sexual health.

Backache

Twenty-four vertebrae. Twenty-three cushioning spinal discs set within 23 spinal joints. Thirty-one sets of nerves, coupled with 140 muscles and hundreds of ligaments and tendons. Put it all together and you have the spine, the incredibly complex structure that enables you not only to stand erect but also to bend and twist and touch your toes.

Because the spine is so complicated, much can go wrong. A staggering 80 percent of the population experiences back pain at some point in life. And although hundreds of reasons can be behind back pain (arthritis, fractures, infection, hereditary conditions, and so on), most cases can be attributed to one of the following causes:

- ✔ **Muscular backache:** Overexertion or injury can mean painfully stretched or torn back muscles.

- ✔ **Facet joint problems:** An injury or breakdown of the bones of the spine can cause them to rub together painfully.

- ✔ **Disc problems:** Spinal discs are the fibrous, fluid-filled rings (think jelly doughnuts) that act as cushions between vertebrae. Pain can occur when a disc moves out of position or becomes damaged.

Recognizing the signs and knowing for sure

If you have back pain, you know it. However, in addition to the agony in your back, you may also experience numbness in your legs and toes or pain in the backs of your legs, called *sciatica*. Both symptoms stem from problems with the spinal nerves. For example, a misplaced disc or damaged joint may be pressing on a nerve and interfering with its function.

Pinpointing the exact cause of back pain is often difficult, if not impossible. Again, the complexity of the back is to blame: So much can go wrong that finding out exactly what's causing the problem is sometimes difficult for practitioners (and treatment is generally similar, anyway). As a result, many doctors simply treat back pain rather than diagnosing its origins.

If your back pain lasts longer than a month — in other words, it has become *chronic* (long-term) rather than *acute* (short-term) — diagnostic tests may be in order. Common tests include

- ✔ **X-ray:** A low dose of radiation is used to create an image of the spine. X-rays help doctors spot spinal abnormalities.

✔ **Bone scan:** A radioactive substance is injected into the body, and a camera takes images of the highlighted bones. Bone scans help doctors diagnose fractures, infections, abnormalities of the spine, and degeneration of the vertebrae.

✔ **CAT (computerized axial tomography) and MRI (magnetic resonance imaging) scans:** A CAT scan is essentially a three-dimensional X-ray. An MRI uses magnetic rays to create a cross-sectional image of the body. Doctors usually use these tests when surgery is being considered.

✔ **Electrophysiologic test:** A needle is inserted into a muscle to monitor its electronic activity. This test helps determine whether spinal nerves are functioning correctly. (A problem with a leg muscle, for example, may indicate a pinched spinal nerve.)

Discography (an invasive test in which dye is injected into a disc to look for abnormalities) and *thermography* (in which temperature differences are used to spot problems) are also used. However, the Agency for Health Care Policy and Research, which assesses different diagnostic techniques, does not consider these tests to be very helpful. If either of these tests is recommended for you, get a second opinion before undergoing the test.

Making it better

When it comes to backache, most care is self-care — the kind you do at home. Still, visiting your family doctor is a wise move, because diagnosing and treating yourself without professional advice is not a good idea. Most back pain resolves itself with conservative measures.

Besides your family practitioner, other doctors who deal with back pain include *orthopedists* (specialists in muscles and bones), *neurologists* (specialists in nerve problems), *physiatrists* (specialists in physical therapy), and *chiropractors* (practitioners who emphasize spinal manipulation). See Chapter 6 for information about choosing a practitioner.

Self-care is the way most cases of back pain are treated, and you can do plenty. Here are the most important considerations:

✔ **Use heat and ice.** Apply an ice pack to the affected area off and on for the first 48 hours after injury. The cold slows blood flow to the area and prevents painful swelling. After 48 hours, apply moist heat or take a hot bath or shower. The warmth brings blood flow back into the area and promotes healing.

✔ **Buy over-the-counter drugs.** Believe it or not, experts say that over-the-counter (OTC) pain relievers do just as good a job at easing your aches as prescription medications do — without harmful side effects.

✔ **Keep to your feet.** When pain strikes, the impulse to crawl into bed and stay there may be strong. However, rest may do more harm than good because it weakens muscles and makes it harder to get them back to normal. Experts say to try to stick to your normal routine. If you do need to take to bed, get up occasionally for a walk around the room.

✔ **Exercise your way back to good health.** After the worst of the pain is over, gradually begin stretching and exercising to fully restore your back. Exercise increases flexibility, strengthens muscles, and helps keep off excess pounds that can put pressure on the spine and back. Stick with walking and other low-impact exercises; stay away from exercise that can twist your back, such as golf or tennis. Take it slowly, and stop if your pain begins again.

If you have persistent back pain or back pain that recurs frequently, see a health care practitioner for a precise diagnosis and medical treatment options, which include prescription drugs and surgery.

Commonly prescribed prescription drugs include antidepressants, muscle relaxants, opioid analgesics, and steroids. However, many people do just as well with OTC drugs as with prescription potions, so you may want to think of these as last resorts.

Surgery should be a last resort as well. Because back pain is so hard to diagnose, it's also hard to treat surgically unless the doctor can find a clear indication of what's wrong. Experts recommend surgery when

✔ A specific cause has been identified and can be treated by surgery.

✔ Pain is constant and significant.

✔ Nonsurgical treatment has been unsuccessful after four to six weeks.

Even if you fit these criteria and surgery is suggested, be sure to get a second opinion! One expert estimates that 50 percent of all back surgeries are unnecessary.

The following complementary therapies may be useful in treating back pain: yoga, biofeedback, massage therapy, acupuncture, and chiropractic therapy. See Chapter 7 for more information about these therapies.

An ounce of prevention

The scary thing about back pain is that after it strikes, it's four times more likely to strike again. For that reason, it's important to prevent back pain before it happens and also to take special care to prevent recurrences. Follow these guidelines to prevent back pain:

✔ Exercise regularly.

✔ Keep your body at a healthy weight.

✔ Adjust your posture. Stand up straight with your shoulders back, align your head over your neck and your neck over your shoulders, tuck your stomach in, and tilt your pelvis slightly backward. Keep your body positioned directly over your feet.

✔ Practice ergonomics. Invest in a back-friendly chair for the office or a car cushion with good lower back support. Get a firm mattress to support your back while you sleep. And follow the cardinal rule when doing heavy labor: Lift with your legs, not with your back.

For more information about getting help with back pain, contact the Back Pain Association of America, P. O. Box 135, Pasadena, MD 21122, 410-255-3633.

Colds and Flu

Colds and influenza, better known as the flu, are caused by viruses. These conditions are spread by physical contact — perhaps from an infected person's hand or mouth to an object that is then touched by another person. The viruses usually spread where groups of people are present (for example, schools and workplaces).

Whether you get a cold or the flu depends on the virus causing the infection. Most colds come from five major virus families, whereas the flu comes from three (the A, B, and C strains). A cold affects the upper respiratory tract (nose, throat, and surrounding air passages). It has a shorter recovery period and a lesser degree of symptoms than does the flu. The flu usually attacks a person suddenly, it lasts longer (usually about a week), and its symptoms include chills and fever, which you don't find typically with a cold.

Recognizing the signs and knowing for sure

Symptoms of a cold usually include sneezing, a stuffy nose, a sore throat, coughing, chest congestion, and general fatigue or aches and pains. Primary symptoms of the flu include a high fever (about 102° F or higher), chills, headache, significant aches and pains, fatigue that can last a couple of weeks after most other symptoms have subsided, and cough and chest discomfort.

If a cold or the flu goes untreated, bronchitis, earache, sinus infection, or strep throat may result.

Making it better

No cure has been found for the common cold or the flu. Medicine may be necessary if the viruses have run their course for a few days and no progress has been made. And some newer medications, if taken early enough, can shorten the course of the flu. Otherwise, rest and relaxation are the key words here.

People who spend a fortune on over-the-counter medications may be upset to learn that many experts advise against them. These drugs relieve symptoms by suppressing the immune system, so you may benefit more by suffering through your illness for the first few days than by quashing your symptoms.

Instead, rely on nondrug ways to fight a cold or the flu. Blow your nose gently, one nostril at a time, for best effects. Inhale steam from a shower or vaporizer and use a salve or rub to help you breathe more easily. Avoid the no-nos: smoking, alcohol, and fatty foods. And the old standbys — drinking plenty of fluids, eating right (including the traditional chicken soup), staying warm, gargling with salt water, taking vitamins, and getting plenty of rest — are also helpful.

If you do decide to use an OTC drug, know what's what. *Analgesics* — namely aspirin, acetaminophen, and ibuprofen — can relieve cold and flu aches and pains (but do not give aspirin to children). *Decongestants* fight nasal congestion (but avoid using nasal sprays for more than three days). Cough medicines should be used sparingly, and take note: Because coughing helps clear away particles in the lungs, water-based warm or hot liquids will do the same job as, or even a better job than, cough medicines in thinning mucus and keeping mucus in the respiratory tract. Finally, throat lozenges are more effective than mouthwashes or gargles in fighting a sore throat.

One word of caution on taking medicine for these viruses. Antihistamines don't do much at all to relieve congestion. In fact, they dry out mucus membranes and can cause the mucus to thicken as it dries out, which can increase congestion.

Antibiotics don't work against viruses. A doctor will more than likely prescribe the aforementioned old standbys as remedies to a cold or the flu. However, if a secondary infection such as sinusitis or strep throat develops, then antibiotics may be recommended.

In the last decade or so, herbal remedies have become very popular in treating various ailments. Herbal and botanical remedies, such as echinacea, Chinese ephedra, and eucalyptus, may help provide cold and flu relief, as may more common herbal preparations such as garlic, ginger, and peppermint. Acupuncture is also thought to provide relief from the aches and pains of colds and flu.

An ounce of prevention

Fight the flu by attacking it before it ever starts — get immunized. The best time of year to be vaccinated is in the fall, and all people over the age of nine should receive a flu shot annually. Flu shots are especially important for seniors, who may have lowered resistance to disease, and for many people with chronic health problems.

Another way to keep away unwelcome cold and flu germs is through simple preventive measures:

- **Wash your hands.** Because viruses travel from person to person through physical contact, washing your hands often deters germs.

- **Let your sneezes and coughs fly.** Covering your mouth when sneezing or coughing traps mucus droplets on the hands, where they'll linger until spread by direct contact to an object or another person. Instead, turn your head — and excuse yourself.

- **Drink lots of liquids.** Drinking fluids, such as water (especially water) and juices, not only rehydrates you but also washes the poisons from your system.

- **Avoid people during flu season.** Restrict your visits to sick loved ones to reduce your chance of getting sick. Also, remember that places where large groups gather are breeding grounds for colds and viruses.

- **Eat well and exercise.** Take plenty of vitamins and minerals, and help yourself to seconds and thirds of fruits and vegetables. By keeping your body active, you serve your mind and your immune system well.

- **Keep stress to a minimum.** Get plenty of rest and sleep, leave work at the office, and let the bills figure themselves out.

For more information about preventing colds and flu, contact the American Lung Association, 1740 Broadway, 14th Floor, New York, NY 10019-4374; 800-LUNG-USA; or on the Web at www.lungusa.org.

Dental Conditions

Dental conditions usually start with the buildup of *plaque,* a mucus containing bacteria and sugar that collects on teeth along the gums. The plaque combines with saliva and forms *tartar* (also known as *calculus*), a hard, chalky substance that collects on teeth along and below the gumline.

That's only the beginning of tooth decay. Experts believe that toxins produced by bacteria within plaque irritate the gums, causing the gums to become infected, tender, and swollen. This inflammation of the gums, or *gingiva,* is called *gingivitis* (see Figure 17-1). A reversible condition, gingivitis can also result from injury to the gums, usually from vigorous toothbrushing or careless flossing. The condition is common in young adults; pregnant women and people with diabetes are also especially susceptible because of changing hormone levels.

Untreated gingivitis may damage gum tissue around the base of the teeth, leading to the formation of pockets in which plaque and calculus can collect. Bacteria within the plaque may cause inflammation to spread, eventually leading to *periodontitis* (see Figure 17-2), in which the supporting tissues of the teeth and the surrounding bone erode. The teeth then become loose and may fall out.

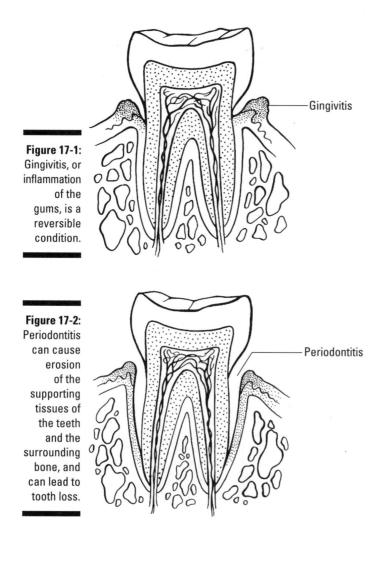

Figure 17-1: Gingivitis, or inflammation of the gums, is a reversible condition.

Gingivitis

Figure 17-2: Periodontitis can cause erosion of the supporting tissues of the teeth and the surrounding bone, and can lead to tooth loss.

Periodontitis

Recognizing the signs and knowing for sure

There's no mistaking a toothache. When you get one, you know it, and you go to the dentist immediately. However, other dental conditions that can result in tooth loss are painless. All the dental conditions we mentioned — the buildup of plaque and tartar, gingivitis, and periodontitis — share the following symptoms: sore gums that bleed easily, halitosis (bad breath), and a receding gumline. With gingivitis and periodontitis, the gums are swollen, too. With periodontitis, the teeth are sensitive and loose.

A dentist will take X-rays and thoroughly examine your teeth and gums to determine your dental health. One of the best preventive measures is regular visits to the dentist.

Making it better

Prevention of and treatment for dental conditions consist of good oral hygiene — those measures that keep the mouth and teeth clean and healthy. Good oral hygiene reduces the incidence of tooth decay, prevents gingivitis and other gum disorders, and helps prevent bad breath. Oral hygiene is broadly divided into personal and professional care.

The most important aspect of personal oral hygiene is daily removal of dental plaque by brushing thoroughly and using dental floss. Using a fluoride mouth rinse or *oral irrigator* (a device that produces a forceful stream of water) may also be helpful, but these aids cannot remove plaque or replace brushing and flossing.

Visit your dentist at least once a year (or more often if recommended) to have calculus and accumulated plaque removed. In cases of periodontal disease, cleanings may be needed more often. The dentist may also prescribe an antibacterial mouthwash for use at home. If a tooth becomes decayed, the dentist may drill out the damaged portion and install a filling to prevent further deterioration. Other procedures may be necessary for advanced decay.

For more information about dental issues, contact the American Dental Association, 211 E. Chicago Ave., Chicago, IL 60611; or on the Web at www.ada.org.

Digestive Disease

The manifestations of digestive disease are many and varied. This section provides a quick introduction to common forms of digestive problems, their symptoms, and their treatments.

- ✔ **Appendicitis:** Inflammation of the *appendix,* a short, narrow organ that dangles from the first section of the large intestine. Symptoms include pain in the abdomen, particularly the lower-right side; nausea and vomiting; lack of appetite; and the urge to pass stool or gas. A doctor can diagnose appendicitis by feeling the abdomen for tenderness and by rectal examination. Treatment involves surgery to remove the infected organ. If the organ is not removed, it may rupture and cause contamination of the abdominal cavity (called *peritonitis,* a potentially fatal condition).

- ✔ **Constipation:** The inability to move the bowels and pass stool, or the infrequent passage of stool. Causes of constipation include obstruction, medications, lack of sufficient fiber in the diet, and insufficient fluid intake. Treatment includes dietary changes and other self-care measures. Constipation also can be treated with glycerin suppositories, laxatives, and purgatives, although their use should be limited and only under a doctor's supervision. Persistent constipation is a sign that further professional medical attention is needed. Chapter 13 addresses constipation in children.

- ✔ **Diarrhea:** Frequent, loose bowel movements. The probable cause is food or water that contains an organism that upsets the delicate balance of the large intestine. When this occurs, the normal process of passing food through the intestines is disrupted, and food passes too quickly through the system. Most cases of diarrhea can be treated with over-the-counter medications; however, if symptoms do not resolve within two or three days, seek professional assistance because of the risk of dehydration.

  Diarrhea in at-risk people — for example, infants and the elderly — is quite serious, and you should seek professional medical attention at the first sign of it. See Chapter 13 for more information about diarrhea in children.

- ✔ **Diverticulosis and diverticulitis:** Conditions affecting the large intestine, characterized by the formation of small pouches called *diverticula* at weak spots on the intestine wall. The condition is known as *diverticulosis* when the diverticula are merely present, and as *diverticulitis* when the diverticula become inflamed or infected. Symptoms of diverticulosis are limited to tenderness or muscle spasms in the lower abdomen. Symptoms of diverticulitis include abdominal pain, fever, and increased white blood cell count. Diagnosis is usually made based on symptoms, but definitive diagnosis may entail a barium enema, in which a contrast material that makes the intestines visible on X-ray is given via enema. At times, a CAT scan may be done. Treatment involves bed rest, stool softeners, and a liquid diet. If infection has occurred, antibiotics are prescribed. In severe cases, a section of bowel may be removed and the remaining portion temporarily attached to a hole in the abdomen to allow for the passage of waste. At a later date, the remaining bowel is reattached. This procedure is known as a *temporary colostomy.*

✔ **Gallstones:** Hard, solid lumps that form in the *gallbladder,* the small organ that stores and secretes the bile needed for the digestive process. (See Figure 17-3.) Stones form when cholesterol and pigments in the organ crystallize and cause intermittent attacks. Symptoms include abdominal pain (often after eating), which may spread to the chest, neck, shoulders, and back, and vomiting during attacks. Indigestion, stomach pain, and constipation may be, but are not necessarily, signs of gallstones. Diagnosis is made through ultrasound and X-ray. Treatment is usually *cholecystectomy,* surgical removal of the stones or the entire gallbladder.

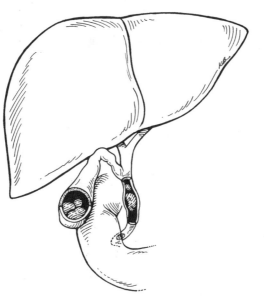

Figure 17-3:
Gallstones
are hard,
solid lumps
that form
in the
gallbladder.

✔ **Gastritis:** Inflammation of the stomach lining. It can be triggered by a number of factors, including smoking, drinking alcohol, excess stomach acid, medications, viruses, and vitamin B_{12} deficiency. In most cases, gastritis is harmless and passes quickly. Rarely, internal bleeding may occur. Symptoms include pain or discomfort in the abdomen, nausea and vomiting, and diarrhea. Diagnosis is made according to symptoms, although a *barium X-ray* (in which a contrast material is swallowed to highlight the digestive system on X-ray) or *gastroscopy* (in which a fiber-optic tube is inserted via the mouth to view the stomach) may also be done. Treatment involves over-the-counter medications such as antacids or acid-reducers (Pepcid AC or Zantac, for example). Vitamin

B_{12} injections may be prescribed if a deficiency is diagnosed. Prevention and treatment also include discontinuation of smoking, drinking alcohol, and taking offending medications.

✔ **Gastroenteritis:** Infection and inflammation of the gastrointestinal tract (also known as "stomach flu"). About half of all cases can be attributed to viruses; other causes include bacteria and parasites. Symptoms include diarrhea, abdominal cramps, nausea and vomiting, fever, and headache. Gastroenteritis usually resolves itself on its own in 36 hours. Although it is generally not dangerous for those in good health, gastro-enteritis may cause death in children, older adults, and people whose immune systems are compromised. Such people should seek treatment immediately if they experience symptoms.

✔ **Heartburn:** A burning pain in the chest that radiates upward toward the neck. It is caused by *acid reflux,* the presence of stomach acid in the esophagus. Chronic heartburn is called *gastroesophogeal reflux disease,* or GERD. Losing weight, not smoking, and avoiding chocolate, pepper-mint, fatty or spicy foods, late-night meals, and caffeine can help. Medical treatment includes antacids, acid reducers (such as Zantac and Pepcid AC), and *proton pump inhibitors* (drugs that slow the production of stomach acid, such as Prilosec).

✔ **Hemorrhoids:** Swollen blood vessels that lie in and around the anus. Symptoms include blood in the stool or toilet bowl, discomfort or pain during a bowel movement, swelling and itching around the anus, a hard lump in the skin around the anus, and mucus discharge from the anus. Diagnosis is made through an examination and sometimes *proctoscopy* (in which a viewing scope is inserted into the rectum). Treatment involves over-the-counter creams or suppositories, sitz baths, ice packs to reduce swelling, and a high-fiber diet. Surgery or laser therapy may be used to remove more serious hemorrhoids.

✔ **Hernia:** A protrusion of an organ or tissue through one of the muscular walls of the body that hold the organs in place. The intestine may push out of the abdomen into the groin (inguinal hernia) or the top of the thigh (femoral hernia), or the abdomen may push through the dia-phragm (hiatal hernia). If the blood supply to the organ or tissue is cut off, that's known as a *strangulated* hernia, which is a surgical emergency. Symptoms include swelling, tenderness, and pain or discomfort in the abdomen, especially while lifting an object.

✔ **Inflammatory bowel disease (IBD):** An umbrella term that covers Crohn's disease and colitis. IBD should not be confused with *irritable bowel syndrome,* or IBS, which is characterized by involuntary muscle movement in the large intestine.

Colitis is a chronic, progressive condition that causes inflammation, small ulcers, and abscesses in the inner lining of the colon, which may lead to obstruction or perforation of the colon. Many people with colitis have no symptoms. If they do occur, symptoms include bloody diarrhea, abdominal pain, frequent bowel movements, joint pain, fever,

Fending off food poisoning

Common types of food poisoning include gastroenteritis, in which unwashed or contaminated food or water is ingested, and the less-common *botulism,* which results from the ingestion of a toxin found in improperly canned foods. Keep these tips in mind to help prevent food poisoning:

✔ **Cook meat thoroughly.** Heat destroys bacteria that may be present in meat.

✔ **Keep food cool.** Food can be safely kept unrefrigerated for up to two hours — one hour if the outside temperature is 85° F or higher. After that, the stage is set for bacterial growth. If you're in doubt about whether something has been out of the fridge too long, throw it away.

✔ **Handle meat safely.** Wash your hands after working with meat, poultry, seafood, and eggs, and don't let their juices touch other surfaces or foods. Wet, warm surfaces promote the growth of bacteria, and hands spread bacteria around. Also, before placing cooked meat on them, wash plates, cutting boards, and any other surfaces that have touched uncooked meat.

For more information about food safety, contact the U.S. Department of Agriculture's Meat and Poultry Hotline at 800-535-4555, or the U.S. Food and Drug Administration's Seafood Hotline at 800-FDA-4010. Operators at these hotlines can answer questions and provide information about food safety.

and weight loss. It is diagnosed by inserting a long, flexible fiber-optic viewing instrument into the rectum to view the inside of the colon. A barium X-ray may be done also. Treatment involves anti-inflammatory drugs, such as sulfasalazine and corticosteroids, and possibly immuno-suppressive medication. Some 25 percent of those with colitis require surgery at some time.

Crohn's disease, or *ileitis,* affects the small intestine, often only the ileum (the final, longest, and narrowest part of the small intestine). Although some people with Crohn's disease have few symptoms, in others it causes chronic diarrhea, abdominal pain, and complications such as bowel obstruction. Other symptoms may include diarrhea, fever, weight loss, fatigue, cramps, and joint pain. It can be diagnosed through barium X-rays and colonoscopy, and perhaps even blood tests and biopsy in doubtful cases. Treatment involves a change in diet, anti-inflammatory medications, and, rarely, corticosteroids to reduce inflammation. If the intestine becomes blocked, surgery to remove the obstruction is necessary.

✔ **Irritable bowel syndrome (IBS):** An involuntary muscle movement in the large intestine; also called *spastic colon* or *irritable colon syndrome.* Symptoms include gas, abdominal pain, diarrhea or constipation (or alternating bouts of each), nausea, feeling full after eating only a small meal, the sensation of urinary urgency, incomplete emptying of the bladder when urinating, fatigue, and pain during intercourse. Diagnosis involves a complete medical history, examination, and stool sample.

Also recommended are sigmoidoscopy or colonoscopy and a barium X-ray. A change in diet, increased fiber, fiber supplements such as Metamucil, and avoidance of lactose (the natural sugar found in milk) may help IBS. Antispasmodic drugs, antacids/antigas medications, antidiarrheal medications, and antidepressant drugs are also used in treating IBS. Because stress is sometimes a factor, mental health counseling and relaxation training can help relieve IBS symptoms.

✔ **Lactose intolerance:** Cramps, bloating, diarrhea, and gas when milk or dairy products are consumed, caused by a deficiency of the enzyme lactase in the digestive system. The enzyme is needed to digest lactose, the sugar in cow's milk. Treatment includes decreasing consumption of dairy products or using an over-the-counter digestion aid. You take these aids before eating or mix them with milk to help convert lactose into simple sugar.

✔ **Polyp:** A tumor, usually noncancerous, that grows from the lining of the large intestine. Symptoms, if they occur, include blood in the stool, mucus discharge from the anus, and a change in bowel movements. They are usually diagnosed during a screening for colon cancer. Although most polyps are not cancerous when they develop, some types may become cancerous — in fact, most colon cancers develop from polyps. For this reason, regular screening via colonoscopy is recommended for those who have polyps. In some cases, surgical removal of the polyps may be recommended to prevent cancer.

✔ **Ulcer:** An open sore or lesion in the lining of the stomach, esophagus, or duodenum. Symptoms include a gnawing or burning pain in the abdomen between the breastbone and the navel, which often occurs early in the morning and between meals. Nausea, vomiting, fatigue, weight loss, and blood in the stool are less-common symptoms. Treatment includes acid-suppressing medications and antibiotics (if the *H. pylori* organisms that are thought to cause ulcers are present). Avoiding smoking and caffeine also may help.

Even if you don't know the nitty-gritty details of all the various digestive conditions, you should know that the following are warning signs that a digestive problem may be present:

✔ Long-lasting stomach pains

✔ Blood in the stools or black stools

✔ Yellowing of the skin and whites of the eyes (jaundice)

✔ Difficulty swallowing

✔ Unexplained weight loss

✔ A sudden change in bowel habits (for example, diarrhea or constipation) that lasts more than a few days

✔ Vomiting

For more information about digestive problems, contact the National Digestive Diseases Information Clearinghouse, 2 Information Way, Bethesda, MD 20892-3570; 301-654-3810; or on the Web at www.niddk.nih.gov.

Eye Conditions

Don't take your eyes for granted. Conditions that may affect your eyes — your windows on the world — range from cataracts and glaucoma to color blindness and farsightedness. Read on to find out about common eye problems.

Age-related macular degeneration (AMD)

The tiny area in the center of the retina, called the *macula,* is responsible for central vision. In AMD, the macula breaks down, resulting in the loss of distance and close vision. AMD is the leading cause of blindness in people over age 60 and often is a normal part of the aging process. Leaking blood vessels under the macula causes the "wet" type of AMD; a slow breakdown of cells causes "dry" AMD.

AMD is painless, and its most common symptom is blurred vision. Straight lines may appear wavy, and blind spots may develop. Diagnosis is made by using an *ophthalmoscope* (the instrument used in eye examinations to look at the retina and macula), an *Amsler grid* (used to detect blind spots or wavy lines in vision), or a *fluorescein angiogram* (in which dye is injected into the arm and then observed as it passes through the eye's blood vessels).

"Dry" AMD cannot be treated; however, it takes many years before vision becomes seriously impaired. "Wet" AMD, the more serious of the two conditions, can be treated with laser surgery if caught early.

To help prevent AMD, maintain a healthy blood pressure, don't smoke, and wear sunglasses that block out ultraviolet rays.

Cataracts

A clouding in the transparent lens of the eye is known as a *cataract.* The most common symptom of cataract is blurred or cloudy vision, as if you're looking through water. In addition, colors may look faded and yellow, or lights may have a glare or halo at night. Cataracts can be diagnosed through a routine eye exam.

Cataracts are treated surgically in one of several ways: The lens may be removed entirely; only the cataract may be cut away from the lens; or vibrations may be used to break apart the proteins that form the cataract in a procedure called *photoemulsification.* After the cataract is removed, a plastic lens is implanted to correct vision. Most people who have cataracts removed wear contacts or glasses after the procedure.

Drinking in moderation and staying away from smoking help prevent cataracts. Wearing sunglasses that protect the eyes from ultraviolet rays is also helpful. Minimizing steroid use is important, too.

Diabetic retinopathy

In diabetes, high levels of sugar build up in the bloodstream. The sugar's presence eventually leads to blood vessel damage. In diabetic retinopathy, the blood vessels in the eye become damaged and may swell or leak fluid, or new, abnormal blood vessels may develop on the retina's surface. This condition results in vision loss and blindness.

Signs of retinopathy include blurred vision, light flashes, changes in color vision, and problems discerning objects from their backgrounds. An eye-care professional can diagnose this condition. People with diabetes should have annual eye examinations to detect any problems early.

When caught early, retinopathy may be treated with laser surgery to seal off leaking or abnormal blood vessels. Advanced stages may be treated with *vitrectomy,* a risky procedure in which the *vitreous humor* (the fluid within the eye) and any scar tissue, blood, and membranes are removed from the eye.

Keeping sugar levels within recommended levels can help prevent damage to blood vessels and therefore prevent retinopathy. See Chapter 18 for more information about controlling that disease.

Glaucoma

Glaucoma occurs when the pressure on the fluid inside the eyes increases and puts pressure on the optic nerves (nerves that carry images from the retina to the brain). The inside of the eye is constantly bathed in fluid that flows into and drains out of the eye. Pressure may increase because fluid drains too slowly out of the eye (called *open-angle glaucoma*) or the drainage canals become blocked (called *closed-angle glaucoma*). Glaucoma usually has no symptoms, and for this reason, it's important to have regular screening for it, especially if you have a strong family history of the disease.

Symptoms of glaucoma include blurred vision, headache, eye pain, nausea and vomiting, and rainbow halos around lights at night. A device called a *tonometer* can be pressed lightly against the surface of the eye to measure the pressure within the eye and diagnose glaucoma. Other diagnostic methods include use of an ophthalmoscope and tests of peripheral vision (which is first affected by glaucoma).

Medications such as beta blockers and epinephine-related drugs may be used to treat glaucoma. Other options include *trabeculoplasty* (a laser therapy procedure that burns tiny holes in the eye to allow fluid to drain faster) and *trabeculectomy* or *sclerostomy* (surgical procedures in which a tiny opening is made in the white part of the eye to aid drainage).

Maintaining proper blood pressure, not smoking, and exercising regularly can help reduce eye pressure and help prevent glaucoma. Also, get plenty of antioxidant vitamins (see Chapter 2).

For more information about diseases of the eye, contact the American Academy of Ophthalmology, P. O. Box 7424, San Francisco, CA 94120-7424; 415-561-8500; or on the Web at www.eyenet.org/.

Refractive errors

When the shape of the eye doesn't permit light to be refracted, or bent, properly, that's known as a refractive error. About 120 million Americans suffer from refractive errors, which include the following:

✔ **Myopia (nearsightedness):** Close objects are seen clearly, but distant objects are out of focus. (See Figure 17-4.)

✔ **Hyperopia (farsightedness):** Distant objects are seen clearly, but close objects are out of focus. (See Figure 17-4.)

✔ **Presbyopia:** The eye's lens becomes less elastic with age, resulting in blurry vision.

✔ **Astigmatism:** An abnormality in the cornea prevents the eye from focusing clearly on near or distant objects.

Headaches and blurry vision signal refractive errors, which an eye professional such as an ophthalmologist or optometrist can diagnose and treat. These conditions generally are treated with eyeglasses or contact lenses, although a surgical option — *radial keratotomy* (RK) — has become available. In RK, incisions are made in the cornea to flatten it out and change the shape of the eye. RK may be helpful for people with nearsightedness or astigmatism.

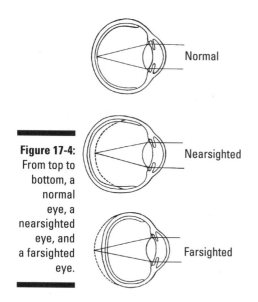

Normal

Nearsighted

Farsighted

Figure 17-4:
From top to
bottom, a
normal
eye, a
nearsighted
eye, and
a farsighted
eye.

Headaches

You may think of headaches as just aches in the head, but there are various types of headaches. Ninety percent of headaches fall into one of two categories:

- **Tension headaches** are caused by constricted (or narrowed) blood vessels. Stress, anger, squinting, and poor posture are among the things that can make you tighten up the muscles in your shoulders, neck, and head. The tightened muscles squeeze the blood vessels, slowing blood flow, irritating the nerves, and causing pain.

- **Vascular headaches** are caused by the abnormal expansion (or *dilation*) of blood vessels on the surface of the brain and the surrounding membranes. *Migraine headaches,* severe headaches that may be accompanied by sensory disturbances, are a type of vascular headache. *Cluster headaches* are a rare form of vascular headache with a pattern; they occur several times a day for 15 minutes to an hour, for several weeks. Then they stop for long periods or perhaps never recur. Vascular headaches are often brought on by triggers, such as too much sun, too much alcohol, or certain foods, such as wine, cheese, hot dogs, or soy sauce. Migraines are often associated with the menstrual cycle.

Recognizing the signs and knowing for sure

Tension headaches bring moderate pain felt equally on both sides of the head. The pain is usually steady and dull. Migraine headaches are often preceded by an *aura,* a set of sensory disturbances that may include flashing lights, distorted vision, temporary speech and hearing impairment, and loss of muscular control and balance. The pain begins after the aura passes. Cluster headaches can be diagnosed by their pattern; they are often accompanied by nasal congestion, discharge, and watering eyes.

If you have frequent or severe headaches, visit your physician. A doctor can not only provide treatment but also rule out any other causes of headaches, such as a brain tumor, a blood clot in the brain, or *meningitis* (an infection of the membranes surrounding the brain and spinal cord).

Making it better

Try these drug-free ways to relieve your headache:

- ✔ **Get up and move around.** This is especially helpful if you've been sitting in one place for a while.

- ✔ **Give yourself a massage.** Stimulating the scalp with your fingertips or a hairbrush can help restore blood flow and ease tension headaches.

- ✔ **Apply heat or ice.** A heating pad or hot shower can help relieve a tension headache; migraines are best helped by holding an ice pack to the forehead.

- ✔ **Relax.** Take a two-minute break and practice a relaxation technique, such as visualization therapy, meditation, or progressive relaxation. (See the section on stress in Chapter 2.)

- ✔ **Practice acupressure.** Gently squeeze the base of the web of skin between your thumb and index finger, an acupressure point for headaches. (See Figure 17-5.)

Tension headaches generally can be relieved with over-the-counter medications such as aspirin, acetaminophen, and ibuprofen. Migraines and cluster headaches may be helped by OTC drugs, but they usually call for prescription medications, such as ergotamine derivatives, isometheptene, corticosteroids, and sumatriptan.

A host of complementary therapies — including massage, acupuncture, and biofeedback — are helpful in relieving headaches. For more information about these and other therapies, see Chapter 7.

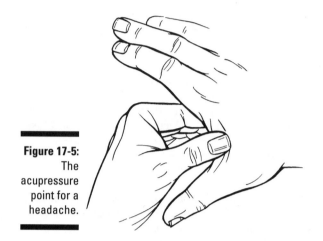

Figure 17-5:
The
acupressure
point for a
headache.

An ounce of prevention

Follow these tips to help prevent headaches:

✔ Get enough sleep.

✔ Avoid substances that you know trigger headaches.

✔ Take regular breaks when working on a computer or reading.

✔ Exercise regularly.

✔ Practice stress management.

For more information about handling headaches, contact the National Headache Foundation, 428 W. St. James Pl., 2nd Floor, Chicago, IL 60614; 800-843-2256; or on the Web at www.headaches.org.

Hearing Loss

Are you always asking people to speak up? Do you have a difficult time holding a conversation on the telephone? If so, you're not alone. More than 28 million Americans suffer from some degree of hearing loss.

A host of different conditions can trigger hearing loss, including the following:

✔ **Acoustic trauma:** Damage to the eardrum. Ten percent of all hearing loss results from sudden loud noises. Sudden blows to the head, damage caused by an object in the ear, skull fractures, and rapid changes in pressure also may result in hearing loss. Often, the eardrum heals on its own, but depending upon the extent of other damage — such as to the nerves or cilia — hearing may not return. However, severe perforations that refuse to heal may require surgery.

✔ **Barotrauma:** A malfunction of the eustachian tube caused by pressure changes. Also called *aerotitis* or "airplane ears," barotrauma results when the external pressure on the eardrum suddenly becomes greater in relation to the inner pressure. Individuals who experience barotrauma suffer from pain and conductive hearing loss when flying in an airplane plane or when diving. Generally, if not immediately, hearing is restored when these people leave these situations.

To combat this problem, try chewing gum, yawning, or sucking on a piece of hard candy. These simple techniques help keep the eustachian tube open, which regulates the pressure. If you're diving, rising slowly from a depth can prevent barotrauma. Also, don't fly too soon after a dive. Decongestants may alleviate the congestion blocking the eustachian tube.

✔ **Congenital hearing loss:** In some instances, a hearing disorder is already present when a person is born; children may be born deaf or impaired due to a genetic deficiency. But congenital hearing loss often results from injury, illness, or other complications during pregnancy. Babies who are born prematurely have a greater risk of hearing impairment at birth. Up to 4 percent of all hearing disabilities are already present at birth.

✔ **Earwax:** One of the most common conditions that affects the outer ear is earwax, or *cerumen*. The ear usually produces a small amount of wax, which gradually works its way out of the ear. However, some people produce a great deal of wax, which can build up in the outer ear, causing conductive hearing loss.

Wax usually works its way out of the ear on its own, but you can place a few drops of baby or mineral oil in the ear twice a day for several days to soften the wax. Then fill a syringe with warm water and, with your head upright, gently squirt some of the water into your ear. Tilt your ear to allow the water to drain out. Repeat this flushing several times. If the wax remains and interferes with your hearing, contact a health care practitioner, who can remove it with suction or a scraping instrument called a *curette*.

✔ **Otitis externa:** Otitis externa, commonly known as swimmer's ear, is an infection of the outer ear canal. It is caused by bacteria, allergies, or fungi and is characterized by itching, pain, swelling, and a feeling that the ear is blocked. Treatment for otitis externa involves antibiotics and eardrops. Generally, if not immediately, hearing will be restored.

If you're often in the pool, a few simple steps can help prevent swimmer's ear:

- Put a few drops of rubbing alcohol in your ears as you're drying off. Doing so dries up any remaining water in the ears.

- Use a hair dryer aimed at the ears to dry up excess water.

- Jump around. If you can feel the water in your ears, tilt your head to one side and jump up and down until the water flows out.

- Pull gently on the earlobe to straighten out the canal and allow the water to run out more easily.

✔ **Otitis media:** Otitis media, or middle ear infection, occurs for many reasons, and the pain associated with it comes from a fluid or pus buildup pressing against the eardrum. Otitis media is common in children.

Middle ear infections are often treated by prescription antibiotics such as amoxicillin, although over-the-counter painkillers, especially acetaminophen (for children, given the risk of Reye's syndrome), can be used to relieve the pain. If medication doesn't help, a *myringotomy* may be done. This procedure is performed by making an incision in the eardrum, which allows the fluid to drain. Tubes may be placed in the eardrum to allow further drainage and the equalization of pressure. (If you haven't read up on kids and ear infections, see Chapter 13.)

✔ **Noise damage:** Noise is another factor that prompts sensorineural hearing loss. Repeated exposure to sources of high-decibel noise such as loud music (often heard through stereo headphones), firearms, airplanes, and loud engines or machinery can lead to permanent damage. According to the National Institute for Occupational Safety and Health, you should wear ear protection if you're exposed to a noise level of 80 decibels or more for eight hours a day; 85 decibels or more for four hours a day; 90 decibels or more for two hours; or 95 decibels or more for one hour. An effective and inexpensive way to combat this problem is to wear earplugs or earmuffs while in the noisy environment. As points of reference, traffic registers somewhere between 70 and 90 decibels; a phone ringing, 80 decibels; a shout, 90 decibels; and a power saw, 95 decibels.

✔ **Presbycusis:** As people grow older, they slowly begin to lose their hearing. This progressive loss occurs when the sensory hair cells within the ear die and are not replaced. Natural hearing loss can begin in the 30s or 40s, and by age 65 one in four people has some degree of difficulty hearing. This type of loss is irreversible, but hearing aids, assistive listening devices, and aural rehabilitation help alleviate the problems associated with it.

Cotton swab no-nos

The old saying is true: You shouldn't put anything in your ear except your elbow. Poking around in your ear with a cotton swab — or anything else — will probably force more earwax or other obstructions deep into the ear than it removes. *Acoustic trauma,* or damage to the eardrum, is an added danger.

✔ **Tinnitus:** For many people, ringing or buzzing is a constant problem. It can be a symptom of hearing loss or an indication of an underlying medical condition. Its causes include ear obstructions, infections, allergies, certain drugs, and injuries.

A number of different methods are used to help people cope with tinnitus. In mild cases, shifting a person's attention away from the ringing may be enough to alleviate the problem. Certain factors such as stress, tension, or fatigue may also aggravate tinnitus, so biofeedback, exercise, relaxation techniques, and an ample amount of rest may also provide relief. In more severe cases, a tinnitus masking device, which produces a sound that absorbs the tinnitus, may be the answer.

✔ **Vertigo:** Vertigo is a *vestibular* disease, or one that affects the inner ear. Vertigo causes balance problems. It is more intense than dizziness because the sufferer feels that his or her surroundings are actually moving. This condition may stem from central nervous system problems, diseases, and certain drugs.

Recognizing the signs and knowing for sure

Although millions of people suffer from hearing impairments, many refuse to seek help or fail to realize that they have a problem. You may have impaired hearing if you

✔ Shout while talking

✔ Turn the radio or television up too loud for others

✔ Often think that people are mumbling when they speak to you

✔ Have a hard time understanding others in noisy environments

✔ Often ask people to repeat what they have said

✔ Experience ringing in your ears

✔ Have difficulty hearing on the telephone

If you think that you have a hearing loss, the first step is to visit your family doctor or an *ear, nose, and throat specialist* (ENT). Otolaryngologists can determine whether you have a hearing loss and what type of loss it is. If the problem is within their purview — such as the result of a rupture, infection, or other disorder — they will treat the problem. Medications are usually prescribed, although in certain circumstances, surgery may be necessary. When the cause is not obvious, a hearing test may be performed to help differentiate the type of hearing loss and determine whether a hearing aid may be helpful. An *audiologist* — a professional trained in the identification, evaluation, and nonmedical rehabilitation of hearing loss — can be helpful at this point.

Making it better

The most common hearing device is the hearing aid. More than 90 percent of those with hearing impairments can be helped by a hearing aid. The degree of benefit, of course, depends on the type and severity of the loss and the nature of the problem. In addition to wearing a hearing aid, aural rehabilitation may help a person to make the best of the hearing that's left. Aural rehabilitative techniques include speechreading (lipreading), learning to discriminate among various background noises when wearing an aid, and using body language and visual cues to improve hearing.

If hearing loss is more profound, assistive listening devices (ALD) may help. Among these devices are closed captioning, telephone amplifiers, telecommunications devices, FM and loop systems, and assistive signaling and alerting devices. Recently, *cochlear implants,* which translate sounds into electrical impulses that are sent to the auditory nerve, have been successful in helping those with extreme sensorineural hearing loss or deafness.

An ounce of prevention

There's no medical way to correct a hearing loss that stems from noise, but you can take certain steps to lessen the damage brought on by noise. For example:

- ✔ Avoid listening to music or the television at a loud volume.

- ✔ Wear earplugs when working around machines, motors, or appliances at work or home.

- ✔ Watch the types of medications you take; some drugs, such as aspirin, may cause hearing loss or ringing in the ears.

- ✔ If you think that you have a loss, get your hearing checked. The loss may become worse if you ignore it.

For more information about hearing loss and hearing problems, contact the American Speech-Language-Hearing Association, 10801 Rockville Pike, Rockville, MD 20852; 800-638-8255 (voice/TDD), 301-897-5700 (voice), 301-897-0157 (TDD); or on the Web at www.asha.org/asha.

Skin Conditions

The skin is the largest organ in the body, but most people take its many roles for granted. After all, the skin protects you from the sun's rays, bacteria, and infection. It also regulates body temperature, stores fat and water, senses the environment, excretes sweat, and aids in the body's synthesis of vitamin D. Yet despite the strength and durability of the skin, more than 1,000 conditions may affect it. Here, in alphabetical order, are some of them:

✔ **Acne:** In acne, the most common skin condition, a sebaceous gland within a hair follicle overproduces oil. Acne is most common in teenagers, so more on this condition can be found in Chapter 14.

✔ **Athlete's foot:** Athlete's foot *(tinea pedis)* is a contagious fungal infection that causes itching, burning, and redness on and between the toes. Affected skin may peel and crack, possibly inviting a secondary skin infection from bacteria. Athlete's foot is common in those who are obese or who perspire a lot, such as athletes (hence the name).

On your own: Use an over-the-counter antifungal product, such as Lotrimin, for the infection. During treatment, wash your feet of all dead skin regularly.

Doctor's orders: In severe cases, oral or injected antifungals may be prescribed.

An ounce of prevention: Keep your feet dry by wearing dry shoes and absorbent cotton socks or by dusting your feet with absorbent powder. Dry your feet thoroughly after washing. Go without shoes and socks whenever possible, but avoid going barefoot in public places, especially locker rooms, where fungus may be present.

✔ **Contact dermatitis:** Contact dermatitis is an allergic reaction that occurs when the skin comes into contact with an allergen — that is, a substance such as poison ivy, wool, chemicals, or detergents that triggers an allergic reaction. Symptoms of a reaction include a red, itchy, scaly rash at the area of contact; cracking and peeling skin; and sometimes blisters.

On your own: Bathe regularly to soothe irritated skin. Apply calamine lotion, hydrocortisone cream, or a similar over-the-counter product.

Doctor's orders: Allergy tests may be done to pinpoint irritating substances. A drug to relieve the itching may be prescribed. Prescription cortisone creams are available for tough cases.

An ounce of prevention: Avoid contact with known allergens. Use a barrier cream, a product applied to the skin to help protect it from allergens. Wash your skin thoroughly with soap and water as soon as possible if you suspect that you've come into contact with an allergen.

✔ **Jock itch:** Jock itch, also called *tinea cruris,* is a contagious fungal infection that affects the groin area and the inner thighs. It often develops on areas of skin that are particularly sweaty because the moisture makes the skin vulnerable to infection. It is most common in men.

On your own: Use an over-the-counter antifungal cream or powder designed for the treatment of jock itch. Keep affected areas clean and dry.

Doctor's orders: For tough cases of jock itch, prescription antifungal creams are available.

An ounce of prevention: Shower and change clothes as soon as possible after working out. Keep vulnerable areas clean and dry. Wear loose-fitting clothes that allow moisture to evaporate.

✔ **Keloids:** Keloids are dark, spreading scars that occur at the site of a skin trauma, such as a cut, scrape, or piercing. The tendency to form these scars is hereditary and is most common among African-Americans.

Doctor's orders: Keloids are treated with cortisone cream or injections. Early treatment increases the chances of improvement. Keloids often recur after treatment. Speak to your doctor about the possibility of keloids if you are about to undergo surgery that entails cutting into the skin. Some evidence shows that an anesthetic administered to the skin before surgery may help prevent such scars.

An ounce of prevention: Take precautions to avoid cuts and scrapes. Do not pierce your ears or any other body parts.

✔ **Psoriasis:** Psoriasis begins as a red, spotted rash that develops into an area of itchy, silvery, scaly skin. The top layer of the rash sheds constantly, while the underlying scales are firmly attached. Psoriasis can be itchy and painful, and the skin may crack or bleed. This recurring condition may be triggered by injury, stress, or infection.

On your own: Use moisturizers, especially during the dry winter months. Because coolness helps soothe itching, put the moisturizers in the refrigerator before you use them. Bathing in hot water can reduce scaling, and oils, powders, and table salt added to the bath water help soften the scales. Gently wash away the softened scales before applying any medication, because the scales can block the medicine from penetrating. Apply moisturizers after you apply medications. You should also expose the affected areas to sunlight, which helps clear psoriasis in some people. Don't allow your skin to burn, though, and remember to cover all unaffected areas with sunscreen. In addition, protect yourself from injury, infection, and stress, all of which can aggravate the condition. Avoid skin contact with harsh soap and chemicals, and never pull at loose skin. Finally, monitor your condition to notice what triggers flare-ups.

Doctor's orders: Prescription medications applied to the skin include steroids, coal tar applications, anthralin, vitamin D_3 (Dovonex), and retinoids. Other treatments include ultraviolet light B (UVB) therapy; psoralen and ultraviolet light A (PUVA) therapy; and the oral prescription drugs methotrexate, Tegison (etretinate), Soriatane (acitretin), and Accutane (isotretinoin). PUVA therapy may increase the risk of skin cancer.

An ounce of prevention: At this time, there are no known methods of preventing psoriasis.

✔ **Rosacea:** Rosacea (pronounced *rose-AY-sha*) is a chronic, progressive skin condition that affects the face. It is sometimes called "adult acne" and is characterized by bumps and pimples, skin inflammation, the development of spider veins, and red, ruddy cheeks.

On your own: Avoid factors that trigger flare-ups, including sunlight, stress, hot and cold weather, alcohol, spicy foods, exercise, hot baths, hot drinks, and irritating skin products.

Doctor's orders: Antibiotics applied to the skin or taken orally are available with a prescription. Laser surgery can be used to treat tiny blood vessels visible through the skin, as well as excess tissue on the nose. Treatment continues indefinitely.

An ounce of prevention: Because there is no known cause for rosacea, currently no method for preventing the condition exists. However, early treatment helps resolve the problem and stops it from progressing.

✔ **Skin cancer:** Skin cancer, the rapid growth of abnormal cells within the skin, is characterized by lesions with a lack of symmetry, irregular borders, varied colors, and a diameter of more than 6 millimeters. Lesions that rapidly change in size and color — no matter what the diameter — may also be cancerous.

Skin cancer is not painful but must be treated immediately to ensure that it does not spread. Have all suspicious lesions examined by a physician as soon as possible. A *biopsy* (removal of a sample of tissue for microscopic examination) may be done to determine whether a lesion is cancerous. For more information, see Chapter 18.

On your own: Perform regular monthly skin self-examinations to spot any cancerous lesions early, when they are most easily cured.

Doctor's orders: Cancers may be removed by using a variety of procedures, including surgery, laser therapy, and cauterization. Radiation therapy may be used to destroy remaining cells. Regular checkups should be performed to spot recurrences.

An ounce of prevention: Because sun exposure puts you at risk for skin cancer, always wear sunscreen, limit your exposure to the sun, and don't visit tanning booths. Eat a diet high in vegetables and fruits containing antioxidant vitamins.

✔ **Warts:** Warts are round, pale, harmless growths that affect the uppermost layers of the skin. They are caused by a virus and can be spread both from person to person and to different areas of the body. They are categorized according to the area of the body where they occur.

- *Common warts* appear on the hands, feet, knees, and face.

- *Flat warts,* which have flat tops, appear on the wrists, arms, legs, and face.

- *Plantar warts,* found on the bottoms of the feet, appear flattened by the pressure of the body.

- *Genital warts* are found on the genitals and require a physician's attention; in women, genital warts may increase the risk of cervical cancer.

Warts (with the exception of genital warts) do not require treatment unless they are causing pain. Plantar warts, for example, may make walking uncomfortable.

On your own: Use an over-the-counter wart remover that contains salicylic acid. Be careful not to apply wart removers to the healthy skin around the warts. Wash your hands before and after touching warts to prevent spreading the warts to other body parts.

Doctor's orders: A physician can remove warts with liquid nitrogen, corrosive agents, or surgery. Genital warts may be treated with the drug podophyllin. All warts may recur because the virus remains in the body indefinitely.

An ounce of prevention: To prevent the transmission of genital warts, use a condom during sexual contact.

For more information about skin disorders and their treatment, contact the American Academy of Dermatology, 930 N. Meacham Rd., P. O. Box 4014, Schaumburg, IL 60173; 847-330-0230; or on the Web at `www.derm-infonet.com`.

Sleep Disorders

Unfortunately, some 222 known sleep disorders can prevent a good night's sleep. The most common include

- ✔ **Insomnia:** The inability to fall asleep or stay asleep. This is the most common sleep disorder.

- ✔ **Snoring:** The noise that occurs during sleep when a partial obstruction of the nasal airway causes the rear, fleshy part of the roof of the mouth, called the soft palate, to vibrate.

- ✔ **Sleep apnea:** A brief absence of breathing during sleep, which can be life-threatening. Sleep apnea occurs when the airway becomes blocked and collapses, disrupting the normal breathing pattern. The disruption of sleep is often so short that the sleeper is unaware of what has happened.

Recognizing the signs and knowing for sure

Obviously, insomnia's main symptom is difficulty sleeping, and snoring's sign is the noise. Sleep apnea is marked by gasping and snorting during sleep and fatigue; this condition is usually noticed by a family member or partner.

Diagnosis of sleep problems is made through a medical examination and history. Family members or partners may also be questioned about the individual's sleep habits, because they may notice symptoms in the person during sleep. Part of the diagnosis should be determining whether a sleep problem is a sign of a more serious medical and/or psychological condition. Many medical conditions — for example, heart disease, diabetes, anemia, and chronic sinus infections — include sleep disorders as secondary effects. Prescription and over-the-counter medications also can affect sleep.

If your practitioner suspects apnea or another sleep disorder after ruling out other conditions, you may be referred to a sleep disorder center — a facility where you're monitored and observed while sleeping. By studying various physiological characteristics that occur when you sleep (known as *polysomnography*), the doctors at the center can obtain a proper diagnosis.

Making it better

A primary care practitioner is not the only physician who can treat sleep disorders. Ear, nose, and throat (ENT) specialists and internists with backgrounds in breathing disorders can treat problems related to snoring or sleep apnea, whereas a neurologist can treat sleep problems related to the central nervous system. Counseling may be an option for people whose sleep problems have a psychological basis.

You can often treat sleep disorders by making simple lifestyle changes. Try these tips to help you get a good night's sleep:

- ✔ **Stick to a regular sleep time.** Don't sleep late on your days off, and avoid napping during the day.
- ✔ **Make your sleeping conditions as comfortable as possible.**
- ✔ **Avoid substances that interfere with sleep — especially in the evening.** Avoid caffeine, nicotine, alcohol, and rich and heavy foods.
- ✔ **Exercise.** But don't do strenuous exercise right before bedtime.
- ✔ **Don't drink a lot of fluid in the evening.** A full bladder will disturb your sleep.
- ✔ **Set aside an hour or so of quiet time before you go to bed each night.**
- ✔ **Use a relaxation technique before you go to bed.**
- ✔ **Drink a glass of warm milk if it helps you sleep.** For some people, though, the amino acid tyrosine in milk acts as a stimulant.

Follow these tips to silence your snores and prevent sleep apnea:

- ✔ **Quit smoking and avoid alcohol or medication such as sleeping pills.**
- ✔ **Lose weight.**
- ✔ **Don't eat a heavy meal before bedtime.**
- ✔ **Sleep on your side or elevate your head.**
- ✔ **Get more sleep.** A study by Stanford University's Sleep Research Center showed that sleep deprivation can increase the amount of time a person spends snoring.
- ✔ **Use a humidifier.** A moist sleeping environment helps prevent mucus from building up in the throat.
- ✔ **Open wide.** Use a mouthpiece or nasal strip to open your airway wider while you sleep.

For insomnia, your doctor may prescribe sleeping pills in association with self-help measures to reestablish good sleep. Sleeping pills are intended to be used for short periods only. Over-the-counter sleeping remedies are also available. These OTC products usually contain antihistamines (drugs mainly used to relieve allergies) that have sedative side effects.

Prescription sleep medications include benzodiazepines and tricyclic antidepressants. Benzodiazepines (which include Valium and Halcion) are prescribed to treat short-term insomnia caused by emotional stress or travel, to relieve anxiety, and to promote sleep, and they are effective for short periods. Tricyclic antidepressants (including Elavil and Tofrantil), which are prescribed for insomnia related to chronic pain or nonrestorative sleep, are effective in very small doses and have mild side effects.

Medical treatments are available for snoring, too. If allergies are causing your snoring, for example, a medication such as a decongestant may be prescribed to help alleviate symptoms. Remember, though, that decongestants provide only temporary relief from congestion and snoring.

Mild sleep apnea may be helped by using the self-care techniques discussed earlier in this section. If those techniques don't help, a nonsurgical option is *continuous positive airway pressure* (CPAP), in which you wear a mask connected to a compressor while you sleep. Oral appliances, which include tongue retainers (to hold the tongue in place so that it doesn't block the airway) and jaw-advancement devices (to alter the position of the lower jaw), are sometimes used to treat mild cases of sleep apnea.

An antidepressant medication called Protriptyline may also be prescribed. This drug works by reducing or inhibiting REM sleep, the phase during which sleep apnea is most likely to occur. The drug may also help increase the tone of the throat muscles.

If these treatments are not effective, or if a physical abnormality such as enlarged tonsils or a deviated septum is causing the apnea, a number of surgical options may be recommended. These surgeries involve removing soft tissue in the throat to open the airway.

Some alternative therapies have been shown to be effective in treating insomnia, including acupuncture, chiropractic care, massage, yoga, self-hypnosis, and relaxation techniques. Herbal teas containing sleep-inducing herbs such as valerian, hops, and wildflowers may help as well. And melatonin (see the sidebar "Melatonin: Miracle cure?") has been touted as a sleep-regulating supplement that can help reset body clocks.

An ounce of prevention

The best way to prevent sleep disorders is to do everything you can to ensure that you sleep restfully. Follow the self-care tips given in the preceding section to help you get a good night's sleep.

For more information about sleep disorders and their treatment, contact the American Sleep Disorders Association, 1610 14th St. NW, Suite 300, Rochester, MN 55901-2200; 507-287-6006; or on the Web at www.asda.org.

Melatonin: Miracle cure?

Melatonin, a hormone produced in the brain's pineal gland, is released into the bloodstream at night and tells the rest of the body that it is time for sleep. Melatonin is plentiful in young people but decreases with age, which may explain why elderly people often find it hard to fall asleep. Because melatonin naturally regulates sleep-wake cycles, supplements of the hormone are being looked at as a cure for insomnia.

But because melatonin is not a drug, it is not regulated by the U.S. Food and Drug Administration. Therefore, there are concerns about effectiveness, correct dosage, and side effects, which may include nausea, headaches, nightmares, depression, and decreased fertility. It has been suggested that melatonin boosts the immune system so much that people with allergies, autoimmune diseases, and immune-system cancers should not take the hormone because it may worsen their conditions.

Researchers and doctors caution that not enough is known about melatonin and its long-term effects to consider it a cure for insomnia. The American Sleep Disorders Association regards melatonin treatments as experimental and does not recommend self-administered doses of the hormone.

Chapter 18

Caring for Chronic Conditions

● ●

In This Chapter

▶ Breaking addictions

▶ Attacking allergies

▶ Adapting to Alzheimer's disease

▶ Alleviating arthritis

▶ Coping with cancer

▶ Controlling chronic pain

▶ Defeating depression

▶ Dealing with diabetes

▶ Halting heart disease (including coronary heart disease, high blood pressure, stroke, and cholesterol and triglycerides)

▶ Handling HIV and AIDS

▶ Preventing osteoporosis

● ●

Some conditions don't just come and go — they keep hanging on. These chronic conditions, which by definition stick around for more than three months, often change the lives of those who have them. Lifestyle changes may be necessary to control the condition (as with diabetes), or long-term treatment may be in order (as with cancer). Either way, if you have a chronic condition, you need to be armed with plenty of information, especially because you must live with your condition every day, in between doctor visits. In this chapter, we provide a jumping-off point for your research, giving you the most important facts about some of the most common chronic problems — as well as where to go for more information.

Addiction

Sipping a beer can be relaxing, and taking a painkiller can relieve discomfort, but if you overindulge in alcohol or another legal or illegal drug, your body may begin to require its presence to function. What develops is an addiction:

the compulsive need for, and use of, a habit-forming substance. Although no one is certain why some people become addicted and others do not, genetics probably plays a role in who gets hooked.

Recognizing the signs and knowing for sure

Addiction is characterized by withdrawal symptoms and tolerance. *Withdrawal symptoms* occur when an addicted person stops taking the drug on which the body has become dependent. The body reacts with symptoms such as aches and pains, trembling, vomiting, sweating, insomnia, and diarrhea. *Tolerance* means that a person needs increasing amounts of a substance to experience the same effects. For example, a person who needs twice as many drinks to feel intoxicated has built up a tolerance to alcohol.

Telling whether a person is struggling with a drug or alcohol problem is often difficult, and a person using drugs or alcohol is likely to hide the warning signs and deny the problem. You may suspect a problem if a friend or family member gets high or drunk on a regular basis, lies about the amount of drugs and alcohol being used, or avoids you to get drunk or high. Other indications include getting into legal trouble, talking constantly about drugs and alcohol and pressuring others to use them, and missing work or school because of drinking or drug use. Mood swings and depression may also signal a problem.

If you're concerned about a drug or alcohol problem, contact a drug and alcohol treatment professional for advice and a definite diagnosis. Common sources of help include community drug hotlines, local emergency health clinics, community treatment services, local health departments, Alcoholics Anonymous, Narcotics Anonymous, Al-Anon/Alateen, and hospitals.

Making it better

Treatment for addiction is accomplished mainly through structured counseling services, which can be done in a group, individually, or in a family setting. You can find help through local hotlines, Alcoholics or Narcotics Anonymous, health clinics, and even your family doctor.

At times, medical care may be appropriate to break the addiction's hold. For example, a person who is addicted to alcohol may take the drug antabuse, which causes vomiting when the person drinks, or Revia, which reduces the desire for alcohol.

Acupuncture and hypnosis are thought to be useful in treating some forms of addiction. See Chapter 7 for more information.

Kicking the smoking habit

An addiction to drugs or alcohol can be enough to break apart a family or marriage. An addiction to smoking, in comparison, hardly seems serious. But the nicotine in cigarettes is highly addictive and can create a dependence that triggers withdrawal symptoms ranging from insomnia and changes in heart rate to chills and fever, anxiety, nausea, and cravings for tobacco (which can last a lifetime for some people). And smoking kills by contributing to a wide range of health problems, including emphysema, heart disease, and lung and other cancers — tearing a family apart just the same.

Quitting smoking is difficult, but many people are able to kick the smoking habit by themselves. The American Cancer Society (800-227-2345) and the American Lung Association (800-LUNG-USA) are excellent sources of support and information for those looking to quit on their own. Smoking treatment programs in your area are listed in the Yellow Pages.

In addition, a number of products — for example, nicotine patches, nicotine gum, and drugs such as Zyban, an antidepressant that has recently been approved for use in smoking cessation — are now available to help break the smoking habit. These products provide a low dose of nicotine that can be used to wean the body away from the drug. Your family practitioner may be a helpful resource for these products.

For more information about managing addiction, contact the National Clearinghouse for Alcohol and Drug Information, Drug Abuse Information and Treatment Referral Line, P. O. Box 2345, Rockville, MD 20847-2345; 800-662-4357 or 301-468-6433; or visit them on the Web at www.health.org.

Allergies

The arrival of spring usually means warmer months, upcoming summer vacations, blooming flowers, baseball, and other life-renewing experiences. For millions of Americans, however, these experiences often are interrupted by sneezing, itchy and/or watery eyes, and other annoying symptoms of allergies. And allergies are by no means exclusive to the spring. In fact, they're easy to come by year-round through a variety of means. Fortunately, most allergies are treatable.

Allergies occur when a person's immune system reacts abnormally to a usually harmless substance (which can be inhaled, ingested, or absorbed through the skin) and attacks it. Such substances, called *allergens,* include various foods, pollen, mold, dust, animal dander, and insect bites.

Recognizing the signs and knowing for sure

Ironically, the first time you come in contact with a substance that will lead to an allergic reaction, no reaction occurs. Instead, your immune system produces antibodies to counter the substance at the next and future contact. When that second encounter occurs (or after a number of subsequent encounters occur), the antibodies release chemicals such as histamines, which inflame body tissues and create the symptoms of an allergic reaction.

Allergies attack in a variety of ways. Most commonly, you develop *allergic rhinitis,* better known as hay fever, which includes sneezing and itchy or watery eyes, as well as a runny nose and nasal congestion. *Allergic dermatitis,* which results when the skin reacts to contact with a certain substance (for example, poison ivy or soap) and produces a rash or some form of irritation, is another common manifestation of an allergy. You can also develop hives, swelling, allergy-related asthma, eczema (an allergic skin disease developed mostly by children), stomach cramps, and diarrhea. There's also a remote chance of *anaphylactic shock,* a severe and possibly fatal reaction to an allergen.

Although finding the cause of an allergic reaction is important, it's not always easy. You may not know what you are allergic to because of previous contact with an allergen without reaction or because of a delayed reaction. You might mistake symptoms of a medical condition for allergies, and vice versa. For example, something as simple as a cold can produce nasal symptoms that resemble an allergy.

The best person to consult when dealing with allergies is an *allergist* — a practitioner who specializes in allergies. An allergist goes over a patient's medical history to learn of previous allergic reactions. Two of the tests most likely to be used are blood tests to look for antibodies and, perhaps more important, skin tests that specifically determine allergens. Skin tests involve taking an allergen and placing a small trace directly on the skin to test for a reaction. Other tests include food elimination and challenge tests, in which specific foods are eliminated from the diet or introduced to the diet to help determine allergic reactions to food.

Making it better

Reducing or eliminating allergies can, in some instances, be as simple as avoiding exposure to allergens. For example, if you're allergic to dogs, you shouldn't get one as a pet. If you're allergic to strawberries, don't eat them.

To lessen allergy symptoms, stay away from irritants that can aggravate your reaction. These include cigarette smoke, perfume, chemicals, and other inhaled irritants. Also, eat a healthy diet, get enough sleep, and exercise regularly; these activities strengthen the body and help ward off triggers such as stress and infection.

Over-the-counter medications such as antihistamines and decongestants are also available to lessen symptoms. *Antihistamines* attack histamine, the chemical that causes swelling and itchiness. These drugs are most effective when you take them before any allergy symptoms appear. *Decongestants* reduce swelling in nasal passages and allow you to breathe more easily.

Antihistamines and decongestants are also available in prescription strength. In addition, another class of drugs, called *corticosteroids* (or simply steroids), are available with a prescription. These drugs treat both respiratory and skin allergies.

If these medicines don't work, consider *immunotherapy* (allergy shots). Immunotherapy involves regular injection of an allergen so that you eventually become desensitized to (thus unaffected by) that allergen. Treatment may last for several years.

An ounce of prevention

Keeping away from allergens is hard to do. Still, avoiding exposure is a good way to prevent allergies. Keep the entire house and its contents clean and dust-free. Use a dehumidifier in the house to cut down on molds and fungus, especially during the summer. Also, wash your hands after being outside, and avoid touching your eyes or nose in case pollen remains on your hands.

Infants have a good chance of developing fewer allergy symptoms if they are breast-fed in the first six months and the mother avoids allergenic foods. That's because breast milk is nonallergenic and provides antibodies that protect the child from infections and future food allergies.

For more information about dealing with allergy problems, contact the National Institute of Allergy and Infectious Diseases, 9000 Rockville Pike, Bethesda, MD 20892; 301-496-5717; or visit them on the Web at www.niaid.nih.gov.

Alzheimer's Disease

Alzheimer's disease is one of the hardest diseases to cope with because it is incurable and irreversible. Although both the victim and the victim's family are taught ways of handling and adapting to the disease, its effects on the victim's mind — memory loss, anxiety, depression, and eventually death — take their toll on everyone involved.

Much has been learned about Alzheimer's over the last 20 years. One of the leading causes of death among the elderly, the disease is a gradual, progressive degeneration of the brain cells that impairs memory, thought, and behavior. Alzheimer's is one of the major causes of dementia, an intellect-depleting syndrome that attacks a person's mental capacity and interferes with the ability to perform daily routines.

Recognizing the signs and knowing for sure

Short-term memory loss is one the first indicators of Alzheimer's. It goes beyond senility, or the degree of forgetfulness that comes with old age, in that the mental capacities diminish to the point that daily activities are affected.

The symptoms for Alzheimer's come in three categories:

- **Cognitive:** Impairment of memory, concentration, judgment, and the ability to calculate and communicate
- **Emotional:** Depression, irritability, fear, emotional outbursts, and apathy
- **Behavioral:** Disinterest, restlessness, impulsiveness, and compulsiveness

Due to a person's disorientation and decline in motor, speech, and behavioral skills, the person becomes more reliant on others for daily functioning. As the disease progresses, a person becomes unable to carry out daily activities as simple as eating or using the bathroom. In the end, death results.

Diagnosing Alzheimer's is more of a process of elimination to weed out possibilities. It begins with a physical exam and a check of the patient's medical history. After doing these tests, the doctor performs neurological tests that measure bodily functions and abilities; the tests may also check a patient's mental status. These tests usually involve a series of questions and exercises that lasts a few minutes. A *neurologist* (a specialist in conditions of the nerves and the brain) may be consulted for a diagnosis.

Next, blood and urine samples are taken and analyzed. Other lab tests involve a chest X-ray or an electrocardiogram (EKG) to check for heart damage. A lumbar puncture (spinal tap) may be performed if the doctor suspects certain causes of dementia, such as meningitis or multiple sclerosis.

Another technique that may be used in testing is an electroencephalogram (EEG), which measures the brain's central activity. Imaging techniques such as computerized axial tomography (CAT scan) and magnetic resonance imaging (MRI), which create distinct images of the brain, and positron emission tomography (PET) and single photon emission computed tomography (SPECT), which show whether the body's systems are working properly, may also be ordered by the physician.

Making it better

Alzheimer's is incurable and irreversible; the only treatments for the affliction are drugs that alleviate symptoms and try to make life comfortable for patients.

Depending on the stage of the disease, people with Alzheimer's may need help bathing, using the bathroom, eating, and running a household. Physical and medical needs may need to be addressed as well. Some people with the condition may not be able to live without assistance. As a result, caregivers become an integral and necessary part of the process.

Care can be provided in the home or in a nursing home if the situation becomes long-term or severe. Home health agencies and adult day-care facilities are also possibilities. Consult a doctor before making a decision on the type of care. Discuss the needs of the person among the family who may provide care, as well as what the family is able to provide not only medically and emotionally but also financially.

The only U.S. Food and Drug Administration–approved drugs specifically for Alzheimer's are Cognex (tacrine) and Aricept. Both drugs slow the progression of dementia and improve cognitive abilities by helping to relay messages through the nervous system, but both have significant side effects, such as nausea, vomiting, and even liver damage in the case of tacrine. Other drugs are currently being developed to aid the fight, but none has yet been determined to prevent or cure the disease.

For more information about dealing with Alzheimer's, contact the Alzheimer's Association, 919 N. Michigan Ave., Suite 1000, Chicago, IL 60611-1676; 800-272-3900; or visit them on the Web at www.alz.org.

Arthritis

Joints, very simply, occur wherever two bones come together. Within the joint, a tough cushioning substance called *cartilage* and a fluid-filled sack led the *joint capsule* keep the ends of the bones from rubbing together. The joint capsule's *synovial membrane* secretes a fluid that functions like the oil in your car; it provides the lubrication that enables your joints to move smoothly.

Arthritis is defined as inflammation of a joint. Although more than 100 types of arthritis exist, the most common types are

 ✔ **Osteoarthritis:** This form is caused by the breakdown of cartilage over time. Any joint in the body can be affected, although hips, knees, fingers, and the spine are frequently affected. The joints may change shape, develop cysts with fluid, and grow bone spurs. Obese people and people who have a family history of arthritis are more likely to suffer from osteoarthritis than the rest of the population.

✔ **Rheumatoid arthritis (RA):** More painful than osteoarthritis, rheumatoid arthritis affects more than just joints. It occurs when the synovial membrane becomes inflamed, causing pain when the joint moves. RA can also cause tiredness, weight loss, and fever. This form of arthritis may affect young people.

✔ **Gout:** Gout occurs when uric acid, found in certain foods and in wine, builds up in the body and forms painful crystals within a joint — usually the big toe. Obesity, diet, and diuretic drugs can increase your chances of developing gout.

Figure 18-1 shows a normal and an arthritic joint.

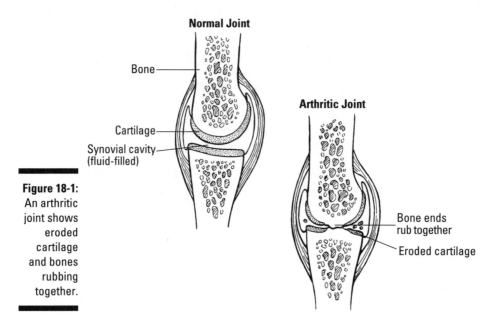

Normal Joint

Bone

Cartilage

Synovial cavity (fluid-filled)

Arthritic Joint

Bone ends rub together

Eroded cartilage

Figure 18-1: An arthritic joint shows eroded cartilage and bones rubbing together.

Recognizing the signs and knowing for sure

Swollen joints, joint pain that lasts for days and recurs frequently, and difficulty performing everyday tasks are signs that it's time to see your doctor. If you suspect that you have arthritis, schedule an appointment now; early treatment may prevent permanent joint damage.

Because there are so many types of arthritis, an exact diagnosis may be hard to make. Still, many tests are available to determine the source of pain. Blood tests, X-rays, and the examination of your joint fluid are some of the possibilities.

If your doctor suspects rheumatoid arthritis, he or she may do a full blood count and a blood test for the "rheumatoid factor," a protein found in the blood of many people with rheumatoid arthritis. This factor indicates the presence of inflammation in the body. To test for gout, a sample of synovial fluid drawn from an affected joint is examined under a microscope to look for the presence of uric acid crystals. Diagnosing osteoarthritis is simpler: Your doctor will examine the affected joint, take your medical history, and possibly order an X-ray to look for joint damage.

Other diagnostic methods include *arthroscopy* (examination of the inside of the joint by insertion of a thin viewing tube), *radioisotopic scanning* (a specialized form of imaging), *electromyography* (examination of the impulses emitted by muscles and nerves), and *biopsy* (removal of a tissue sample for microscopic examination).

Making it better

Arthritis has no cure, but you can lessen the pain of its symptoms and slow its progress. You may feel better if you follow these suggestions:

- ✔ **Exercise.** Exercise is a great way to loosen up your joints, send pain packing, and build muscle. Your best bets are walking, stretching, swimming, riding a stationary bike, and exercising in water — activities that don't strain the joints.

- ✔ **Try a change in diet.** Some experts say that milk, cheese, eggplant, chili peppers, tomatoes, and potatoes may make your symptoms worse. Fried foods also can cause inflammation. But do add more mackerel, sardines, and salmon — fish high in omega-3 fatty acids — to your diet.

- ✔ **Take vitamins and minerals.** Vitamins A, B₆, and C and the minerals selenium, pantothenic acid, and copper are thought to be helpful.

- ✔ **Get hot and cold.** Heat therapy increases the flow of blood to your joints, and cold therapy can relieve pain. If possible, spend time in a whirlpool to loosen your joints and relieve pressure. Heating pads accomplish the same results.

- ✔ **Have a massage done by a therapist.**

- ✔ **Baby yourself.** Avoid doing too much, get enough sleep, and buy tools designed especially for people with arthritis.

- ✔ **Turn to over-the-counter drugs for relief.** Aspirin, acetaminophen, and nonsteroidal anti-inflammatory drugs (such as ibuprofen) can ease pain.

Medication is the main form of treatment for arthritis. Nonsteroidal anti-inflammatory drugs (called NSAIDs) — such as aspirin, acetaminophen, and ibuprofen — help relieve joint pain. In addition, steroid drugs such as cortisone and prednisone may be prescribed for rheumatoid arthritis, although they're not helpful for osteoarthritis. Finally, remittive agents (gold salts, penicillamine, and methotrexate) may help alter the disease's course.

Among the surgical options are *osteotomy,* a procedure to correct bone deformity; *arthroscopic debridement,* the removal of floating bits of cartilage that cause pain; and *arthroplasty,* a joint replacement operation.

Your doctor may recommend that you see a *rheumatologist,* who specializes in rheumatoid arthritis, or a physical therapist to restore better motion in your joints.

Acupuncture provides pain relief for some arthritis sufferers. Other nonconventional approaches include Swedish massage and use of arnica, meadowsweet, cayenne pepper, devil's claw, feverfew, and other herbs.

An ounce of prevention

Your best defense against developing arthritis is a healthy lifestyle that combines exercise with good nutrition. Exercise keeps joints flexible, but be careful to choose a form that's easy on your body. (Running, for example, is not.) Protect your knees with kneepads while inline skating, and always wear a seat belt when riding in a car. Staying on the lean side makes life easier on your joints, too.

For more information about managing arthritis, contact the Arthritis Foundation, 30 W. Peachtree St., Atlanta, GA 30309; 800-283-7800 or 404-872-7100; or visit them on the Web at www.arthritis.org.

Cancer

We can't give you all the details about the many different types of specific cancers and their treatments in a few short pages. But we *can* give you information about cancer in general: what it is, what triggers it, how it's diagnosed, and how it's treated, plus where to find more information if necessary.

We'll start with a basic definition. Cancer occurs when cells divide and multiply without order. To stay healthy, the body makes new cells to replace old ones. But when cells begin to reproduce without control or order, normal cells may malfunction or be crowded out and starved by the new cells. As a result, the body no longer functions as it should.

The rapidly multiplying cells may form a mass of tissue, called a growth or tumor. Three different types of tumors exist:

- ✔ **Benign (noncancerous) tumors** don't spread to other parts of the body and are rarely life-threatening.

- ✔ **Malignant (cancerous) tumors** are made up of cells that can invade other organs and affect their proper function. They can spread by invading neighboring tissues or by entering the bloodstream through the lymph nodes (glands that are part of the immune system) and traveling to various parts of the body. The spread of cancer is called *metastasis*.

- ✔ **Precancerous lesions** are limited areas of the body that show abnormal, but not necessarily cancerous, changes. For example, a lesion may consist of rapidly growing normal cells. Lesions can result from an injury or disease. If left untreated, they have the potential of becoming malignant.

Recognizing the signs and knowing for sure

The American Cancer Society lists seven basic warning signs of cancer:

- ✔ A change in bowel or bladder habits
- ✔ A sore that does not heal
- ✔ Unusual bleeding or discharge
- ✔ Thickening or a lump in any part of the body
- ✔ Indigestion or difficulty swallowing
- ✔ An obvious change in a wart or mole
- ✔ Nagging cough or hoarseness

If you or a member of your family has any of these symptoms, talk with a practitioner as soon as possible. Early detection and treatment greatly increase the chances of being cured, so listen to the body's warning signals. Don't wait until you have pain. Pain is not an early indication of cancer; on the contrary, it's usually a late symptom. Remember that these symptoms can also be related to other conditions that are not cancerous. A trip to the doctor can put your worries to rest.

Imaging techniques are often used for diagnosis. These methods produce pictures of the inside of the body to determine whether a tumor is present. Imaging techniques include

- ✓ **X-rays:** X-rays involve the use of radiation to create an image of the body.

- ✓ **Radionuclide scanning:** The patient swallows a radioactive substance, and a scanner measures the radioactivity in certain organs and provides a picture of any abnormal areas on paper or film.

- ✓ **Ultrasound:** Sound waves are used to create an image of internal structures.

- ✓ **Magnetic resonance imaging (MRI):** Magnets and computers are used to create a picture that can show the size, shape, and location of a tumor and whether the cancer has spread to other parts of the body.

- ✓ **Computerized tomography (CAT scan):** A beam that rotates around the body is used to create a three-dimensional X-ray. CAT scans can show the relationship of a tumor to other structures, the size of the tumor, and whether it has spread to other organs.

- ✓ **Endoscopy:** A thin, lighted scope (called an endoscope) is inserted through an incision or opening in the body. The scope provides a view of the interior of the body.

- ✓ **Lab tests:** Lab tests, such as blood and urine tests, are also commonly performed and may show whether cancer has affected the body.

If an imaging technique reveals that cancer may be present, a *biopsy* is done. A biopsy is the collection of a sample of tissue from the suspicious area or growth for microscopic examination. In most cases, a biopsy is the only sure way to diagnose cancer.

The tissue that is removed is examined by a specialist in the examination of human tissue, known as a *pathologist.* The pathologist determines whether cancer is present, and if so, what type it is and at what stage it is. A positive biopsy indicates the presence of cancer, and a negative biopsy means that no cancer has been found. Biopsies are not always accurate, however. They may detect cancer when none is present (false positive) or find no cancer when cancer is actually present (false negative).

Making it better

Several basic methods of treating cancer are used individually or in combination. The type of cancer, its stage, and the age and overall health of the patient determine the method used.

✔ **Surgery** is used to remove cancerous tissue and any affected lymph nodes. For most forms of cancer, surgery is the primary treatment, although other treatments may be used along with — or instead of — surgery.

✔ **Radiation therapy** (also called radiotherapy) involves the use of high-energy rays to destroy the reproductive material of cancerous cells and prevent them from multiplying. It is generally used after surgery as an *adjuvant,* or supplemental, therapy to destroy any cancer cells that may remain.

✔ **Chemotherapy** uses anticancer drugs to kill cancer cells. The drugs are administered orally or through an injection and travel through the bloodstream and throughout the body. Although the prescribed dose is chosen to try to limit damage only to cancer cells, chemotherapy affects normal cells as well. Chemotherapy is given in cycles of a treatment period that is followed by a recovery period, then another treatment period, and so on.

✔ **Hormone therapy** can be used to fight types of cancer that depend on hormones to grow — prostate cancer and breast cancer among them. This therapy is designed to prevent cancer cells from getting the hormones that they need by surgically removing the hormone-producing organs (such as the testicles) or by using drugs that stop hormone production or change how the hormones work.

✔ **Biological therapy** (also called immunotherapy) is the injection of a substance into the body — for example, the protein interferon — to enhance the body's natural defenses against cancer. It's a relatively new form of treatment, and it's still considered experimental. It can also be used to help protect the body from some of the side effects of treatment, such as infections that occur during chemotherapy.

✔ **Bone marrow transplantation** may be used for particularly aggressive or recurrent forms of cancer (such as lymphoma, lung cancer, leukemia, and breast cancer). Bone marrow is the tissue that produces new cells and helps to maintain the immune system, and it can be damaged by the high doses of chemotherapy and radiation that may be needed to treat some forms of cancer. In a bone marrow transplant, the bone marrow is removed, stored, and then replaced after the high-dose treatment is completed. In this way, the cell-producing bone marrow is preserved rather than destroyed by the cancer treatment.

A number of alternative therapies are thought to help slow the progress of cancer or help relieve its symptoms or the side effects of treatment. Macrobiotics, a form of nutritional therapy, is thought to detoxify the body and slow cancer damage. Acupuncture may be used to relieve pain, boost energy levels, and reduce depression. Homeopathy, Bach flower remedies, and aromatherapy are also thought to be helpful. See Chapter 7 for more information about complementary care.

An ounce of prevention

The following general recommendations are thought to help reduce your risk of cancer:

- ✔ **Don't smoke.** Smoking is the most preventable risk factor for cancer.

- ✔ **If you drink alcohol, do so in moderation.**

- ✔ **Shun the sun.** Avoid the sun between 11 a.m. and 3 p.m., when it's high overhead and its ultraviolet rays are strongest. Wear protective clothing or sunscreen rated SPF 15 to 30 to block most of the sun's harmful rays.

- ✔ **Eat a high-fiber, low-fat diet.** Be sure to get at least five servings of fruits and vegetables per day.

- ✔ **Watch out for health risks in the environment.** If you work around harmful substances, follow safety rules to keep your risk of cancer to a minimum.

- ✔ **Get regular examinations by your practitioner.** Checkups and preventive screenings go a long way toward catching cancer early, when it's most easily cured. Screening is especially important if you're at high risk for cancer — for example, if it runs in your family.

- ✔ **Practice self-examination regularly.** Women should learn how to do breast self-examinations, and men should learn to do testicular self-examinations. Both men and women should examine their skin regularly to spot skin cancer.

For more information about cancer and treatments, contact the American Cancer Society, 1599 Clifton Rd. NE, Atlanta, GA 30329-4251; 800-ACS-2345 or 404-320-3333; or visit them on the Web at www.cancer.org.

Chronic Pain

Few people can imagine what it's like to live with chronic, unremitting pain that makes carrying on a normal life nearly impossible. Yet many men, women, and children struggle with chronic pain, as well as the feelings of hopelessness and isolation that come with living with a problem that few people can understand or empathize with.

Headache, cancer, arthritis, osteoporosis, and lower back problems are the most common causes of chronic pain, but sometimes an actual cause is difficult to pinpoint. Any pain that lasts for more than three months is considered chronic.

Recognizing the signs and knowing for sure

If you have constant or recurring pain for three or more months, see your doctor for an evaluation. Begin with your family doctor, who will attempt to determine why you are experiencing constant pain and what your treatment options are. Keep in mind that pain is a tricky business, with psychological factors sometimes coming into play.

Making it better

Your physician may refer you to a specialist, such as a neurologist, orthopedist, or neurosurgeon, for treatment. Still another possibility is a referral to a pain clinic, which can provide physical therapy, biofeedback, hypnosis, imagery, occupational therapy, psychotherapy, and family counseling.

Prescription drugs such as morphine, demerol, and some antidepressants (which relieve nerve pain) may be recommended. Another, less well-known method of pain relief is transcutaneous electrical nerve stimulation, or TENS. TENS devices stimulate nerves with a current of low-level electricity that "turns off" the pain.

On your own, exercise can increase the endorphins — the chemical messengers in your brain that promote feelings of well-being — in your body. Heat, ice, and massage therapy also can make pain disappear for a time. Over-the-counter pain relievers help, too.

Some people find relief by using herbal therapy. Capsaicin, ginger, arnica, hypericum, sarapin, and bromelain are reputed to reduce pain. In addition, acupuncture can be an effective treatment for neck, head, arm, and shoulder pain. Biofeedback, self-hypnosis, guided imagery, meditation, yoga, and other relaxation techniques can also play a role in pain management.

For more information about combating chronic pain, contact the American Chronic Pain Association, P. O. Box 850, Rocklin, CA 95677; 916-632-0922.

Depression

For most people, feelings of depression are temporary and short-term. For hundreds of millions of others, though, these feelings don't go away and can lead to more serious problems. Clinical depression is a serious disorder that requires treatment. Depression can affect a person's entire physical and emotional well-being, altering feelings, thoughts, and behaviors.

Depression comes in many forms. The most common type is major depressive disorder, which includes

- **Melancholic depression:** A person who loses interest in activities once held to be enjoyable and who can't enjoy circumstances when good fortune strikes is suffering from melancholic depression.

- **Psychotic depression:** A person who experiences delusions and hallucinations is suffering from psychotic depression. The risk of suicide is high with a person who has this condition.

- **Atypical depression:** A person who eats more, sleeps more, or gains more weight than usual is suffering from atypical depression. The opposite is usually true for people who suffer from depression.

Another type of clinical depression is *manic-depressive disorder,* which can best be described as an emotional roller coaster. A person suffering from this disorder often has high levels of energy and in the process can act recklessly and impulsively. The person's emotional state can shift drastically from heightened or exaggerated optimism to severe, self-punishing pessimism.

Recognizing the signs and knowing for sure

Because the causes of depression are largely biochemical or psychosocial, recognizing them may be difficult. Biochemically, a lack of chemicals called neurotransmitters (for example, dopamine and serotonin) in the brain, endocrine disorders, some medicines, and even genetics are all possible explanations for depression. Psychosocially, life experiences such as death, divorce, childhood tragedies, and daily hardships that create stress can trigger depression.

According to the American Psychiatric Association, a person must exhibit daily at least five of the following nine symptoms over a two-week period to be diagnosed as having a major depressive disorder:

- Depressed mood
- Significant loss of interest in most or all activities
- Significant weight loss without dieting or decrease/increase in appetite
- Sleeplessness (insomnia) or excessive sleep
- A speeding up or slowing down of physical or mental activities

✔ Sluggishness

✔ Feelings of worthlessness or unnecessary guilt

✔ Lack of concentration or decisiveness

✔ Frequent thoughts of death or suicidal tendencies

Making it better

The good news for people who recognize the need to seek help is that depression is very treatable. Like many conditions, early diagnosis and treatment of depression can lead to significant reduction in its duration and intensity.

Along with primary care physicians, the practitioners who treat depression are mainly mental health professionals: psychiatrists, psychologists, clinical social workers, family therapists, and psychiatric nurses. Not all caregivers who treat depression are allowed to prescribe drugs, however. Check first.

Depression shouldn't be treated through self-care alone, although steps can be taken to fight the condition. A person with depression should try to be social, participate in pleasant activities, and avoid taking on overwhelming or stressful responsibilities. People with depression rarely "snap out of it," so they shouldn't expect too much from themselves or blame themselves for not feeling up to par.

Four main treatments for depression are available. The most well-known is psychotherapy, or talk therapy. The two types of psychotherapy are *psychodynamic* (in which the doctor helps the patient find and understand the root of his or her problem or at least gain awareness of it) and *cognitive/behavioral* (in which the doctor helps the person address the problem by suggesting ways of changing behaviors, patterns, and so on).

Another type of treatment is *pharmacotherapy,* or the use of drugs such as antidepressants to prevent or relieve depression. Tricyclics (TCAs), monoamine oxidase inhibitors (MAOIs), and selective serotonin reuptake inhibitors (SSRIs) are the three main types of antidepressants. Other medications, such as Ritalin and lithium (primarily used for manic depression), are used to treat depression.

Another form of treatment is ECT, or electroconvulsive therapy. Used frequently in the past as a means to control unruly mental patients, ECT involves sending a low-voltage current through electrodes to the brain, inducing a convulsion that helps alleviate depression.

An ounce of prevention

Although being happy and mentally healthy all the time is virtually impossible, you can do some good things to keep a positive mind. One effective tactic is exercise, which can improve your physical as well as psychological well-being. Another is to regulate sleeping patterns. Although some doctors prescribe limited sleep time in order to alleviate symptoms of depression, getting a good night's rest on a regular basis can only be positive.

For help with mental health issues, contact the National Mental Health Association, 1021 Prince St., Alexandria, VA 22314-2971; 800-969-6642; or visit them on the Web at www.nmha.org.

Diabetes

Diabetes mellitus is caused by the body's inability to handle the breakdown of carbohydrates into sugars, which fuel the functions of metabolism. This inability is caused by low levels of insulin, a hormone produced in the pancreas. Insulin enables cells to remove sugar from the blood and create energy within the cells. In patients with diabetes, either the pancreas does not produce enough insulin or the insulin produced does not function properly.

Millions of people have the condition and don't know it. It seems unlikely that such a serious condition could go unnoticed, but diabetes comes on slowly over a number of years, so its effects aren't always recognized. In fact, most people don't find out that they have diabetes until they develop a complication because of it (see the sidebar "The complications of diabetes" for more information).

The two most common types of diabetes are type 1 and type 2.

- ✔ **Type 1 diabetes** can occur at any age but is most commonly found in patients under age 30. It is sometimes called insulin-dependent diabetes or juvenile diabetes.
- ✔ **Type 2 diabetes,** sometimes called non-insulin-dependent diabetes, can also occur at any age but is usually found in people older than 40.

Although both types of diabetes are treatable, type 2 has fewer complications and a better prognosis than type 1. Type 2 diabetes accounts for 85 to 90 percent of all cases of diabetes.

A third type of diabetes is found only in women: gestational diabetes. Gestational diabetes occurs during pregnancy, when the body's ability to handle glucose is thrown off by the growth of the fetus and the changes in the hormonal balance. Gestational diabetes usually resolves after the birth of the child. However, having this condition puts the woman at risk for development of type 2 diabetes for five to ten years after the pregnancy.

Recognizing the signs and knowing for sure

As we said before, it's possible to have diabetes and not know that you have it. Symptoms include

- ✔ Sudden, unexplained weight loss

- ✔ Frequent urination

- ✔ Excessive thirst

- ✔ Frequent and/or excessive hunger

- ✔ Vision problems

- ✔ Slow healing of cuts or bruises

- ✔ Frequent infections

- ✔ Circulation problems, including tingling and numbness in the arms, hands, legs, or feet

- ✔ Genital and skin itching

A positive diagnosis for diabetes can be made by using a blood test to measure the sugar levels in the blood. In normal adults, blood-sugar levels range between 60 and 100 milligrams per deciliter (mg/dl), when a person is fasting (defined as not having eaten for three or more hours).

A fasting plasma glucose level measures the blood sugar level when a person hasn't eaten for 8 to 12 hours. Several of these tests are given on different days to determine the range for the individual; diabetes is diagnosed if the levels are more than 126 mg/dl on two consecutive tests.

An oral glucose tolerance test is a fasting blood sample taken after a person has eaten a high-carbohydrate diet for three days. After the sample is taken, the person drinks a glucose solution, and new blood samples are taken on a regular basis over the next three to five hours to show how the body is handling the glucose. Normally, blood sugar levels rise after glucose is consumed, and then return to normal levels after the glucose has been metabolized. If the glucose readings remain high more than one to two hours after the glucose solution was consumed, diabetes can be diagnosed.

The complications of diabetes

Left unchecked, diabetes hastens the failure of several bodily functions. As the body is unable to process the excess sugar, the kidneys are forced to pass sugar out of the body, having first dissolved it in water (urine). This is the cause of the excess urination and excessive thirst as the body uses the fluids to get rid of the excess sugar. The kidneys are stressed as they attempt to pump out the excess sugar, and, over time, the exertion and vascular damage lead to kidney failure. Diabetes is the leading cause of end-stage kidney disease.

Another effect of diabetes is on the circulatory system. As the kidneys take fluid from the body, the circulatory system has to work harder to pump blood through the veins and arteries. This can lead to stroke, coronary heart disease, and circulation problems in the hands and feet (which can cause gangrene if the circulation drops too low). Erection problems may also develop. These conditions are two to four times more common in people with diabetes and account for most of their hospitalizations.

Another problem of diabetes is retinopathy. The delicate membrane that lines the eye and responds to light, forming the images you see, can be damaged by the circulatory problems caused by diabetes. This damage can lead to blindness. In addition, an as-yet-unknown link exists between the buildup of excess sugar in the body and the formation of cataracts, which can also lead to blindness.

Neuropathy, or nerve damage, is also an effect of diabetes. The nerves in the hands and feet are usually affected first, due to the changes and the decrease in circulation in the extremities. The symptoms of numbness and tingling are a sign that diabetic neuropathy is occurring. Also, in some cases, pain occurs in these nerves as the lack of circulation damages them.

By maintaining a normal blood-sugar level through treatment, complications often can be avoided. Work with your doctor to devise a treatment plan that works for you.

Making it better

Treatment of diabetes is becoming more sophisticated each year. Although no cure for the condition has been found, effective management of the condition is possible, depending on the stage of the disease at diagnosis. With proper care, most people with diabetes live long, normal lives with little or no effect from the disease.

Type 1 diabetes is the most severe form of the condition and requires the highest level of treatment. Insulin, in the form of self-administered injections or an implanted insulin pump, is used to regulate the body's sugar to an acceptable level. An improper level of insulin can cause too much sugar (*hyperglycemia*) or too little sugar (*hypoglycemia*) to be in the bloodstream, and both problems affect the body. The person is required to maintain an organized review of blood sugar levels by taking samples from a fingertip on a regular basis.

People with type 2 diabetes produce insulin, but for some reason it does not function properly in their bodies. Most of these patients are able to maintain control of their blood sugar levels without insulin injections. Because four out of five people with type 2 diabetes are overweight, a simple dietary program, combined with proper exercise, may be sufficient to remedy their problem and maintain proper insulin and blood sugar levels. In more severe cases, prescription medications, combined with diet and exercise, are usually sufficient to maintain control. If type 2 diabetes is left unchecked, insulin may be recommended.

Gestational diabetes symptoms are usually mild and not life-threatening, but the condition can have serious effects on the developing fetus. About 3 percent of all pregnant women are at risk for gestational diabetes, mostly pregnant women over age 25. As a result, these cases are usually classified as high risk and monitored closely. In these cases, for unknown reasons, the child tends to be large and have oversized organs. Babies are usually born premature, cause difficult labors because of their size, and have respiratory problems, low blood calcium, jaundice, low blood sugar, and infections. Proper management by medication, insulin injection, or dietary control can maintain a proper blood sugar level in pregnant women with gestational diabetes and prevent problems.

If you have a family history of diabetes, you should have regular checkups to make sure that you are not developing some of the same problems. Regular blood sugar tests can determine whether you are diabetic and whether you can control the condition with diet and exercise alone or whether other measures are required. If you are pregnant, a blood-sugar screening should be a standard part of your prenatal workup, with regular follow-ups throughout the pregnancy. If gestational diabetes develops, the condition may be treated with diet and exercise alone, or with oral medications.

Early detection is the main aid in proper treatment of any type of diabetes. Long-term lack of treatment for diabetes greatly increases the risk of complications and permanent damage to the kidneys and the rest of the body.

An ounce of prevention

Type 1 diabetes cannot be prevented at present. To reduce your risk of type 2 diabetes, maintain a healthy weight, eat low-fat foods, and get regular exercise that helps you lose weight and build muscle mass. Evidence shows that exercise that builds muscle mass may help trigger the muscles' use of insulin and help prevent diabetes.

For more information about dealing with diabetes, contact the American Diabetes Association, 1600 Duke Street, Alexandria, VA 22314; 800-232-3472; or visit them on the Web at www.diabetes.org.

Heart Disease

Heart disease can mean more than just a heart attack. In this section, we talk not only about the evils of myocardial infarction (a fancy name for heart attack) but also the dangers of high blood pressure and stroke, two other common forms of heart disease. We also discuss cholesterol and triglycerides, which are contributors to heart disease.

Coronary heart disease

Coronary heart disease (CHD), also called coronary-artery disease (CAD) or coronary vascular heart disease (CVHD), is caused by a buildup of fatty deposits, called *plaque,* on the walls of the arteries (see Figure 18-2). These buildups cause a degeneration of the artery and obstruct the flow of oxygen- and nutrient-rich blood through the body, especially to the heart. When the heart fails to receive sufficient oxygen-rich blood flow, the heart muscle starves and becomes damaged. A minor blockage can trigger chest pain, called *angina.* In more severe cases, the heart suffers a myocardial infarction and possibly sudden death.

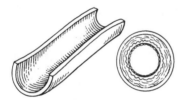
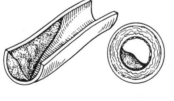
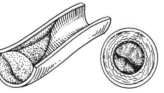

Figure 18-2:
Coronary heart disease occurs when plaque builds up on the walls of the arteries.

Angina pectoris: Breaking the silence

Too often, heart attacks are silent, without symptoms, and go unnoticed until sudden death occurs. But angina, the pain felt when the heart is deprived of oxygen, breaks that silence and gives warning that a heart attack may be in the not-too-distant future. It's usually triggered by physical exertion or excitement.

Symptoms of angina include heavy, strangulating chest pain; pain that begins under the breastbone on the left side of the chest; and pain that radiates to the throat, neck, jaw, and left shoulder and arm. Angina episodes usually last less than 15 minutes. Any chest pain that lasts longer may be a sign of a true heart attack.

Men tend to have a greater risk of suffering heart attacks and suffer them earlier in life than women. However, after menopause, women's death rate from heart disease increases to equal that of men. Children of parents with heart disease tend to have a greater risk of developing the condition themselves, especially if the parent suffered a heart attack at an early age (earlier than age 55 for men and earlier than age 65 for women).

Recognizing the signs and knowing for sure

Symptoms of a heart attack may include

- ✔ Subtle but constant pressure, fullness, squeezing, or pain in the chest that lasts for more than a few minutes or goes away and then comes back
- ✔ Pain in the shoulders, neck, or jaw that runs down the arms or back
- ✔ Dizziness, fainting, sweating, nausea, unusual shortness of breath, or weakness with chest discomfort during minimal exercise (such as climbing stairs)
- ✔ Chest pain during exertion or stress that subsides during a period of rest
- ✔ Indigestion that antacids cannot relieve
- ✔ Difficulty breathing

Not all of these warning signs accompany every heart attack, so be sure to seek help immediately if you suspect that an attack is occurring.

Heart attack help

If you are with someone having a heart attack, follow this plan of action:

✔ Call for help immediately.

✔ Help the person into a comfortable sitting or partially reclining position.

✔ Loosen the person's collar, belt, cuffs, and shoes.

✔ If you're trained, perform cardiopulmonary resuscitation (CPR) if the person's heart and breathing have stopped. See Chapter 5 for more on CPR training.

Coronary heart disease and angina can be diagnosed even before a heart attack occurs. The simplest test is an electrocardiogram (EKG or ECG). This test uses electrodes placed at specific points on the chest and limbs to measure the heart's electrical output. It is used by physicians to uncover evidence of suspected heart disease or as a routine informational step in a regularly scheduled physical examination. Among the problems an EKG can show are irregular heartbeat rhythms and signs of heart muscle damage caused by a blocked coronary artery.

In a similar test called a stress test or treadmill stress test, an EKG reading is taken while a person exercises. This test determines whether the heart is working properly while under stress. If the stress test is "positive," meaning that some signs of ischemia (lack of blood flow to the heart muscle) are present, additional testing is required to determine the exact nature of the problem. But not all heart problems can be diagnosed with a stress test.

Angiography is a test that uses an X-ray, combined with dye injected into the heart, to determine the blood flow to the heart muscle. Any blockages in the blood flow show up as the dye follows the blood vessels through the heart.

Cardiac catheterization is a variation of angiography in which a plastic tube is inserted through a blood vessel in the groin and then threaded into the heart in order to inject dye into specific places to monitor the blood flow. During catheterization, the pressure in the heart chambers can be monitored and blood samples can be taken, all of which provide the doctor with additional information.

In addition, new variations of CAT (computerized axial tomography) scans or MRI (magnetic resonance imaging) scans can be used to create a three-dimensional image of the heart in a noninvasive manner (a way that does not enter the body). However, these tests are expensive and are not always available in all areas.

Making it better

If you experience a heart attack, *thrombolytic drugs* — known as clot-busting drugs because they break up obstructions in the arteries — may be administered at the hospital. Blood pressure medications, painkillers, or other drugs may be given as well. After your condition has stabilized, treatment of heart blockage becomes the main concern.

Depending on the degree of buildup of plaque in the arteries and whether you've already experienced an attack, heart disease may be treated in several different ways. If the problem is just starting and the buildup is small, medication may be recommended.

- ✔ **Vasodilators** relax the arteries and increase blood flow. Nitroglycerin, a common drug for treating angina, is a vasodilator.

- ✔ **Angiotensin-converting enzyme (ACE) inhibitors** interfere with the body's production of angiotensin, a chemical that causes the arteries to constrict. They are used to lower blood pressure and strengthen the pumping action of the heart.

- ✔ **Calcium channel blockers** help open blood vessels and encourage blood flow.

- ✔ **Beta blockers** are used to lower blood pressure.

- ✔ **Aspirin** helps thin the blood and prevent clots.

- ✔ **Diuretics** (also called thiazides) are used to lower blood pressure by drawing water and salt out of the body via the urine.

- ✔ **Digitalis** (also called digoxin or digitoxin) strengthens the heartbeat and reduces the size of an enlarged heart.

If a heart attack has occurred or if testing determines that the degree of coronary artery blockage is severe, surgical techniques can be used to open, bypass, or even replace clogged arteries.

An initial approach is to open the arteries. In *angioplasty* (also called *balloon angioplasty* or *percutaneous transluminal coronary angioplasty,* or *PTCA*), a catheter is inserted into the narrowed artery, and a balloon at the tip is inflated to push aside any blockage. Angioplasty is effective, but the blockage often recurs.

Bypass surgery (also called *coronary artery bypass graft,* or *CABG, surgery*), in which the blocked artery is bypassed by using a graft taken from the person's leg or thigh, is the recommended treatment for people who are at higher risk and have one or more blocked arteries. Although the mortality rate is higher for this procedure than for angioplasty (5 percent as opposed to 1 percent) the long-term effects are better, and fewer additional procedures are required after the bypass.

Coronary-stent placement combines the balloon angioplasty procedure with placement of a small metal tube in the artery. The tube, or stent, is placed on the end of a balloon catheter and moved into position in the blocked artery. The balloon is then expanded, and the stent is left to push the blockage out of the way and prop open the artery. This procedure carries about the same risk as an angioplasty but has a better long-term effect, requiring fewer additional procedures.

An ounce of prevention

Although you can do little about some risk factors for heart disease, such as age, gender, and family history, you can still affect many factors to lower your risk of a heart attack.

- **Stop smoking.** According to the American Heart Association, smoking more than doubles your chance of a heart attack, and smokers are more likely to die from a heart attack than nonsmokers. Within ten years of quitting smoking, your risk of heart disease drops to the same level as other people with your same medical risks who have never smoked.

- **Control your blood pressure.** High blood pressure means that the heart is working harder than it should be to push blood through your arteries and veins. This can cause the heart to enlarge and can cause atherosclerosis (the buildup of plaque in the arteries). We talk more about high blood pressure later in this section.

- **Practice relaxation.** Stress is a large factor in heart attacks. If you're more relaxed, you lower your risk of a heart attack. Time management and stress management techniques (discussed in Chapter 2) can lower your overall stress level.

- **Exercise.** Regular exercise can help you lose weight, reduce stress, lower your cholesterol level, and lower your blood pressure — all factors that can affect your cardiac health. However, certain types of exercise, such as isometric exercise and weight lifting, can trigger heart attacks. Talk with your doctor about what kind of exercise is right for you.

- **Drink moderately.** Although a drink or two a day may have a beneficial effect on your cardiovascular system, more than that can cause damage.

- **Ask you doctor about aspirin.** Studies have shown that a small amount of aspirin daily may reduce your chance of a heart attack by thinning the blood and preventing clots from forming. It can also reduce the severity of heart attacks if they do occur. But aspirin is not safe for everyone and may increase the risk of hemorrhagic stroke in some people.

- **Monitor your cholesterol levels.** Cholesterol, a fatlike substance that plays a large part in the formation of plaque, has been found to raise heart attack rates by 2 percent for every 1 percent rise in the cholesterol level. Read the section "High cholesterol and triglycerides" for more on cholesterol.

✔ **If you have diabetes, monitor it carefully.** One of the effects of uncontrolled diabetes is cardiovascular complications, caused by the excess urination and the changes in the body's fluid levels.

High blood pressure (Hypertension)

Blood pressure is the force that the blood exerts on the walls of the vessels as it passes through the body. The pressure can increase or decrease according to two factors: the force with which the heart is pumping and the size of the arteries through which the blood must pass. Narrow or constricted blood vessels lead to an increase in blood pressure.

High blood pressure, or hypertension, is a chronic condition that puts both the heart and the blood vessels under great strain because it causes them to work harder to meet the body's needs. It can lead to stroke, heart attack, and kidney failure, as well as an enlarged heart and scarred or hardened arteries.

In 90 to 95 percent of cases, the cause of hypertension is unknown. In the remaining cases, a congenital heart defect, kidney problem, or other problem may be the cause.

Hypertension is called "the silent killer" because it has no symptoms. You could have it for years without knowing it — and estimates say that about 35 percent of people with the disease don't know that they have it.

Recognizing the signs and knowing for sure

As we said before, high blood pressure often has no symptoms. However, signs that sometimes do occur include

✔ Headaches

✔ Heart palpitation

✔ Flushed face

✔ Blurry vision

✔ Nosebleeds

✔ Difficulty breathing after exercise

✔ Fatigue

✔ Frequent need to urinate

✔ Ringing in the ears

✔ Dizziness

Blood pressure is measured with a *sphygmomanometer,* or blood pressure cuff. Healthy blood pressure levels range from person to person — there's no such thing as an ideal level. However, doctors usually feel that the lower your rate, the better. Table 18-1 lists the guidelines that physicians usually use to diagnose high blood pressure. Remember, though, that blood pressure normally elevates under stress. To have elevated blood pressure, you must have elevated readings on repeated attempts. Being in a physician's office may be stressful, and your blood pressure may be normal outside that office.

Table 18-1	Blood Pressure Guidelines	
	Systolic (mm/Hg)	*Diastolic (mm/Hg)*
Optimal	<120	<80
Normal	120 – 129	80 – 84
High normal	130 – 139	85 – 89
Stage 1 hypertension	140 – 159	90 – 99
Stage 2 hypertension	160 – 179	100 – 109
Stage 3 hypertension	180 – 209	110 – 119
Stage 4 hypertension	>210	>120

Making it better

The recommendations for self-care should come as no surprise. If you have hypertension, begin a moderate exercise program (with your doctor's advice), quit smoking, and avoid alcohol, salt, and caffeine. Also try to shed any excess weight. Eat foods high in potassium and calcium, too.

Medications are often used in treating high blood pressure — in fact, some experts believe that drug therapy should be started even before self-care tactics are tried. Common drugs for hypertension (called, appropriately, antihypertensives) include

- Angiotensin-converting enzyme (ACE) inhibitors
- Calcium channel blockers
- Diuretics
- Beta blockers
- Vasodilators

These drugs are explained more fully in the section "Coronary heart disease," earlier in this chapter.

Stroke

When the blood supply to the heart is cut off, it's known as a heart attack. A stroke, which occurs when the blood supply to the *brain* is cut off, is also known as a brain attack.

Stroke is nothing to take lightly. When blood can't reach the brain, the brain's cells begin to die. Some strokes result in death; others leave the victim severely disabled because the brain can no longer function fully. Stroke is the third leading cause of death and the leading cause of serious disability in the United States.

Strokes occur in two different ways. If the blood flow through vessels in the neck or head becomes blocked, that's called an *ischemic* stroke. If a blood vessel in or near the brain ruptures, that's called a *hemorrhagic* stroke. Not exactly a type of stroke, a *transient ischemic attack,* or *TIA,* is a temporary blockage in blood flow to the brain. These so-called ministrokes often precede more serious attacks.

Recognizing the signs and knowing for sure

Stroke and TIA have the following symptoms:

- Sudden weakness or numbness of the face, arm, or leg
- Sudden loss of vision
- Sudden difficulty speaking or understanding speech
- Sudden severe headaches with no cause
- Unexplained dizziness, unsteadiness, or sudden falls, especially occurring with other signs

The faster a stroke is diagnosed and treated, the fewer brain cells die. Immediate emergency care is essential if symptoms of a stroke occur.

Stroke is diagnosed through a physical exam, neurological testing, and blood tests. Also, imaging tests, such as CAT scans, X-rays, and MRIs, can be used to determine the type of stroke suffered and the extent of the damage to the brain. Tests may also be done to detect blockages and narrowing of the arteries.

Making it better

Again, immediate treatment may help reduce the effects of a stroke. After a stroke occurs, treatment focuses on stabilizing the patient and preventing additional brain damage.

Self-care, of course, isn't an option during a stroke. However, after the stroke itself has passed, rehabilitation may be necessary to overcome some of its effects. Clinics, hospitals, and nursing facilities often have rehabilitation programs, and home-based programs are available as well.

Blood pressure medications may be prescribed to lower pressure slowly. With ischemic stroke, clot-busting drugs called *thrombolytics* are used to restore blood flow to the brain. One such drug, called tissue-plasminogen activator (TPA), is commonly administered, although it needs to be given within three hours of the stroke's onset. *Anticoagulant,* or blood-thinning, drugs also may be used to improve blood flow and prevent the formation of clots in narrowed arteries. Surgery may also be performed to open blocked passages. With hemorrhagic stroke, the source of the bleeding must be stopped — perhaps through surgery or medications.

An ounce of prevention

Again, preventing stroke and other forms of heart disease is pretty straightforward: Eat a low-fat, low-salt diet, exercise regularly, don't smoke, and maintain a healthy weight. Also take steps to control the stress in your life. Cholesterol levels should be watched as well. And if you have high blood pressure, remember to take your blood pressure medication.

High cholesterol and triglycerides

Cholesterol is a soft, waxy, fatlike substance found in the body's cells. It's not a fat, but is a related substance called a *sterol.* Cholesterol doesn't dissolve in water or blood, and it's carried through the bloodstream by a protein shell called a *lipoprotein.*

The primary lipoproteins are high-density lipoprotein (HDL) and low-density lipoprotein (LDL). HDL is responsible for ushering cholesterol to the liver, where it is removed from the body. Because it gets rid of excess cholesterol in your system, it's known as the "good" cholesterol. LDL, on the other hand, carries cholesterol to cells within the body. If too much LDL is in a person's system, it simply circulates through the bloodstream, eventually sticking to artery walls and contributing to heart disease. For this reason, LDL is the "bad" cholesterol.

If you have trouble keeping your cholesterols straight, just associate the H in HDL with "healthy" and the L in LDL with "lousy."

Triglycerides have a different chemical structure than cholesterol, but they also provide fat for energy and transport it throughout the body. Triglycerides are a risk factor for heart disease, although experts are not yet sure why that is, because they don't stick to artery walls. Some experts believe that trigylcerides may thicken the blood.

Knowing for sure

No symptoms exist for high cholesterol and trigylceride levels — unless you consider resulting heart disease a symptom. The only way you can detect these levels is through a blood test. Recent research suggests that blood tests that measure the ratio of HDL cholesterol to LDL cholesterol to total cholesterol, which provide the most accurate picture of heart disease risk, should be performed. With a high cholesterol level due to high amounts of HDL, you're much better off than if the high level is caused by LDL.

In studies, a total-cholesterol-to-HDL ratio of less than 6:1 seems to protect against heart disease, while a ratio greater than 6:1 increases risk. In an LDL-to-HDL ratio, less than 4:1 is protective, and greater than 4:1 increases risk.

If you know your total cholesterol, HDL, and LDL levels, you can calculate these ratios yourself. Your total-cholesterol-to-HDL ratio is simply total cholesterol divided by HDL. The same goes for LDL-to-HDL; simply divide the first figure by the second. Following are the Cholesterol Classification Guidelines for Adults from the National Cholesterol Education Program:

Total cholesterol

Desirable: <200 mg/dl

Borderline high: 200 – 238 mg/dl

High: >240 mg/dl

HDL cholesterol

Desirable: >50 – 75 mg/dl

Borderline low: 35 – 49 mg/dl

Low: <35 mg/dl

LDL cholesterol

Desirable: <130 mg/dl

Borderline high: 130 – 159 mg/dl

High: >160 mg/dl

Triglycerides

Safe: 200 mg/dl or less

Borderline: 200 – 400 mg/dl

High: 400 – 1,000 mg/dl

Very high: >1,000 mg/dl

Making it better

High cholesterol and trigylceride levels themselves don't indicate disease. However, lowering your levels also lowers your risk of coronary heart disease.

Most doctors believe that eating fat contributes to high cholesterol levels. However, controversy is raging over whether dietary cholesterol (the kind you eat) has an effect on blood cholesterol levels (the amount in your blood vessels). Still, the American Heart Association recommends getting less than 300 milligrams of cholesterol from food daily, and less than 200 milligrams if you have heart disease. Food sources of cholesterol include meat, eggs, milk, yogurt, and cheese.

Other self-care tips for lowering cholesterol and triglycerides include losing excess weight, limiting fat intake to less than 30 percent of daily calories, eating plenty of fiber, avoiding saturated fats, and getting regular aerobic exercise. Research shows that regular aerobic exercise increases HDL levels. Avoiding alcohol reduces trigylceride production.

Medications may be prescribed to lower cholesterol and trigylceride levels. These include bile acid sequestrants (such as cholestryamine — brand name Questran), which reduce the amount absorbed from foods, and HMG CoA reductase inhibitors or statins (such as simvastatin — brand name Zocor), which inhibit the body's ability to produce cholesterol. Other statins are pravastatin (Pravachol) and fluvastatin (Lescol). The drug fenofibrate (Tricor) helps lower triglyceride levels and boost HDL levels.

For more information about heart disease and treatments, contact the American Heart Association, 7272 Greenville Ave., Dallas, TX 75231-4596; 800-AHA-USA1 or 214-373-6300; or visit them on the Web at www.amhrt.org.

HIV and AIDS

Acquired immune deficiency syndrome (AIDS) is the final stage of a progressive disease resulting from infection by human immunodeficiency virus (HIV). This virus, which can remain dormant in the body for many years before becoming active, weakens the body's immune system, the body's ability to fight infections and other diseases. AIDS has no cure and eventually results in death.

Recognizing the signs and knowing for sure

Despite the fact that HIV affects each person differently, most affected persons pass through some general stages as the disease develops.

First, the body produces infection-fighting substances known as *antibodies* in response to the HIV virus in the bloodstream. Usually within six months of infection, these antibodies can be detected in the blood, thereby confirming the presence of HIV in the individual. Just after infection, symptoms including fatigue, malaise, swollen lymph glands, rash, night sweats, and diarrhea may appear. However, after these initial, mild symptoms pass, HIV can lie dormant in the body for years — up to ten years — before additional symptoms appear. During this time, an HIV-positive individual can still pass along the infection to others, even though he or she appears perfectly healthy.

HIV: How you get it, how you don't

The AIDS virus is present in blood, semen, vaginal secretions, and breast milk of infected people. Transmission occurs when one of these fluids comes into contact with a cut or sore or with the mucous membranes of the vagina, penis, rectum, or mouth. Usually, this contact occurs through unprotected intercourse; the virus can also be transferred through the sharing of infected drug needles. Health care workers who get stuck or cut with contaminated needles or exposed to blood also may contract the disease. The risk of contracting AIDS through a blood transfusion or donor sperm is very low; these fluids are screened for the disease before they're used.

Many activities do *not* result in HIV exposure. You cannot get HIV from visiting, socializing with, working with, or going to school with someone who is HIV positive. You cannot get HIV from being sneezed on or coughed on by someone who is HIV positive. You cannot get HIV by sweating with or crying with someone who is HIV positive. Being bitten by a mosquito or other insect cannot transmit HIV to you. Touching objects that a person with HIV has touched does not transmit the disease. And most important, giving blood does not put you at risk for HIV.

The best way to avoid contracting AIDS is to avoid unprotected intercourse and intravenous drug use. Chapter 19 contains more information about safer sex and protecting yourself against AIDS.

In the second stage, the HIV virus becomes active and attacks and cripples the immune system. The virus attacks the antibodies known as *T cells,* which are responsible for attacking and destroying antigens. When the T cells are destroyed, the immune system does not function, and the body becomes vulnerable to a variety of infections and diseases. These diseases take advantage of the weakened immune system.

The third stage of the disease is marked by the development of AIDS-related complex (ARC). As the HIV infection progresses and the immune system weakens, symptoms of ARC appear. These include severe rashes, arthritis, intellectual impairment, pneumonia, kidney infections, personality changes, yeast infections of the mouth, and neurological disorders.

In the final stage, full-blown AIDS occurs as the immune system is severely impaired and diseases and infections plague the body, eventually causing death.

Many people who have AIDS have no symptoms and may not even know that they are infected. Unless you have tested negative for HIV or have not engaged in any high-risk activities, you cannot know for certain, without testing, whether you are free of the virus.

A blood test can be done to test for HIV antibodies. However, these antibodies generally do not show up in the bloodstream for at least one to three months after infection, and it may take as long as six months for the antibodies to develop sufficiently to show on a blood test.

You can get an HIV test at many health care facilities, both public and private. Usually, HIV testing is done with a blood test. However, an oral kit is also available that uses an absorbent pad to collect a saliva sample for analysis. In addition, a urine test for HIV was approved by the U.S. Food and Drug Administration in June 1998. Because AIDS can be transmitted through blood, these alternatives to blood tests are thought to be safer for health care professionals performing the tests.

Home testing kits are also available for use in total privacy. These kits contain a special paper that is used to absorb a drop of blood from the finger and then mailed to a certified testing laboratory. The results, which remain anonymous, are provided a week later by telephone. These kits are available over-the-counter in drugstores and by mail-order.

Making it better

There is currently no cure for AIDS. But treatments can slow the progression of the disease and its symptoms, thereby prolonging the life of people with AIDS. At the present time, treatment of AIDS focuses on three main areas:

✔ **Arresting the progression of the virus:** This has been attempted with the use of drugs called *nucleoside analogues,* which prevent the replication of the virus. Initially, the drug AZT is used, and then other similar drugs, such as ddI, ddC, and d4T, are added to the regimen when AZT loses its effectiveness.

✔ **Treating the opportunistic infections and diseases that attack the body in its weakened state:** Antimicrobial drug therapy is used to treat such infections.

✔ **Attempting to restore the health of the immune system:** Methods such as bone marrow transplants and immunoglobulin therapy are used.

In July 1996, researchers announced that a class of drugs called *protease inhibitors,* in combination with nucleoside analogues, can reduce the levels of HIV in the blood to below detectable levels. In addition to slowing the growth of the virus, this treatment also increases the number of T cells. Although this is not a definitive cure, it does provide hope for the future. One of the biggest problems with the treatment is its cost of $10,000 to $15,000 per year.

Alternative therapies can help ease the symptoms of HIV and/or AIDS, although these should still be considered part of the treatment program under the direction of a doctor. Treatments such as acupuncture, use of herbal medicines, massage, dietary modification, chiropractic therapy, homeopathic medicine, and body and mind relaxation exercises have had an effect with some patients. Normally, these therapies are used in combination with other traditional drug therapies and are intended to help the body strengthen the immune system. See Chapter 7 for more on complementary treatments.

An ounce of prevention

Preventing HIV and AIDS is fairly straightforward: Don't have unprotected sex, and don't share intravenous drug needles.

Also be careful if you're considering a tattoo. The needles used in tattooing can transfer HIV just as drug needles can. Make sure that the tattoo artist uses new needles and sterile ink for each customer.

Of course, if you have HIV, avoiding intravenous drug use, abstaining from sex, and practicing safe sex are essential to keep from transmitting the deadly disease to others. You can find more information about safer sex and protecting yourself in Chapter 19.

For more information about HIV and AIDS, contact these organizations:

✔ **Centers for Disease Control and Prevention, National AIDS Clearinghouse,** P. O. Box 6003, Rockville, MD 20849-6003; 800-458-5231 or 800-243-7012 (deaf access)

✔ **Centers for Disease Control and Prevention, National AIDS Hotline,** 800-342-AIDS, 800-344-7432 SIDA (Spanish), 800-243-7889 (TTY)

Osteoporosis

If your body were a house, it would always be under construction. Each of the 206 bones that make up your skeleton is constantly being built up and broken down. This ongoing cycle stars the mineral calcium as the home improvement expert. As long as you're getting enough calcium — and precious few of us are, studies show — your skeleton remains strong. Osteoporosis occurs when bones become weakened, porous, and likely to break. It can lead to death.

Besides helping to build and rebuild living bones, calcium also regulates your blood pressure, maintains your heart rate, and allows your muscles to contract. When calcium is in short supply, your body can always find some by borrowing it from your bones.

One in two women over age 50 and one-third of all men over age 75 develop the condition. Women are at a higher risk for osteoporosis than men because their bones are less dense to begin with. That risk increases after menopause, when the body's production of the protective hormone estrogen decreases.

Other risk factors include smoking, a small stature, a sedentary lifestyle, a low calcium intake, a family history of the disease, testosterone deficiency, and use of certain drugs, such as steroids.

Recognizing the signs and knowing for sure

Sometimes it's easy to spot someone who has osteoporosis: The classic "dowager's hump" and stooped way of walking are unmistakable signs of advanced osteoporosis. However, early changes in bones are not visible to the naked eye. Some symptoms to watch out for are

✔ Pain in the lower back

✔ Bone fractures

✔ Poor posture

✔ Bad gums (Your dentist may be the first professional to suspect that you have osteoporosis.)

✔ Gradual loss of height

Your physician has several ways to measure the strength of your bones. The good news is that testing for this condition is painless and usually involves passing a scanner over your spine, wrist, or hip. Bone density tests include single-beam and dual-beam densitometers and dual-energy X-ray absorptiometry (DEXA). DEXA scans are thought to be the most accurate, although they are expensive.

Bone-density tests produce a figure that is compared with a measurement of peak bone mass done at age 30. If the figure is more than 2.5 times lower than peak bone mass, osteoporosis is diagnosed.

Your insurance company may not pay for a bone-density scan, so be sure to check whether you're covered before you go for the test. In July 1998, Medicare began covering scans for some individuals who have osteoporosis or are at high risk for developing it. Experts are predicting a wider availability of cheaper tests in a year or two.

In addition to bone tests, blood and urine tests may be done to detect calcium levels in the body.

Making it better

Treatment is focused largely on stopping bone loss rather than reversing it. Your family practice physician or ob-gyn may prescribe hormone replacement therapy or one of several available drugs.

If you have osteoporosis, lifestyle changes are in order. If you smoke, stop, because smoking is bad for your bones. You want to increase your calcium intake, too. Even people who hate milk or can't tolerate it can find extra calcium in soy products, peppers, beets, nuts, fish, bananas, apples, nectarines, and whole grains. Taking vitamin D supplements helps move calcium into your bloodstream and into your bones.

Walking, jogging, bicycling, hiking, karate, bowling, and jumping rope can help keep bones healthy, as can various other forms of physical activity. During times when you feel achy, aspirin or a heat massage can make you more comfortable.

Strength training (lifting weights) is a very effective way for people of all ages to improve their bone density. And studies show that you're never too old. Seniors especially benefit from working with weights. A 1994 study that looked at the effects of strength training in nursing home residents (average age 87) found that muscle strength increased 113 percent in those who exercised, walking speed increased 12 percent, and the ability to climb stairs increased 28 percent. Researchers speculated that the increased strength and mobility would decrease the number of falls and hip fractures of the residents.

The most widely prescribed treatments for osteoporosis are medications, including

- **Sodium fluoride:** Sodium fluoride can reduce bone fractures and build bone mass. It may be a good choice for men, who can't benefit from estrogen replacement therapy.

- **Estrogen replacement therapy:** ERT boosts the body's levels of protective estrogen and can cut bone fractures in half. Many forms of estrogen are available to women.

- **Etridronate:** Etridronate, better known for its role in treating Paget's disease, shows promise as an osteoporosis drug because it increases bone mass and slows bone loss.

- **Calcitonin:** Calcitonin improves the cellular level of bones, slows the progression of osteoporosis, and in some cases may even increase bone density.

- **Alendronate:** This drug increases bone strength and reduces fracture risk. It does not contain hormones.

- **Calcitriol:** Calcitriol, with the active ingredient vitamin D, cuts fractures by helping the body absorb more calcium.

- **Thiazide:** Thiazide's advantage is that it prevents the body from excreting calcium.

Boron, a mineral frequently found in multivitamins, has been shown to help women over age 50 retain bone density. Calcium products such as calcium citrate, Cal Apatite, Fern Osteo, and Bone Builder can also help keep bones strong.

An ounce of prevention

Exercising and healthy eating habits go a long way toward protecting your bones from losing density as you age — this goes for women and men. Don't smoke or drink alcohol regularly. And if you're a woman who is over 50 and postmenopausal, ask your doctor about bone-density screening. Not all physicians recommend it to their patients, but the earlier you notice the problem, the sooner you can begin blunting its damage.

For more information about osteoporosis and preventing it, contact the National Osteoporosis Foundation, 1150 17th St. NW, Suite 500, Washington, DC 20036; 800-223-2226; or visit them on the Web at www.nof.org.

Chapter 19

Not Just Fooling Around: Sexual Health

Sexual health is an important part of overall health, affecting both physical and emotional well-being. Concerns range from infertility and sexual dysfunction to contraception and the prevention of sexually transmitted infections — issues that touch us all, whether we are just facing puberty, have already started a family, or are facing life after retirement.

Preventing Pregnancy

Love, romance, furious passion: They may seem to be at odds with contraceptives, which are devices and methods that prevent pregnancy. But if you're sexually active and not interested in conceiving a child, then you need to think about your contraceptive options, their benefits, and their drawbacks. Without contraception, 85 of every 100 sexually active women will become pregnant each year.

When choosing a contraceptive, think about

- ✔ **Its effectiveness against pregnancy:** Effectiveness is measured according to *typical use* (a rate that takes into account that people usually use birth control inconsistently or incorrectly at least some of the time) and *perfect use* (the rate if the method is used correctly and consistently all the time).

- ✔ **Its effectiveness against sexually transmitted diseases (STDs):** Male and female condoms and spermicides help reduce the risk of

STDs. However, other methods provide no barrier against transmission when used alone. Your choice depends on your preferences and the nature of your sexual relationships.

✔ **Your physical needs:** Due to side effects or health concerns, not all people can use all methods. For example, women over 35 who smoke shouldn't use oral contraceptives because of a risk for blood clots and stroke.

✔ **Your and your partner's personal preferences:** Maybe you like a method that allows you to be spontaneous. Maybe you don't want to use a messy liquid or an applicator. Maybe you have religious objections to certain methods. Or maybe you want a method that's easily reversible should you decide that you want to have a child.

Choosing a reversible method

Contraception can be reversible or permanent. This section lists the most common reversible birth control methods, along with some background information. Talk with your partner and your doctor about options that you think may be right for you.

Abstinence

Abstinence is not having vaginal intercourse. This is the only method that is 100 percent guaranteed not to cause pregnancy. Granted, it may be hard to stick to, but it's free and available without a prescription. *Periodic abstinence* (about 80 percent effective with typical use and 98 percent with perfect use) calls for couples to refrain from intercourse during a woman's fertile period, which can be determined through a number of methods. Abstinence and periodic abstinence are often preferred by religious groups that frown on contraception.

Norplant

Norplant is the surgical implantation of six soft capsules underneath the skin of a woman's upper arm. The implants gradually release hormones that prevent ovulation and thicken the barrier that the sperm must overcome to pass into the uterus. Norplant is more than 99 percent effective, and protection from pregnancy lasts for five years, but it doesn't prevent STDs. Norplant may cause some side effects, including irregular bleeding and absent periods. It's available by prescription only. The cost is $500 to $750 for insertion; insurance coverage is unlikely but is offered by some plans.

Depo-Provera

Depo-Provera is a contraceptive injection for a woman. Like Norplant, Depo-Provera is more than 99 percent effective. It works by preventing ovulation and by thickening the cervical mucus. Its effects last for 12 weeks, but it doesn't protect against STDs. The method has some side effects, including irregular bleeding, absent periods, nausea, and sore breasts. It's available by prescription only. The cost is $20 to $40 per injection, plus the cost of the office visit; insurance coverage is unlikely but is offered by some plans.

Oral contraceptives (The Pill)

Oral contraceptives involve doses of estrogen and/or progestin taken daily by a woman to prevent ovulation. The Pill is 97 percent effective with typical use and 99 percent effective with perfect use. Drawbacks include having to remember to take daily pills, plus short-term side effects such as nausea, weight gain, bloating, and breast tenderness. Rarely, the Pill contributes to blood clots, stroke, and heart disease. On the upside, it protects against ovarian and endometrial cancers — protection that can last up to 15 years after stopping the Pill. Plus, protection against endometrial cancer increases with each year of use; women who use the Pill for eight years reduce their risk by up to 80 percent. In addition, it usually lessens menstrual flow and cramping. It doesn't protect against STDs. The Pill is available by prescription only. The cost is $15 to $25 per month, sometimes covered by insurance.

Intrauterine device (IUD)

An IUD is a plastic device that is placed within the uterus to prevent fertilization and implantation of an egg. IUDs got a bad rap in the 1970s, when they were taken off the market because of safety concerns. However, they are now considered to be very safe and can be up to 99 percent effective (depending on the type selected). IUDs do have some side effects, and they're no barrier to STDs. They're best for women who have already had a child. IUDs are available by prescription only. The cost is $150 to $300 for insertion; insurance may cover the cost.

Condom

Here's one for the guys — a latex sheath worn over the penis during intercourse to catch semen and prevent pregnancy. Condoms are good protection against STDs when used properly and have no side effects, except possible allergic irritation, but they do interfere with spontaneity. They are 88 percent effective with typical use and 98 percent effective with perfect use. No prescription is necessary. Condoms cost about $0.30 each.

Diaphragm and cervical cap

A soft rubber cup (diaphragm) or thimble-shaped cap (cervical cap) is worn over the cervix to prevent sperm from penetrating the womb. Both are often used with spermicide. With typical use, these are 82 percent effective. With perfect use, they're 94 percent effective. The device must be inserted shortly before intercourse, which interferes with spontaneity. They rarely cause side effects. These devices provide no protection against STDs, and are available by prescription only. They cost $13 to $25; insurance may cover the expense.

Withdrawal

Withdrawal is the removal of the penis from the vagina before ejaculation. Because this method calls for a great deal of experience and self-control to be done right, it's quite risky. Plus, enough semen to cause pregnancy may be released prior to withdrawal. It's 82 percent effective with typical use and 96 percent with perfect use. It doesn't protect against STDs, but it's free and available without a prescription.

Spermicides

Spermicides come in many forms — creams, jellies, films, and foams — and are inserted into the vagina to block and inactivate sperm. With typical use, they're 79 percent effective; with perfect use, they're 97 percent effective. They can increase the effectiveness of another method if used in conjunction with that method, such as a diaphragm. They can be messy, may interfere with spontaneity, and may cause allergic irritation. They provide no protection against STDs. No prescription is necessary. The cost is $8 for an applicator kit, plus $2 to $5 for refills.

Vaginal pouch

The female version of the condom, a vaginal pouch is a latex sheath worn within the vagina. Effectiveness is 76 percent with typical use and 90 percent with perfect use. The pouch is the only method available to women that protects against STDs. However, the pouch is bulky and may slip and squeak (yes, squeak) during intercourse. No prescription is necessary. Vaginal pouches cost $2.50 each.

Opting for a permanent method

All the methods discussed in the preceding section are reversible, meaning that after their use has stopped, pregnancy is possible. Some methods are more immediate than others — for example, a condom is instantly reversible, whereas Depo-Provera takes three months to leave the system — but they are all temporary.

Tubal sterilization (for women) and vasectomy (for men) are two forms of permanent contraception — surgical procedures done to prevent pregnancy for the rest of a person's lifetime. Sterilization means freedom from pregnancy and contraception for a one-time cost.

Whether you're a man or a woman, you need to think twice — and then think again — about whether permanent contraception is for you. If you're sure that you don't want children, you have health concerns, or you're afraid of passing on a hereditary disease to a child, a permanent method may be the right choice. But think how your situation may change if one of your children died or you divorced and remarried. Would you want more children then?

For men only: Vasectomy

A vasectomy is a surgical procedure in which the *vas deferens,* the small tubes within the male reproductive system through which sperm travels, are blocked. The interruption keeps sperm from getting into the semen (and therefore from getting into the vagina and causing pregnancy). Vasectomy has no effect on erections, hormone production, or the amount of ejaculate. It is more than 99 percent effective (in rare cases, the tubes may reconnect by themselves).

In a traditional vasectomy, a small incision is made in each side of the scrotum. The tubes are located and cut (see Figure 19-1), and the ends are tied off, cauterized, or blocked with clips. Then the incision is stitched shut. Side effects from this method are rare; possibilities include pain, infection, swelling, and skin discoloration. Surgery is usually done in a doctor's office using local anesthesia.

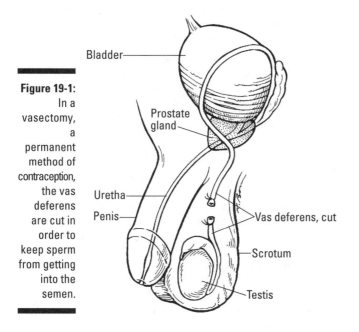

Figure 19-1:
In a vasectomy, a permanent method of contraception, the vas deferens are cut in order to keep sperm from getting into the semen.

A new method, no-scalpel vasectomy (NSV), recently made its debut. In an NSV, a single small hole is punched in the center of the scrotum. Both tubes are drawn out through the hole and cut and tied as in the traditional method. No stitches are required, and little bleeding occurs. The risks of pain, infection, and discomfort are even less than with a traditional vasectomy.

Both procedures take 15 to 20 minutes and cost about $1,000.

For women only: Tubal sterilization

Various methods are used to reach the fallopian tubes, which are then cut and sealed off in various ways (cauterization, clips, clamps, or ties) to prevent the egg from meeting the sperm. Surgical sterilization is about 99.6 percent effective (with problems attributed to surgical error, regrowth of the tubes, or existing pregnancy before the surgery). Women's options for permanent contraception include

- ✔ **Laparoscopy:** A laparoscope is inserted through a small abdominal incision, and gas is pumped into the abdominal cavity to raise the skin and tissues away from the organs to make them visible. A second instrument is inserted through a second small incision to cut and tie the tubes.

- ✔ **Culdoscopy:** A fiber-optic instrument is inserted through an incision in the vagina to locate, cut, and tie the tubes.

- ✔ **Laparotomy:** A long incision is made to open the abdomen, expose the fallopian tubes, and cut and seal them off. Laparotomy is used only when existing scar tissue would interfere with a simpler procedure.

- ✔ **Mini-laparotomy:** A slender tool is inserted into the vagina and used to push the uterus and the fallopian tubes up toward the surface of the abdomen, where they are more accessible. Then a small incision is made in the abdomen, and the accessible tubes are lifted through the incision, cut, and tied.

Hysterectomy (or removal of the uterus) also results in permanent contraception. However, because it carries a number of risks and side effects, hysterectomy should not be performed for sterilization alone.

The procedures listed here take between 10 and 45 minutes to complete, are done under general or local anesthesia, and usually take place at a hospital or outpatient center. Because these procedures are more invasive and more involved than a vasectomy, permanent contraception tends to be riskier and more costly for women than for men.

For more information about reversible and permanent contraception, contact these organizations:

- ✔ Planned Parenthood Federation of America
  810 Seventh Ave.
  New York, NY 10019
  800-230-PLAN

- ✔ National Family Planning and Reproductive Health Association
  122 C St., NW, Suite 380
  Washington, DC 20001-2109
  202-628-3535

✔ Access to Voluntary and Safe Contraception International
(AVSC International)
79 Madison Ave., 7th Floor
New York, NY 10016
212-561-8000

Safeguarding against STDs

Sexually transmitted diseases are the stuff of high school health class filmstrips and locker room jibes, but if you've got one — or suspect that you do — you know that they're no laughing matter. More than just embarrassing and uncomfortable, STDs may lead to serious health conditions, including infertility and mental disorders. Pregnant women with STDs may suffer miscarriage or have children with birth defects. In some cases, STDs may lead to death.

And STDs don't discriminate: They can affect anyone who's exposed, regardless of social status, race, gender, sexual preference, or income. Some 12 million Americans become infected with STDs each year, and about one of every two Americans will become infected at some point in life.

STDs are transmitted through sexual contact. That includes vaginal, as well as oral and anal, intercourse. Some STDs can be transmitted through kissing and touching, too, as well as sharing contaminated needles (usually a risk for intravenous drug users). However, STDs are not spread through contact with toilet seats, door handles, handshakes, or the like: The bacteria and viruses that cause STDs can't live for long outside the body. In addition, some of them require friction to gain entry into the skin and mucous membranes. The skin on the hands and buttocks is not especially susceptible to infection. All these factors make it *highly* unlikely that an STD would spread through such contact.

Recognizing the signs

The symptoms of STDs vary according to the condition, and some have no symptoms at all. But common signs include

✔ Unusual discharge from the penis or vagina

✔ Discharge from the rectum

✔ Sores, lumps, or a rash on the genitals

✔ Pain or burning during urination

✔ Itching around the genitals

Common STDs

Chancroid: A bacterial infection spread through vaginal, anal, and oral intercourse. The primary symptom is a small boil or ulcer on the genitals that develops into an open sore. Untreated, this STD can swell glands in the groin area.

Chlamydia: A bacterial infection spread through vaginal and anal intercourse. It can cause sterility in both men and women and can also lead to arthritis, bladder infections, pelvic inflammation, and ectopic pregnancy. It often has no symptoms. Chlamydia is the most common STD in the United States.

Cytomegalovirus (CMV): A virus transmitted in saliva, semen, blood, vaginal secretions, urine, and breast milk. It's prevalent in infants, causing disability, mental disorders, and blindness in young children. CMV has no cure, although drugs can control symptoms.

Gonorrhea: A bacterium transmitted by vaginal, anal, and oral intercourse. It can cause sterility, arthritis, heart problems, and nervous system disorders, plus stillbirth and premature labor in pregnant women.

Hepatitis B (HBV): A virus transmitted through intimate and sexual contact and intravenous drug use. HBV is very contagious, and it has no cure. In rare cases, HBV causes liver disease and death. A vaccination is available and is recommended for health care workers, people with multiple sex partners, men who have sex with men, IV drug users, and certain international travelers. Unvaccinated teenagers are also encouraged to get the vaccine.

Herpes: Herpes simplex virus (HSV) type-1 is primarily associated with cold sores; type-2 generally affects the genitals, causing a recurring rash of painful, itching blisters. However, the conditions sometimes overlap; HSV-1 may cause genital sores, and HSV-2 may cause cold sores. Both types are spread through contact with open sores. Herpes has no cure, and sores continue to recur over a lifetime, often in response to stress.

Human immunodeficiency virus (HIV): The virus that causes acquired immunodeficiency syndrome (AIDS), a deadly STD for which there is no cure. See Chapter 18 for more on AIDS.

Human papillomavirus (HPV): A group of 60 viruses that cause genital warts and other conditions. It is spread through vaginal and anal intercourse. Some subgroups of HPV are thought to contribute to the development of cervical cancer.

Molluscum contagiosum: A virus spread through vaginal, anal, and oral intercourse. It affects the skin and mucous membrane, causing small pimples on the genitals and thighs.

Syphilis: A bacterium (called a *spirochete*) spread through intimate contact. Syphilis has a number of stages; if left untreated, it can cause damage to the nervous system, heart, brain, and other organs. It can also cause death.

Making it better

If you experience any symptoms of an STD, put aside any embarrassment and see your doctor. STDs call for a practitioner's attention: Some are difficult to diagnose without laboratory or microscopic tests, and if left untreated, serious consequences may arise.

STDs caused by bacteria may be treated with antibiotics. Viral conditions are harder to control and may stay in the body for life, with symptoms flaring up now and again. However, medications are becoming available to help suppress viral symptoms; for example, the drug acyclovir helps suppress herpes outbreaks.

An ounce of prevention

You can't tell by looking at someone whether he or she has an STD, and you may not know if you have one yourself. After all, many STDs don't have symptoms. Plus, many people who know that they have an infection aren't honest with themselves or with their partners and won't admit it. As we said before, STDs don't discriminate — anyone can be affected. For all these reasons, STDs continue to spread.

To keep them from spreading to you, you have two choices: You can practice abstinence and refrain from sex, or you can practice safer sex, which means taking precautions to prevent the spread of infection. Sex is safe when it is between two monogamous partners who have had sex only with each other, or between monogamous partners who have tested negative for STDs.

Outside those circumstances, a latex condom or vaginal pouch should be used correctly and consistently during intercourse to prevent STDs. Stay away from intravenous drugs — contaminated needles can spread disease. And don't be afraid to talk with your partner about the issue of safer sex: If you're intimate enough to have intercourse, you should be able to overcome the embarrassment of talking about condoms.

For more information about sexually transmitted diseases, call one of the following numbers:

- ✔ **National Herpes Hot Line:** 919-361-8488
- ✔ **National STD Hot Line:** 800-227-8922
- ✔ **National AIDS Hot Line:** 800-342-AIDS (Spanish: 800-344-SIDA; hearing-impaired: 800-AIDS-TTY)

Surviving Sexual Dysfunction

Sexual dysfunction refers to a group of disorders that prevent the enjoyment of sex. Stress and psychological factors are the most common reasons for a disorder, but effects of prescription drugs and physical conditions are sometimes responsible, too. The disorder may require treatment, but many times help from a partner and understanding and intimacy between a couple resolve the problem.

Loss of libido

The most common form of sexual dysfunction is a decreased *libido,* or sex drive. First of all, realize that there is no "appropriate" or "normal" amount of sexual desire. Only you can determine the "right" amount, and only you can decide whether you have a sexual desire problem. You may find that you have less sexual desire than your partner, but this doesn't indicate that you have a problem with sexual desire — only that a difference exists in how much sex each of you desires.

When a lowered libido causes problems with sexual satisfaction, it should be treated as a sexual dysfunction. Loss of libido can occur for many reasons — stress, fatigue, the birth of a child, or relationship problems, for example. In addition, a medical condition such as kidney or liver disease may cause it, and the side effects of medications taken for high blood pressure and depression include loss of libido. In a small percentage of men, the levels of the male hormone testosterone drop with age, and with the drop in hormone level comes a drop in sexual desire. In women, hormone fluctuations that affect sex drive may occur with pregnancy, menopause, and the use of oral contraception.

If you think that your libido needs a boost, visit your practitioner to rule out any medical conditions. Although sexual desire changes with age, life circumstances, and the state of a relationship, most decreases in desire pass with time and open communication with your partner. If your problem continues for more than three months and has no physical cause, consult a sex therapist, who can teach you ways to boost your libido.

Discomfort during intercourse

Intercourse should not be painful, although pain can be caused by a wide range of conditions. Physical problems such as sexually transmitted diseases can cause pain, as can emotional factors — guilt or memories of traumatic events such as rape, for example. At times, an inattentive partner or sexual inexperience can contribute to pain.

If you experience painful intercourse, visit your practitioner; it may be a sign of a physical condition. Men may choose to visit a urologist, a specialist in the male reproductive system, while women may choose a gynecologist, a specialist in women's reproductive health.

Erection problems

The health problem that men fear most but are least likely to discuss, let alone admit having, is impotence. This condition involves having trouble getting or keeping an erection, or both. Despite its moniker, impotence has little to do with lack of power — one reason most doctors and therapists now refer to the condition as an erection problem or erectile dysfunction. Although such problems are highly treatable, men too often put off seeing a doctor for erection difficulties.

At least half of all men between ages 40 and 72 have experienced erection problems at one time or another, perhaps because of fatigue or another temporary circumstance. But for at least 20 million American men, the problem is chronic. Those who have high blood pressure, diabetes, or heart disease are four times more likely to suffer erection problems than men without these conditions. Smoking increases the risk of problems even more.

Not in your head: Physical erection problems

Until about 20 years ago, erection problems were thought to be the result of mental or emotional conditions. Now, doctors and therapists know that in 75 to 80 percent of cases, chronic erection problems have a physiologic, or physical, cause. Physical causes can be treated more predictably. Chronic physical erection problems may be caused by one or more of the following:

- **Circulatory problems:** Heart disease and cholesterol buildup in the arteries can restrict blood flow to the penis, making erections difficult.

- **Hormonal imbalances:** Imbalances in hormones such as insulin and testosterone can cause problems.

- **Medications:** Antidepressants and blood pressure drugs, as well as other prescription medications and even many over-the-counter drugs, list erection problems as a possible side effect.

- **Nerve disorders:** Alcoholism or diabetes may damage nerves.

- **Trauma:** Pelvic trauma caused by events that seem harmless enough, such as a fall during sports or a long ride on an uncomfortable bike seat, may be responsible for erection problems.

The mind-body connection: Psychological erection problems

Twenty to 25 percent of erection problems have a psychological or psychogenic cause rather than a physical one. This doesn't mean that the problem is "only in your head." It means that what's in your head is causing a problem that affects your penis.

Fear of performance failure is probably the most common cause of psychogenic erection problems. This can be a vicious cycle: A temporary erection problem makes you self-conscious; you start to worry that the problem is not temporary, and the worry itself causes the problem again. Other factors that may trigger psychogenic erection problems are low self-esteem, depression, premature ejaculation, marital difficulties, and a history of sexual abuse.

Even stress can cause erection problems. Seek treatment if the problem persists, and use relaxation and time-management techniques to control stress that interferes with your sexual functioning.

Making it better

Experts recommend seeking treatment for erection problems if they persist for more than five weeks. The specialist who treats erection problems is a urologist. The doctor takes a thorough medical history, looking for signs of problems such as heart disease and diabetes, and may even measure blood pressure in the penis to evaluate blood flow and determine whether a circulation problem exists. The doctor also asks a lot of detailed questions about your sex life. Answer openly and honestly. Erection failure that starts suddenly is most likely psychogenic, whereas problems that build slowly probably have physiologic causes.

Depending on your history, the doctor may order tests. Some of these tests help determine whether the problem has its base in physical or psychological conditions. Another test checks for nerve damage to the penis itself.

In the past decade, great strides have been made in treating physiological erection failure. Erection problems are usually relieved when the underlying physical condition is treated, although in some cases (such as with diabetes), the damage may be irreversible. Your urologist can review with you and your partner the treatment that's most appropriate for you. In most cases, you should try the least invasive treatment first.

The following are the current medical treatment options available:

- **Bypass:** If blood flow to the penis has become blocked, surgery may be done to reroute the vessels around the blockage.

- **Hormonal treatments:** In a small number of cases (about 5 percent), testosterone replacement — through either monthly injections or a patch worn on the skin — solves erection problems.

- **Implants:** This treatment involves surgically implanting either a semi-rigid, bendable rod or an inflatable tube into the penis. With the rod implant, the penis is always rigid, and the implant is noticeable. With the inflatable device, a pump is surgically placed in the scrotum, and inflatable tubes are placed in the penis. When an erection is desired, the pump is squeezed and the tubes are filled with a gel, causing an erection.

- **Injection therapy:** This treatment involves injecting a drug into the base of the penis.

- **Oral medications:** The U.S. Food and Drug Administration recently approved an oral drug called sildenafil (brand name Viagra) for erection problems. The drug is expected to become one of the all-time best-selling drugs on the market.

✔ **Topical drugs:** Early tests of a three-drug cream applied to the penis to create an erection have been promising, but additional testing must be done before the drug becomes available.

✔ **Vacuum devices:** In this treatment, a small, sealed vacuum pump is used to draw blood into the penis before intercourse.

Premature ejaculation

Who decides whether an ejaculation is premature? You and your partner. If an ejaculation happens before it's desired, then it's premature. This problem is most common among younger men who are overeager or anxious about their sexual performance. Rarely is premature ejaculation due to a physical problem. Mainly, it's a matter of learning control.

Reliable medications aren't available for this problem, but a number of nonmedical techniques may work. Condoms may be worn to decrease sensitivity and delay orgasm. Masturbation to orgasm before intercourse may help as well, because a second erection usually lasts longer than a first. Some experts recommend squeezing the tip or base of the penis for several seconds just before orgasm. This "squeeze technique" softens the erection slightly, and sexual stimulation can be continued. A sex therapist may be able to teach you other techniques to delay ejaculation.

Retarded ejaculation

This is the opposite of a premature ejaculation: That is, when you want to achieve orgasm, you can't. Ejaculation is delayed or never happens. This condition can be frustrating, cause physical discomfort, and make you lose interest in sex.

Seeking counseling

Counseling is virtually mandatory for erection problems, no matter what their cause. Even the most loving couple experiences great stress during a period without intercourse, and they must understand that resuming sexual relations is also rather stressful, especially if it involves the use of injections or devices.

Counseling focuses on communication between partners. Exercises in communication can help solve relationship problems, restore self-esteem, and relieve negative emotions that may be contributing to erection problems. Therapy may also include exercises in lovemaking that are designed to improve sexual function, relieve performance anxiety, and improve sexual communication.

Men with retarded ejaculation often brag about how long they can have intercourse without achieving orgasm. However, if you can't have an orgasm when you want — and we don't mean that you're refraining from orgasm in order to please a partner; that's a different situation — you may want to visit a sex therapist for treatment.

For more information about handling erection problems, contact these organizations:

✔ American Association of Sex Educators, Counselors and Therapists
P. O. Box 238
Mount Vernon, IA 52314-0238

✔ Impotence Information Center
10700 Bren Road W.
Minnetonka, MN 55343
800-328-3881

Coping with Infertility

Infertility is defined as the inability to conceive after a year of unprotected intercourse. About 40 percent of fertility problems are found in the woman, and another 40 percent are found in the man. The remaining 20 percent are caused by both partners or are unexplained.

The cause of infertility in men usually can be traced to the sperm, the microscopic cells contained in the semen that penetrate the woman's egg to cause pregnancy. Sperm may be malformed, may be slow swimmers, or may not be abundant enough.

A problem with the reproductive system, such as a blocked tube or an erection problem, may keep sperm from reaching its intended destination. A *variocele,* a varicose vein within the testicles, may lower sperm counts because the collection of blood increases the temperature within the glands, which kills the sperm. Injury to the testicles, infection, hormonal imbalances, and physical and chromosomal problems all may contribute to male infertility.

Infertility in women can be caused by any number of factors, ranging from blocked fallopian tubes or a problem with the shape or lining of the uterus to antibodies in the cervical mucus and problems with ovulation. Hormonal imbalances, thyroid disorders, and conditions such as diabetes may also contribute.

Knowing for sure

Diagnosing infertility in men is much simpler, less invasive, and less expensive than diagnosing it in women, so start there when a problem arises. The main way to diagnose male infertility is through a sperm analysis. The sperm are collected and analyzed for speed, number, and shape.

In women, infertility can be diagnosed through

- ✔ Urine and blood tests
- ✔ Pelvic exam
- ✔ Endometrial biopsy (in which a sample of the uterine lining is taken and examined)
- ✔ Hysterosalpingogram (in which dye is injected into the uterus to highlight the organ as X-rays are taken)
- ✔ Laparoscopy (in which a fiber-optic viewing scope is inserted through a small incision in the abdomen)
- ✔ Hysteroscopy (in which a fiber-optic viewing scope is inserted through the vagina into the uterus)

These tests check for hormonal imbalances, problems with ovulation, abnormalities of the uterus or fallopian tubes, scar tissue, or any blockages of the reproductive system.

Making it better

Infertility usually requires treatment by a specialist. For men, this specialist is a urologist, who specializes in the male reproductive system. A gynecologist is the specialist for women. Women may also choose to see a reproductive endocrinologist, a doctor who focuses on female hormonal and infertility problems.

Traditional treatments

In men, hormonal treatments may be prescribed if levels are unusually low. Any sexually transmitted infections or sexual dysfunction that contributes to infertility is treated as well. Surgery may also be recommended to remove a varicocele. In this procedure, the vein is tied off or opened. Surgery can also open blockages within the epididymis or vas deferens.

Women have much the same options. Hormonal treatments may be used to regulate menstruation and prompt ovulation. If the fallopian tubes are blocked, they may be able to be opened surgically. Scar tissue may also be removed with surgery. Again, any STDs should be treated accordingly.

Advanced treatments

Modern technology has brought pregnancy to new levels in the form of advanced infertility treatments. Artificial insemination, in vitro insemination, and embryo transfer are three methods of causing pregnancy when traditional infertility treatments fail.

✔ In *artificial insemination,* a donor (usually the woman's partner or an anonymous donor) provides a sample of sperm, which is prepared in a way that concentrates the healthiest, strongest sperm. The sample is placed within the cervix, and the sperm go forth to do their thing. Artificial insemination is the easiest and least expensive advanced procedure.

✔ Women whose fallopian tubes are blocked but whose ovaries still function have the option of *in vitro fertilization,* literally "fertilization in glass." In this procedure, drugs are used to stimulate the ovaries to release several eggs. The eggs are collected in a minor surgical procedure and then placed in a glass dish, along with sperm from a partner or donor, where they are fertilized. Then the fertilized eggs are inserted into the uterus, where it is hoped that they will plant themselves and grow. In a variation on this procedure, the eggs may be collected, mixed with sperm, and reinserted into the fallopian tubes, where it is hoped that fertilization will occur in its natural environment, so to speak.

✔ A woman who cannot conceive but who can carry a pregnancy to term may choose *embryo transfer,* in which an egg provided by a surrogate is fertilized with a partner's or donor's sperm and then implanted into the woman's uterus.

Advanced fertility treatments are not for everyone. Infertility is a highly emotional issue, and advanced methods of achieving pregnancy are, too. The procedures are expensive, complicated, and sometimes painful, and they're not guaranteed to work, so couples need to prepare themselves for possible failure. To complicate matters further, methods may involve hormonal treatments, which cause wild mood swings. Moral issues may arise as well — for example, concerns about the use of anonymous donor sperm. Counseling is available for those who seek it.

For more information about dealing with reproductive problems, contact these organizations:

✔ American Society for Reproductive Medicine
1209 Montgomery Hwy.
Birmingham, AL 35216-2809
205-978-5000
www.asrm.com

✔ RESOLVE
1310 Broadway
Somerville, MA 02144
617-623-1156
www.resolve.org

Part VI
The Part of Tens

The 5th Wave   By Rich Tennant

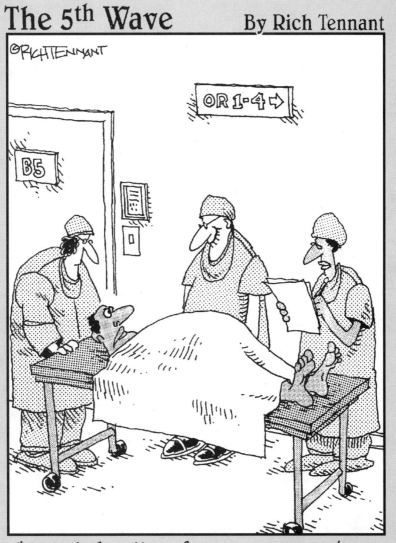

"Included with today's surgery, we're offering a manicure, pedicure, haircut, and ear wax flush for just $49.95."

In this part . . .

David Letterman wows audiences nightly with his Top Ten Lists. His lists tell you everything from the top ten ways to eat peanut butter and jelly to the top ten worst Halloween costumes. We give you more practical information in our top ten lists, but we still have the wow factor. We tell you ten easy ways to improve your health, ten questions to ask your parents about your past health (it affects you more than you may know!), and ten ways to make the most of your money in medical matters.

Chapter 20

Ten Things You Can Do Today to Improve Your Family's Health

. . . .

In This Chapter

▶ Keeping illness at bay

▶ Protecting your family from injury

▶ Incorporating health into everyday life

. . . .

*O*n a stereotypical day in family life, you rise early, get the kids ready for school, and pack off to work for eight hours of whatever you do to earn your keep. Later, at home, you put dinner on the table, the dishes in the dishwasher, the laundry down the chute, and the kids in the bunk beds before tucking in your own tired self. Where, you ask, can you find room for health in this routine?

Fortunately, boosting health doesn't take as much time as you may think. In fact, just a few tweaks to your regular routine can mean better health for your entire family. In this chapter, we tell you about some adjustments that you can make right now.

Wash your hands regularly

If, like some sort of bizarro superhero, you had microscopic vision, you would be able to see the microorganisms on all the surfaces around you: telephones, toys, every doorknob you pass. You'd also be able to see how they've set up housekeeping on your skin: growing, feeding, and dying right under (and on and around) your very nose.

Before you panic, though, let us tell you that most of these organisms are harmless — and some are even necessary to your health. But those that aren't benign can make the rounds easily enough, and the hands help them do their dirty work by picking up microorganisms and passing them on to other people. You might consider the hands to be a form of public transportation for germs.

Having everyone in the family wash their hands on a regular basis — and especially after using the bathroom and before meals — helps prevent the spread of infectious illness. We're not just talking about colds and flu. Chicken pox, measles, mumps, and a host of other conditions spread through hand-to-hand contact. Plus, the bacteria that may cling to the hands after you use the bathroom can lead to especially nasty *e. coli* infections. (And studies show that about one-third of adults in the United States don't wash after using a public restroom.)

Does handwashing work? Experts say yes. One four-month study of elementary school kids found that students who washed their hands four times a day had fewer stomachaches, colds, and flu episodes than kids who were allowed to do as they pleased.

For best results, you need to do more than just run your hands under the faucet. Lather up and rub your hands together for a minute or two. Make sure to get the areas under your fingernails, between your fingers, and on the backs of your hands. Then rinse your hands thoroughly. If you wear rings, make sure to wash well around and underneath them: They give germs a place to hide. Finally, dry off thoroughly on a clean hand towel. Hand towels should be washed regularly to keep bacteria from hanging around. To be extra safe, use disposable towels.

When washing, you may want to use antibacterial soap, which is said to kill germs better than ordinary soap and even to inhibit the growth of bacteria after you dry off. However, some researchers worry that the product will make the bacteria that it doesn't eliminate even stronger, contributing to antibiotic resistance.

Drive slower

As the driver of a car, *you* are responsible for the safety of your passengers. And it's a simple fact: Drivers who exceed the speed limit have more accidents than those who obey the law. In 1996, the most recent year for which statistics exist, speeding was a factor in 30 percent of all fatal crashes, says the U.S. Department of Transportation. Also in 1996:

- ✔ 12,998 lives were lost because of speeding.
- ✔ 624,000 people received minor injuries in speed-related crashes.
- ✔ 41,000 people received critical injuries in speed-related crashes.

Do yourself and your family a favor by sticking to the speed limit and adjusting your speed to road conditions. You may get there a little later, but you'll get there in one piece.

Take a breather

Good things happen to your body when you relax. Your muscles become less tense, and your alpha (or relaxed) brain waves increase. Your heart and breathing rates slow down. Your metabolism slows, and your digestive system cuts back on the amount of acid it's secreting. Your brain steps up production of feel-good hormones called *endorphins*.

Fortunately, you don't have to escape to a tropical island to unwind; you can practice a relaxation technique. Granted, a relaxation strategy isn't quite as enticing as a vacation, but it can boost your health with only one or two 10- to 15-minute sessions every day.

Techniques range from mediation and visualization (imagining yourself on that tropical island, for example) to aromatherapy and hydrotherapy (taking a warm, scented bath). We talk about these methods and others in Chapter 2. Many books with more specifics are available at your local library.

The important thing to remember is that there's a distinction between relaxing and doing nothing. The health benefits of these techniques come only when you reach a state of true relaxation — not a state of boredom.

Apply sunscreen

How does sunscreen pop up on a list of daily activities? Isn't it just for days at the beach or the amusement park? Nope. Sunscreen is important all the time. Ninety percent of sun exposure comes from everyday outdoor activity. And sunburns can occur even on cool and cloudy days — and even in the shade if light reflects off water, sand, or snow.

The problem of sunburn, and even suntans, goes beyond the temporary pain of lobster-red skin. Sun damage contributes to wrinkles, age spots, and sagging skin, as well as skin cancer.

Both sunblock and sunscreen protect the skin; they just do it in slightly different ways. Sunblock reflects the sun's rays off the skin; sunscreen absorbs the harmful rays. When choosing a product, look for one marked *broad-spectrum*. That term indicates that the product repels both ultraviolet A (UVA) and ultraviolet B (UVB) wavelengths of light. At one time, experts thought that only UVB rays were harmful; now, it is known that both forms cause damage.

You also want to read the label if you have sensitive skin. A common sunblock ingredient, para-aminobenzoic acid (or PABA), can trigger allergic reactions. To prevent problems, look for products labeled *PABA-free*. In addition, put the product on a small patch of skin before applying it all over, and then wait an hour or two to see whether a reaction develops. If the sunblock fails this test, switch to another brand.

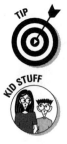

Apply sunscreen liberally to all exposed skin 15 to 30 minutes before you go outside; the delay gives the product time to be absorbed into the skin for maximum effectiveness.

Kids need sunscreen, too. Children and teens who get sunburns or blisters are more likely to get skin cancer later in life. However, do not apply sunscreen to babies under six months of age because the chemicals can be easily absorbed into the child's system. Ask your pediatrician about using sunscreen on young children.

Spend time with your pets

Sure, Lassie saved Timmy every time he fell into a well. But what can your dog (or cat, or hamster, or lizard, for that matter) do to boost your family's health? Quite a bit, say experts.

A study by Johns Hopkins Medical Center, for example, found that 50 out of 53 people with pets were alive a year after their first heart attacks, while only 17 of 39 people without pets survived the year. At the University of California at Los Angeles, a 12-month study of Medicare enrollees showed that the one-third of subjects who owned pets visited their doctors less often than the pet-free group did. And that's not all. A study from the State University of New York at Buffalo found that elderly women with pets, but no human companionship, had significantly lower blood pressure than elderly women who lived alone without pets. Plus, older women with pets had blood pressure nearly as low as young women with family and friends around.

All these statistics imply that pets are great stress-relievers, and — as Chapter 2 tells you — the more relaxed you are, the better your health tends to be. Stress taxes the body's systems by boosting heart and breathing rates, and it also depresses the immune system, leaving you more open to infection or disease.

So take a few minutes out of your day to spend with your favorite pet. Toss the tennis ball around with the dog, tease the cat with a piece of string, or just sit and stare at the graceful tropical fish in your aquarium. If you have an outdoorsy pet (we're thinking dog, mainly, but with llamas and pigs out there as pets now, we don't want to limit you), you can double your relaxation and better your health by taking your pet for a walk or run or by playing an energetic game of Frisbee or the like. Exercise energizes and tones the body and also helps get rid of stressful impulses (clenched teeth, for example).

If you don't have a pet, consider getting one. However, choose wisely: Taking care of a rambunctious puppy could very well cause more stress than the dog will relieve.

Get your family on the move

The family that plays together stays together, right? That family is also probably very healthy, too. Guidelines say that everyone — kids included — should get at least 30 minutes of continuous exercise on most, if not all, days of the week for maximum health. Follow these tips to help make family exercise fun:

- ✔ **Practice togetherness.** Choose group activities such as hiking, swimming, or cross-country skiing. And don't leave out the older generation: Exercise is especially helpful for seniors.

- ✔ **Pick something that's satisfying for everyone.** Small children can get frustrated with games and activities that are too complex, and older kids can get bored just as easily with simpler fare. Choose an activity that everyone enjoys.

- ✔ **Don't exercise just for exercise's sake.** Instead of dragging the family out for a lap around the block, invite them for a neighborhood nature walk. Or teach them to dance instead of pushing an aerobics video.

- ✔ **Involve friends.** Have your children invite their friends and classmates for a bowling or skating party or camping trip to make exercise a social event.

Change your perspective on dinner

The U.S. Department of Agriculture's Food Guide Pyramid (see Chapter 2) is all well and good, but most people don't take it to heart when preparing meals for their families. Americans have a love affair with protein: We plop down a big piece of meat or fish, beans, or eggs and back it up with a few spoonfuls of potatoes or broccoli or flavored rice.

To boost your family's health, start thinking of your main dish as a side dish and vice versa. All those proteins rank high on the food pyramid, meaning that you should eat less of them than of vegetables, grains, rice, and breads, all of which rank in lower, larger tiers.

To figure out how your plate should be divided, picture it as a typical pie chart. Devote about a quarter of it to your traditional "main-dish" protein. Then fill up the rest with low-fat vegetables and grains.

Turn off the television or computer

A study published recently in *The Journal of the American Medical Association* reported a relationship between the amount of television children watch and how fat they are. Specifically, researchers found that boys and girls who watch four or more hours of television each day have greater body fat and a greater body mass index than those who watch fewer than two hours per day.

Of course, you don't need rocket science to tell you that if your kids are watching Nickelodeon or surfing the Net, they're not getting the exercise they need. (The same goes for adults!) Another complicating factor is food. In plenty of households, snacking and watching television are inseparable activities. So if you turn off the tube, you also encourage better eating habits.

Brush and floss

Do you take good care of your teeth and gums? If not, you're neglecting one of the simplest tasks that can boost your health. Brushing and flossing — although widely regarded as chores — prevent the development of tooth decay and gum disease, which can cause problems ranging from bad breath to tooth loss. And these activities take a measly three minutes twice a day. If you don't do it already, make brushing and flossing part of your daily routine.

Encourage (that is, force) your kids to brush and floss, too! Although national statistics show that children's dental heath is improving, 50 percent of kids still get cavities in their permanent teeth.

Go to sleep early

Sleep is as important to your health as nutrition and exercise are. Despite the fact that 98 percent of Americans agree with that statement, says the National Sleep Foundation, one of every three Americans sleeps 6 hours or less a night during the work week. The average American gets about 7 hours of sleep a night — the low end of the 7-to-9-hour stint that experts say the average person needs. (Babies, by the way, need 18 hours; children need 10 to 12 hours; teens need 10 hours; and seniors need 8 hours.)

We all know the truth in the statement "There aren't enough hours in the day." So we turn to those hours during the night, when we should be in bed, to finish what we need to get done, and we're aided by ingenious inventions ranging from the electric light to all-night grocery stores.

To improve your health, stop thinking of sleep as a luxury and make an honest attempt to get a good night's sleep — even if it means not catching the end of *Late Night with David Letterman* or waiting until morning to finish the laundry.

Chapter 21

Ten Ways to Make the Most of Your Doctor Visit

● ●

▶ Preparing for your visit
▶ Using your time effectively
▶ Holding your own with your doctor

● ●

*E*xperts say that doctor-patient communication leaves a lot to be desired. Too often, doctors rush patients through examinations, one hand on the doorknob, one eye on the wristwatch. Too often, they speak in terms that their patients don't understand. And too often, they don't really listen to their patients' concerns. Studies even show that doctors spend a mere 18 seconds listening to their patients before interrupting with a question.

Consumers aren't innocent, either. They devote their precious office time to vague and half-remembered symptoms. They rattle on about subjects unrelated to their health, jump from complaint to complaint, or plague doctors with personal theories of what may be wrong. They leave the doctor's office with unanswered questions, confused about their condition but embarrassed or afraid to admit that they don't understand.

To get the information that you need to make the best decisions possible for your family's health, you need to bridge this communication gap and make the most of every moment you have with your doctor. The tips in this chapter are designed to do just that.

Keep track of everyday health

Symptoms are often the keys to finding out what's wrong with you. To help your doctor help you better, keep track of your health between visits. It may seem like unnecessary drudgery, but if you give your physician information quickly and accurately, you get more out of your office visit.

Your best bet is to keep a small notebook handy in which to record symptoms, when they occur, and under what circumstances. For example, if you're having heartburn, does it come on after a spicy dinner, when you're lying down, or first thing in the morning? Where do you feel the pain? Is it mild, moderate, or severe? Is it a sharp pain, a burning pain, or an ache? How often do you get it, and how long does it last? You get the idea. Write down as many details as possible, and then share them with your doctor. You can even make a copy of your notes for the office medical records.

Keeping track of your children's health issues in a notebook is a good idea, too. For an infant, jot down developmental milestones, such as when your baby first rolled over, responded to your voice, or sat upright without your help. For older kids, record any injuries or over-the-counter medications being used. Keep track of eating habits, bathroom habits, and, of course, any symptoms or complaints. When you take your child in for a visit, your doctor will quiz you on these matters, so you can save time (which is precious during a ten-minute visit) and get more information across because you have it all at your fingertips. A notebook ensures accuracy, too, because you don't have to count on your memory (although we're sure that it's outstanding).

Do your homework

If you have an existing condition, asking logical and informed questions about it during an office visit will help you become a major partner in your health care decisions.

Try to read up a little bit about your condition before you see your doctor. Don't neglect to take advantage of a free service right in your own community: the public library. If you haven't discovered all the resources, ingenuity, and helpfulness that a reference librarian has to offer, then by all means do so. Even if you live in a small community with a modest library — one with a limited catalog of medical and health books — interlibrary loan is always available. In addition, hospitals often let people use their medical libraries.

A word of caution, however, about health information in cyberspace: Be careful of the sources of information. Because the Internet is essentially a large bulletin board without supervision, anybody can put any kind of information on it. That means that you must determine whether the information you read is valid, sound, and worthy of your consideration.

Make a list

Who hasn't left a doctor's office at least once without thinking, "Oh, wait! What about . . . ?" To avoid wanting to kick yourself after the visit, think *before* you go to the doctor. Make a list of all the questions and concerns you want to ask the doctor while you're there. A list keeps you from being distracted from the task at hand, helps you remember all your concerns, and organizes your thoughts so that you can be sure to get all your questions answered.

Don't be afraid to pull out the list and fire away after you have your doctor's attention. If a doctor seems agitated about your questions or the fact that you have a list, explain how important it is that you understand what's going on. Also note that, ultimately, you must make your own medical decisions, and the only way that you can do so is with information. Your list is a valuable tool in getting that information. If your doctor simply refuses to respect you and your wishes, consider finding a new doctor who will.

Anticipate your doctor's requests

When making your doctor's appointment, be sure to ask what's expected of you and plan ahead. For example, don't go to the bathroom before your appointment if you know a urine sample will be requested. If you're having a blood sample taken, find out whether you will be able to eat beforehand — some tests require that you fast for a certain number of hours in preparation. You may also want to wear short sleeves if your blood pressure will be taken—or shorts if your knees are going to be examined.

Keep in mind, too, that some medications interfere with test results or mask symptoms. A drug might increase your blood pressure, for example. And taking an over-the-counter cold medication before you visit your practitioner might relieve your sniffles, but it might also affect your diagnosis. So again, when you make your appointment, alert the office to the medications you're using and ask whether any of them might interfere with your visit.

Call ahead

Just as a savvy traveler calls the airport to see whether a flight is on time, you can save a lot of time (and money if you must take time off from work) by calling your doctor's office the day of your appointment to see whether they're running on schedule. If you see your doctor regularly, ask the receptionist to call *you* if appointments are running late. Doing so enables you to adjust your schedule or change the appointment if necessary.

Bring a friend or family member

Going to the doctor can be an intimidating experience. Not only are you likely to be sick and far from your best when you visit, but you may also be worried about what could be wrong. For these reasons, take another set of ears along with you when you visit the doctor. When you're nervous, you're more likely to miss something important that the doctor says. A friend or family member can also verify what the doctor has said and ask questions that you are too upset to ask.

If your doctor or a nurse gives you a hard time about your companion, explain that you need that person's assistance. If the doctor absolutely forbids you to bring your companion into the office, think about finding another doctor.

Remember, though, that just as you may want to have someone along during an appointment, you can go alone if you want. Think about whether you'd be afraid or embarrassed to be examined or answer questions in front of another person. Some doctors discourage "guests" during visits because they fear that their patients won't tell the whole truth. Some practitioners, for example, sometimes don't allow partners into gynecological examinations so that women can be honest about issues such as sexual habits and domestic violence.

If you can't take someone along you with or you wish to go alone, think about taking a tape recorder instead to make sure that you hear and understand everything the doctor says.

Stick to the subject

We're sure that your doctor loves to hear about your cat, your job, and the thousands of details about your life, but to get the most from the few minutes you have in the doctor's office, focus on communicating your health concerns. After a few formalities, get right down to business by relating your symptoms. Also resist the temptation to speculate on what you think is wrong with you; leave that to the professional in the room. Most doctors with tight schedules (which is all of them, these days) appreciate straightforward patients and take them seriously.

One caveat here: We're not saying that your doctor should know nothing about you personally; we're merely saying that you shouldn't ramble on. Lifestyle and environment are many times intertwined with health concerns. For example, constant headaches may be caused by a chemical in the home or workplace; or a stressful situation such as a divorce could contribute to back pain. If you think that a personal situation may relate to your health condition, certainly relate it to your doctor!

Ask for a translation

During office visits, doctors often lapse into medi-speak — their own technical language of medical terms and phrases. You may be told about your risk of *myocardial infarction* (heart attack), *cerebrovascular accident* (stroke), or *syncope* (fainting), for example. Or you may be told to take your medication *postprandial* (after a meal).

In their defense, physicians' training drills this language into them — it becomes second nature, and they may not even realize that you don't understand. So it's up to you to make sure that you do. If your doc hits you with a term that you're not familiar with, ask for a definition. Don't be afraid of embarrassing yourself or having your doctor think less of you. You're taking a much greater risk if you leave the office not understanding your physician's instructions.

You may also want to check out Appendix A for a rundown of common medical terms, and Appendix B for help with common medical abbreviations.

Say "no" if you don't understand

Somewhere in the course of history, doctors took on something of a godlike status. As a result, patients are often too willing to go along with whatever their doctors say, even if they're not quite sure what that means.

Don't fall into that trap. Doctors exist to serve you, the consumer. If you don't understand a test, treatment, or procedure that's recommended to you, don't submit to it! You should be able to answer four questions about any treatment that your doctor recommends before you agree to it:

- ✔ What is the purpose of this test/procedure/medication?
- ✔ How will it help my condition?
- ✔ Are there less costly and equally safe alternatives to what is proposed?
- ✔ What are the possible side effects, and what is the likelihood that a side effect will occur?

Don't let yourself be intimidated by comments such as, "Who's the doctor here?" or "It's to make you better." You have a right to know what's going to happen to you. Every test or procedure costs you money, not to mention time and possible discomfort.

Update your medical record

At home after your trip to the doctor, take a few minutes to write down what went on while it's fresh in your mind. You should record the reason for the visit, what the doctor did and said, the results of any tests that were taken (including routine tests such as blood pressure and weight measurements), what treatments were recommended or prescribed, doctor's instructions, and any comments that you have. If a friend or family member went along with you, ask that person to review your notes to make sure that you didn't leave anything out or make any mistakes. If you used a tape recorder, listen to the tape of the visit again.

Add your notes to your medical record to keep it as up-to-date as possible. Not only is it wise to have such a record for the long-term, but it helps in the short-term, too, to refresh your memory whenever you need it. ("Did the doctor say to take two pills once a day or one pill twice a day?") If you don't have a medical record, turn to Chapter 3 for information about creating one.

Chapter 22

Ten Ways to Stretch Your Medical Dollar

• •

• •

Clipping coupons, comparison shopping, and searching for bargains are all part of family life. Why not apply your price-savvy tactics to health care, too? As a smart medical consumer, never forget that health care is a business. In fact, it's the largest business in the United States. In this chapter, we offer advice on how to get your money's worth from the medical system — and maybe some freebies, too.

Negotiate charges and fees

People should haggle with car dealers and flea market vendors, not their doctors, right? Wrong. The truth is, most doctors will adjust their standard fees for patients with limited incomes or special circumstances. Of course, doctors don't usually admit that they negotiate fees, but in fact, doctors negotiate fees all the time — with insurance companies. Every time a doctor contracts with an insurance company, that doctor is allowing someone else to set the price of services. And today, with so many doctors available and comparatively few patients, doctors may be eager to negotiate fees to keep your business.

Here's the strategy: If a fee seems too high or is more than you can pay, tell your doctor. Say that you feel the fee is wrong or that you can't afford the cost, and then ask if the fee can be lowered in your case or if other arrangements can be made. If you've been seeing the physician for many years, use your loyal patronage as leverage. A doctor's financial security over the long haul is based on your repeat business.

You might also try negotiating a fee for a particular problem. For example, a typical child's ear infection calls for two doctor's office visits: one to prescribe an antibiotic and one for a quick glance-in-the-ear follow-up to make sure that the drug is working. Instead of paying for two office visits, ask if the fee for the second visit can be waived if all is well with your child.

Or if you get weekly allergy shots, negotiate a fee that includes only the cost of the shot and not the cost of the office visit. Same goes for routine blood pressure checks: Negotiate a low fee — say, $5 — instead of the standard charge.

Even if you have insurance, negotiating fees pays off — for your insurance company directly, and for you indirectly. The more money you save your insurance company, the less likely it is that your premiums will increase in the future.

Get to know your doctor's office staff

The people on a physician's staff, for the most part, control what goes on in the doctor's office, so become familiar with them. If you know who does what, you can seek out the right person to answer your question, make an emergency appointment for you, or solve your billing problem. This advice goes for office nursing staff as well. Patients generally are not charged for brief consultations with the office nurse, by phone or in person.

Look for free and low-cost community services

For free or inexpensive immunizations, flu shots, simple screening tests, vision and hearing checks, cholesterol tests, and the like, keep an eye open for health promotions in your area. Clinics, your local health department, and nearby hospitals are likely sponsors, as they work to boost community health and awareness.

You can also find bargain services at local health fairs. During these events, hospitals or clinics invite people in to check out the place, all the while showing off the latest, top-of-the-line equipment. Along the way, you find free health screenings and other services.

Although it's great of them to give away their services, hospitals that sponsor health fairs have ulterior motives. Most health fairs are pure marketing, designed to attract new customers. Today, more than ever, hospitals are competing for patients, so you need to discern whether a particular hospital really cares about your health or is trying to make a buck.

Also, by giving away screening tests at fairs, hospitals figure that they get to treat whatever they find to be wrong with you (and reap whatever profit comes with that). If you have a test or service performed by a hospital or clinic, keep a record of the results and follow up with your own physician as soon as possible if a problem is found.

Test-drive your drugs

Physicians regularly receive samples of prescription and over-the-counter medications from pharmaceutical company representatives hoping to make sales. Ask your doctor to pass on some of these samples to you — especially if you're just beginning a new prescription. That way, you can "test-drive" a drug to make sure that it works for you. You can make sure that it doesn't cause any nasty side effects before you spend the money on a one-month supply of the stuff.

If getting samples from your physician isn't an option, turn to your pharmacist. Some pharmacists are willing to fill a new prescription only partially, giving you a one- or two-day supply to check for side effects. If all is well, you can pick up and pay for the remainder of the prescription the next day.

And one more thing: Many drug companies offer free or reduced-price drugs for those who need them but can't afford them. To find out whether a manufacturer has such a program in place for a drug you need, ask your doctor or pharmacist.

Bring your own medications and vitamins to the hospital

Everyone knows that candy costs three times more at the movie theater than at the supermarket, and few of us are above stashing a Milky Way in a coat pocket to savor during the feature presentation. Unfortunately, such markups are not unique to the cineplex. Hospitals are notorious for their astronomical drug prices. For example, a Motrin in the hospital costs a consumer $4, although the hospital's cost is only 15 cents. That's a markup of 2,667 percent!

The solution? Bring your own — an especially good idea if you take a number of medications and vitamins on a daily basis and intend to keep to your regimen while in the hospital. Prior to your hospital stay, tell your doctor that you want to bring your own medications and vitamins with you, and make sure that your condition doesn't call for care that will change your regimen. When you get to the hospital, make arrangements with the staff to store your supplies until you need them. Mark everything with your vital information and, in all cases, make sure that you get what's yours.

"Brown-bagging" your hospital stay may take some doing — hospitals don't like you to bring your own any more than movie theaters do. But if you stand your ground, you're likely to get your way. Make sure, too, that you're not charged for what you're not getting. If possible, meet with a hospital administrator and get approval for your plan put into writing.

Donate blood

In recent years, blood supplies around the world have dwindled. For example, someone in the United States needs a unit of blood nearly every two seconds. Each year, 12 million units are transfused to more than 4 million people.

You can do a good deed *and* stretch your medical dollar by adding your own blood to the stockpile. A number of blood banks offer insurance coverage for blood supplies to donors (and sometimes their families) in exchange for a certain number of donations each year. In other words, if you give blood, you can get what you need for free should the need arise.

Join an ambulance service

For a small yearly donation, volunteer and private ambulance companies offer unlimited services to families in their areas. Ambulance service is a pretty good deal. You get to support health care in your community, and you also get a free ride to the emergency room if necessary — no small peanuts, considering that ambulance rides cost hundreds of dollars and often aren't covered by insurance.

In most cases, you're required to use that specific ambulance company, which may not always be possible, depending on availability and the number of companies servicing your area. Some companies, however, reciprocate with other local services, picking up each other's patients. Be sure to find out whom you should call in an emergency to receive covered service.

Borrow medical equipment when possible

Crutches, adjustable beds, and blood pressure monitors are all examples of medical equipment. If you're recovering from an injury or surgery and need a piece of equipment for only a short period of time, think about borrowing it. After all, why should you invest in something that you (hopefully) will never need again after you've healed?

Most home health aids can be borrowed from community organizations; call your local home health organization or visiting nurse association. If borrowing medical equipment isn't possible, try renting. Medical equipment companies and many local pharmacies rent equipment. Shop around for the best price.

Purchasing equipment is your best bet in two situations, however: first, if the equipment is needed indefinitely, and second, if your insurance company will cover the cost.

Make a living will

A living will is a document that informs your family and medical personnel of your wishes concerning medical care if you are unable to make your wishes known yourself. Most often, a living will limits the types of care you receive if you are facing a terminal stage of illness. For example, you may request not to be put on an automatic ventilator or another artificial life-sustaining treatment.

End-of-life care is extremely expensive — more than 50 percent of medical costs are incurred in the last five days of life. If you know that you don't want to undergo life-sustaining procedures or treatment, a living will can help save your family money by giving them a tool with which to call off the host of doctors and staff who are going to try to save you. By law, every hospital must ask you whether you have a living will or another such document that can be followed if the circumstances arise.

If you have a living will, make sure to discuss it with your family and your doctors, and make sure that all these people have a copy of the document.

For more information about living wills, turn to Chapter 12, or contact Choice in Dying, 200 Varick St., New York, NY, 10014; 800-989-WILL.

Avoid weekend hospital admissions

Don't allow yourself to be admitted to the hospital on a nonemergency basis on a Friday. You will simply languish, expensively and in no particular comfort, until Monday. Most laboratories that perform diagnostic workups don't do those things on weekends. Only basic care is performed on weekends, so a weekend admission means one or two extra days in the hospital — at your expense.

Wait until Monday — or better yet, Tuesday, some experts say. By Tuesday, the hospital is back in gear after the weekend.

Appendix A
Glossary of Medical Terms

Acquired immunodeficiency syndrome (AIDS): A condition that develops after the human immunodeficiency virus has sufficiently destroyed the immune system. It is marked by a series of opportunistic infections (infections caused by viruses or germs that are usually not harmful to people) and eventually ends in death.

Adhesion: Scar tissue that forms after infection or surgery.

Adjuvant therapy: Therapy used in conjunction with another treatment to ensure its success.

Adverse reaction: A reaction to a drug that becomes a serious condition or even a hazard in and of itself, and occurs at normal doses.

AIDS: See *Acquired immunodeficiency syndrome*.

Allergy: An abnormal reaction to stimuli (allergens), such as dust mites, pollens, milk, or cat hairs. Common allergy symptoms include hay fever, rashes, upset stomach, and breathing difficulties.

Alopecia: Hair loss.

Alpha-fetoprotein test: A diagnostic blood test given early in pregnancy to detect fetal abnormalities.

Alzheimer's disease: A pattern of forgetfulness, disorientation, and loss of memory that usually afflicts the elderly but is not an inevitable part of the aging process. Previously referred to as *senile dementia*.

Ambulatory: Walk-in, same-day, or outpatient (usually referring to surgery, and distinct from inpatient or hospital care).

Amenorrhea: Absence of menstruation.

Amniocentesis: A diagnostic test done during pregnancy in which a sample of amniotic fluid (the fluid within the womb) is removed and analyzed to detect fetal abnormalities.

Amniotomy: A procedure in which the amniotic sac surrounding a fetus is surgically ruptured to trigger or speed labor.

Analgesic: A pain-relief medication.

Androgen: A male hormone, such as testosterone.

Androgenic alopecia: Male-pattern baldness.

Angina pectoris: Chest pain that is the most common symptom of heart disease. It results when the amount of blood flowing to the heart is insufficient to accomplish the work demanded of the heart.

Angiogram: An X-ray picture of a blood vessel made after injecting an opaque substance or dye through a thin tube *(catheter)* into the blood vessels to make them visible on X-ray film.

Anorexia nervosa: An eating disorder characterized by an obsession with thinness.

Antibiotic: A medication that is effective against bacterial organisms. Antibiotics are not effective against viruses.

Antibody: A substance made by the immune system to neutralize foreign or invading substances in the body.

Antigen: A foreign or invading substance within the body that triggers an immune system reaction.

Antioxidant: A molecule that helps limit potentially harmful oxidative reactions by neutralizing free radicals. Nutrients that act as antioxidants include vitamins C and E, beta carotene, and selenium.

Arteriosclerosis: Hardening of the arteries caused by deposits (called *plaques*) of fats (especially cholesterol), calcium, and smooth muscle cells that restrict the flow of blood and facilitate the forming of blood clots.

Arthritis: The inflammation of one or more joints.

Asthma: An obstructive lung disease characterized by sudden attacks of coughing, breathlessness, and wheezing that can sometimes result in suffocation.

Atherosclerosis: A condition in which the inner layers of artery walls become thick and irregular due to deposits of fat, cholesterol, and other substances.

Barium enema: X-ray pictures of the large intestine (colon) made after injecting barium sulfate into the rectum; used to locate abnormalities in the colon. Often called a *lower GI (gastrointestinal) series.*

Barium meal: X-ray pictures of the esophagus, stomach, and first part of the small intestine made after the patient swallows barium sulfate on an empty stomach. Used to locate abnormalities. Often called an *upper GI (gastrointestinal) series.*

Benign prostatic hyperplasia (BPH): A condition in which the prostate becomes enlarged, squeezing the urethra, the tube that carries urine out of the body. BPH causes frequency of urination at night (nocturia), difficulty urinating, dribbling after urination, and possibly an inability to urinate. Also called *enlarged prostate.*

Binge eating disorder: An eating disorder in which a person consumes large amounts of food frequently and repeatedly.

Biopsy: The removal of a portion of body tissue for microscopic analysis. It is used to determine the status of growths that may be cancerous.

Bronchiolitis: An infection of the small breathing tubes of the lungs. A common condition in infants.

Bronchitis: A common inflammation of the bronchial tubes, or air passages, caused by infection or exterior irritation, often including cigarette smoke.

Bulimia: An eating disorder that involves eating large amounts of food (bingeing) and then vomiting or using laxatives to remove the food from the system (purging).

Cancer: A general term for a malignant tumor or for forms of new tissue cells that lack a controlled growth pattern.

Cardiac catheterization: The insertion of a thin, flexible tube (a *catheter*) through a vein or artery into the heart. Used to collect information about the heart's structure and performance and to inject an opaque substance (dye) so that an X-ray can be made.

Cataract: A condition that occurs when the normally clear eye lens hardens and clouds with age, blocking light waves to the retina and obstructing vision.

Catheterization: The passage of a flexible surgical tube into an opening.

Cauterization: The application of a caustic substance, hot instrument, electric current, or other agent to destroy tissue.

Cerebral palsy: A neuromuscular disorder in infants caused by damage to the brain during pregnancy or shortly after birth. Signs include inability to control arms and legs, speech impairment, and jerky head and torso movements.

Cesarean section: A surgical procedure in which the uterus is surgically cut to deliver a baby.

Chicken pox: A highly contagious viral disease caused by a herpes virus and occurring mainly in children, marked by a rash of pink spots that usually begin on the abdomen and spread to the face and extremities. Sometimes called *varicella.*

Chlamydia: A sexually transmitted organism that attacks the urinary and reproductive tracts of men and women. Chlamydia is the most prevalent sexually transmitted disease.

Chorionic villus sampling: A diagnostic test done during pregnancy in which the fingerlike projections of the placenta (the organ that develops to nourish the fetus) are sampled and analyzed to detect fetal abnormalities.

Chronic fatigue syndrome: A variety of at least eight unexplained symptoms — including sore throat, muscle pain and weakness, chills or low-grade fever, headaches, extreme fatigue, tender lymph nodes, joint pain, neurological problems, and sleep disorders — that cause a 50 percent reduction in physical activity for at least six months. The cause is unknown. The disease is not contagious or fatal.

Cirrhosis: A degenerative disease of the liver, usually associated with alcoholics and heavy drinkers.

Colposcopy: A procedure that uses a magnifying instrument called a colposcope to examine the surface of the cervix and vagina for lesions.

Complete blood cell count (CBC): An examination of blood samples to get a count of the number of red cells, white cells, and hemoglobin in the blood and to determine the percentage of red cells in the blood. Used to check for infection or screen for blood disorders.

Computerized axial tomography (CAT) scan: A diagnostic procedure that uses X-rays to create cross-sectional images of internal body parts. Frequently used to locate disease, tumors, or abnormalities in the scanned part of the body.

Conception: The process in which sperm penetrates the female ovum and creates a zygote; the beginning of pregnancy.

Conjunctivitis: Inflammation of the thin membrane lining the eyelid and covering the front of the eye. Commonly called *pink eye,* conjunctivitis can be caused by bacteria or viruses, an allergic reaction, or an ingrown eyelash in the lower lid.

Contraindication: A condition or disease that renders a particular line of treatment improper or undesirable.

Copayment: A cost-sharing requirement of many types of health insurance policies that requires the insured person to assume a portion or percentage of the costs of covered services. Also called *coinsurance.*

Croup: An inflammation of the airways that makes breathing noisy and difficult; its best-known symptom is a distinctive, seal-like bark. Young children are most susceptible to the condition.

Culture: A test used to diagnose many kinds of bacteria and viruses. It involves the growth of bacteria or other cells in a special growth broth.

Cyst: A noncancerous, fluid-filled cavity or sac.

Cystic fibrosis: A condition often diagnosed in infancy or early childhood that's caused by an inherited defect of the glands affecting the respiratory and digestive systems.

Cystitis: Inflammation of the bladder.

Cystocele: A condition in which the bladder bulges through the vaginal wall. Also known as a *cystic hernia.*

Cystogram: An X-ray of the bladder made by inserting a thin tube through the urethra into the bladder.

Cystoscopy: A procedure in which a slender, hollow tube with a lens at each end (called a *cystoscope*) is passed into the urethra and bladder, allowing a visual examination of the urinary tract.

Deductible: The amount a policyholder must pay before the insurance company begins to make payment for services provided.

Depression: A chronic psychiatric disorder characterized by feelings of helplessness, hopelessness, and guilt; diminished self-worth; and a loss of pleasure from usual activities.

DES (diethylstilbestrol): A synthetic hormone prescribed to millions of pregnant women in the U.S. between 1941 and 1971, usually to prevent miscarriage. In the children of the women who took it, DES has been found to cause abnormalities of the reproductive system and, in some cases, cancer at an early age.

DHEA: The supplement dehydro-epiandrosterone, a "building block" of the hormones estrogen and testosterone. Some experts think that DHEA combats aging.

Diabetes mellitus: A chronic disease marked by excess glucose in the blood and urine, caused by the failure of the pancreas to release enough insulin (or any at all) into the body.

Diagnosis: The identification of a disease or condition.

Diastolic pressure: The measure of blood pressure when the heart is between beats; the bottom number in the blood pressure fraction. See also ***Systolic pressure***.

Dilation: Expansion or widening, as of a blood vessel, body opening, or tube.

Dilation and curettage (D&C): The removal of a layer of tissue from the wall of the uterus. As a diagnostic test, it is used to determine the cause of excessive bleeding or other problems.

Diverticulitis: An inflammation of the *diverticula* — small, mucus-lined sacs that form on the walls of the large intestine.

Down syndrome: The most common form of inherited mental retardation, caused by defective chromosome development in the embryo.

Drug-drug interactions: Drugs can affect each other's activity when more than one drug is taken at a time. The activity of one drug may be decreased or increased when a second drug is taken, or the combination of two drugs may cause an entirely different effect than intended.

Dysmenorrhea: Painful menstrual periods; most common is the uterine cramping associated with menstruation.

Dysplasia: Abnormal development of cells.

Earache: Pain in the ear caused by teething (in small children); by the eruption of wisdom teeth (in adults); by dental disease; by infection or congestion of the nose, throat, and jaw; or by the blocking of the eustachian tube (which joins the nose-throat cavity and the inner ear).

Echocardiogram: An ultrasound recording of the heart's internal structures. Used to locate heart valve problems or heart deformities.

Ectopic pregnancy: A life-threatening condition in which a fertilized egg implants outside the uterus, usually in the fallopian tubes.

Eczema: A noninfectious and usually chronic inflammatory skin disease that may cause blistering and/or scaling.

Electrocardiogram (ECG or EKG): A diagnostic test in which electrodes attached to the chest measure the heart muscle's electrical activity. Used to detect heart damage, as after a heart attack, and to monitor the effects of certain drugs.

Electroencephalogram (EEG): A recording of the brain's electrical impulses and brain patterns that is collected by electrodes placed on the scalp. Often used to detect brain damage, diagnose epilepsy, or confirm brain death.

Emphysema: A lung disease characterized by enlargement of the lungs and progressively worsening breathlessness.

Endometriosis: A condition in which tissue from the lining of the uterus (called the endometrium) implants outside the uterus, causing pain, cysts, and the development of scar tissue.

Endoscopy: The use of a hollow tube containing a light source and a viewing lens to examine interior parts of the body. In some cases, tiny instruments can be threaded through channels in the scope to facilitate surgical procedures.

Epilepsy: A condition characterized by seizures lasting from a few seconds to 15 or 20 minutes. Epilepsy is a symptom of overactive brain impulses and excitability of the brain.

Episiotomy: A procedure in which an incision is made in the tissue between the vagina and anus during childbirth to widen the birth canal.

Estrogen: The female sex hormone produced chiefly by the ovaries in women.

Fallopian tubes: The tiny, muscular tubes that carry eggs from the ovaries into the uterus.

FDA (Food and Drug Administration): The U.S. federal agency responsible for approving all prescription and nonprescription medicines on the basis of safety, effectiveness, and proper labeling.

Fibroids: Solid, usually benign tumors that grow on the outside, inside, or within the wall of the uterus. Technically known as *leiomyomas* or *myomas*.

Food poisoning: An acute illness, usually gastrointestinal, caused by eating contaminated or poisonous food. Symptoms include nausea, vomiting, diarrhea, and abdominal cramps.

Food-drug interactions: Foods can interact with drugs in a variety of ways, by either slowing down or speeding up the time the medication takes to travel to the part of the body where it's needed, or by preventing a drug from being absorbed properly. Also, natural and artificial chemicals in foods can render drugs useless or even dangerous.

Free radical: A molecular fragment that attempts to steal electrons from other molecules, possibly contributing to cancer and other conditions.

Gallstones: Hard, solid lumps that form in the gallbladder.

Gastritis: Inflammation of the stomach lining.

Gastroenteritis: Infection and inflammation of the gastrointestinal tract.

General anesthesia: Anesthesia that affects the entire body for a long period.

Generic drug: A drug with a condensed version of the original chemical name, which is suggested and filed for by the pharmaceutical company that invented the drug. A generic drug does not have to be the same size, shape, or color as the brand-name product, but it does duplicate the active ingredients of the brand-name drug.

Genitourinary: Pertaining to the area around the genitals and urinary tract.

Gestational diabetes: A temporary form of diabetes that develops during pregnancy.

Gingivitis: Inflammation of the gums.

Gland: An aggregation of cells, specialized to secrete or excrete materials.

Glaucoma: A painless illness that results when fluid pressure inside the eye presses on and damages the optic nerve.

Gonorrhea: A sexually transmitted disease residing in the mucous membranes and spread through unprotected intercourse. It often has no symptoms.

Gout: A form of arthritis that causes swelling of one or more joints (usually the big toes). It is caused by an accumulation of uric acid, a waste product, in the blood.

Gynecomastia: The abnormal swelling of one or both breasts in a male.

Halitosis: Bad breath.

Health maintenance organization (HMO): A managed care plan that provides a range of services in return for fixed monthly premiums.

Heart attack: An event that results when the blood supply to the heart is blocked by a clot or by plaque in one or more coronary arteries. The part of the heart that is deprived of blood dies, or *infarcts*. Also called *myocardial infarction*.

Heartburn: A burning pain in the chest caused by the presence of stomach acid in the esophagus.

Heat exhaustion: The accumulation of large amounts of blood near the skin in an attempt to cool it, and the simultaneous deprivation of blood to the interior organs.

Heat stroke: An emergency condition in which blockage of the sweat glands results in dangerously high body temperatures.

Hemoglobin: The oxygen-carrying pigment found in red blood cells.

Hemophilia: An incurable, gender-linked genetic blood disorder in which the blood is unable to clot.

Hemorrhoids: Swollen blood vessels in and around the anus.

Hepatitis: A condition characterized by inflammation of the liver, involving yellowing of the skin, stomach discomfort, abnormal liver functioning, and dark urine, which may be caused by a virus, bacteria, parasites, alcohol, drugs, poison, or transfusions of problematic blood.

Hernia: The protrusion of all or part of an organ or tissue through a weak spot in the surrounding muscular wall. Hernias commonly occur in the groin, near a surgical incision, and in the diaphragm.

Herpes: Any of a group of recurring viral illnesses marked by outbreaks of blisters in the genitals, anus, cornea, mouth, and brain. Herpes can be transmitted sexually.

Hodgkin's disease: A chronic, malignant cancer of the lymph nodes that usually strikes people between the ages of 15 and 35, and 50 and 60.

Hormone: A substance produced by a gland that influences how the body works.

Hormone replacement therapy (HRT): The use of synthetic or naturally occurring hormones to replace those that the body is no longer producing.

Human immunodeficiency virus (HIV): A usually sexually transmitted viral disease that attacks the immune system, triggering an onslaught of opportunistic infections. See also ***Acquired immunodeficiency syndrome***.

Human papillomavirus (HPV): A large group of sexually transmitted viruses that cause all forms of venereal warts and lesions. Some types of this virus have been linked with cervical cancer.

Hypertension: A common disorder (often without symptoms) characterized by blood pressure consistently exceeding 140/90 mm/Hg.

Hypoglycemia: An abnormally low level of blood sugar. It can be the precursor of diabetes or signal another disease, or appear as a symptom in those who have diabetes.

Hypogonadism: A medical condition in which the body does not produce sufficient testosterone.

Hysterectomy: The surgical removal of the uterus.

Hysterosalpingogram: An X-ray picture of the uterus and fallopian tubes.

Hysteroscopy: A diagnostic and surgical procedure in which a thin, tubular viewing scope is inserted through the cervix into the uterus.

Immunity: The ability of the body's immune system to resist disease.

Immunization: The process of creating immunity to certain viruses and bacteria by exposing a person to weakened or inactive organisms.

Impotence: The inability of a man to develop or maintain an erection sufficient to copulate. Also called *erectile dysfunction* or *erectile difficulty.*

In situ: In place; cancer that has not yet spread.

In vitro fertilization: The process of joining egg and sperm outside the body in a laboratory-controlled environment, and then injecting the newly fertilized egg into the mother's womb.

Incontinence: The inability to control urination or defecation.

Infertility: Diminished or absent capacity to produce offspring.

Influenza: A contagious respiratory disease, also called *flu* or *grippe,* caused by one of a group of airborne viruses and spread by coughs, sneezes, and exhaled breath. Sometimes occurs in epidemics.

Insomnia: The inability to fall asleep or to remain asleep through the night.

Ischemia: Lack of blood flow, especially to the heart.

Laparoscopy: Examination of the interior of the abdomen by means of a laparoscope (a thin, metal viewing scope), which is inserted through a small incision.

Laryngitis: Inflammation of the mucous membranes lining the larynx, characterized by the swelling of the vocal cords and hoarseness or loss of voice.

Laser surgery: The process of using a laser (a concentrated beam of light that can produce a tremendous amount of heat) to cut or destroy tissue.

Leukemia: Any of a group of diseases characterized by a proliferation of white blood cells in the bone marrow that impedes the manufacture of red blood cells.

Local anesthesia: Anesthesia used for procedures in which only a small part of the body needs to be anesthetized for a short period.

Lyme disease: A tick-borne, inflammatory illness characterized by fatigue, fever, and chills. It may result in heart, joint, brain, and nerve disorders if not treated promptly.

Lymph nodes: A number of small glands located throughout the body that work as part of the immune system to defend the body against harmful foreign particles.

Macronutrients: Nutrients such as carbohydrates, protein, and fats that the body needs in large quantities each day.

Magnetic resonance imaging (MRI): An imaging technique that produces detailed pictures of areas inside the body by linking a computer with a powerful magnet.

Male menopause: A condition in which testosterone levels gradually decline, possibly leading to fatigue, loss of libido, erection problems, and osteoporosis.

Mammogram: A diagnostic test in which X-rays of the breasts (mammary glands) are taken to detect lumps or thickened tissue that could be cancerous.

Managed care: A method of delivering, supervising, and coordinating health care, often through health maintenance organizations and other networks of doctors and hospitals. The purpose is to eliminate inappropriate services, control costs, and assure access to effective treatment.

Mastectomy: The surgical removal of the breast.

Measles: A highly contagious respiratory infection caused by a virus. Symptoms include a red rash, runny nose, coughing, fever, and irritability.

Medicaid: A government program that provides health care assistance to the poor.

Medicare: The government's medical insurance program for people ages 65 and over, those who are permanently and totally disabled, and those with end-stage renal disease.

Menarche: The first menstrual cycle.

Meningitis: Inflammation of the membranes covering the brain and spinal cord caused by bacteria or a virus. It can occur in epidemics and in isolated cases.

Menopause: The natural and permanent cessation of menstruation. Menopause usually takes place between the ages of 45 and 55.

Menstruation: The shedding through the vagina of the uterine lining, consisting of blood and tissue.

Metastasize: To spread, as in the case of cancer, to distant organs or tissues.

Micronutrients: Nutrients such as vitamins and minerals that the body needs in small quantities each day.

Mineral: A nonorganic compound, one that does not contain carbon and does not originate from living organisms.

Miscarriage: The spontaneous end to a pregnancy before the fetus is capable of survival.

Mononucleosis: A viral infection that causes swelling and tenderness of the lymph glands in the armpits, groin, elbows, and neck. Symptoms include jaundice, sore threat, fever, headache, and aching joints.

Multiple sclerosis (MS): A nonfatal disease of undetermined cause that strikes when nerve cells lose *myelin,* the fatty substance essential for normal conduction of electrical impulses.

Mumps: A viral infection marked by swelling of the glands within the mouth and neck.

Muscular dystrophy: A neuromuscular disease in which the muscles enlarge and then begin to separate, with muscular tissue being replaced by fat and connective tissue.

Myomectomy: The surgical removal of fibroid tumors from the uterus.

Necrosis: The death of living tissue.

Neonatal-perinatal medicine: A subspecialty of pediatrics that deals with disorders of newborn infants, including premature ones.

Nonprescription medicine: Medicine that can be bought without a doctor's prescription; also known as *over-the-counter medicine.*

Obese: Weighing 20 or more percent over your healthy weight.

Oophorectomy: The surgical removal of one ovary, also called *ovariectomy.* Bilateral oophorectomy indicates removal of both ovaries.

Osteoporosis: A condition in which the bones lose mass and become porous, resulting in weak bones that can fracture easily.

Otitis media: Inflammation of the middle ear, the area located behind the eardrum. Such ear infections commonly affect children.

Ototoxic: A medication or other substance that contributes to hearing loss.

Outpatient: Someone who is not officially admitted to a hospital for an overnight stay but who is treated in other health care settings. Outpatient care is provided in clinics, hospital outpatient departments, and physician offices.

Ovaries: Olive-shaped glands connected by the fallopian tubes to the uterus. They secrete estrogen, the main female hormone, and, in fertile women, release an egg each month.

Over-the-counter (OTC) medicine: See *Nonprescription medicine.*

Ovulation: The phase of the female menstrual cycle during which an ovary releases an egg. Ovulation occurs approximately two weeks prior to the onset of menstruation.

Ovum: The egg, or reproductive cell, of a woman.

Palliative: Capable of reducing the symptoms of a disease and slowing its growth, but unable to wipe it out.

Pap test: A test in which cells are scraped from the cervix, smeared on a glass slide, and examined under a microscope. Used to detect signs of cancer or infection. Also called a *Pap smear* or *cervical smear.*

Parkinson's disease: A progressive disorder of the central nervous system that causes a deficiency of the neurotransmitter (or brain chemical) dopamine.

Pelvic inflammatory disease (PID): A sexually transmitted infection of the uterus, fallopian tubes, and/or ovaries that can result in sterility.

Periodontitis: An advanced form of gum disease in which the tissues that support the teeth begin to deteriorate. It may result in tooth loss.

Phlebitis: The swelling of a vein, often with the formation of a clot, especially in the legs and in areas afflicted with varicose veins.

Plaque: Fatty buildup on the lining of a blood vessel; in dental terms, mucus that contains bacteria and sugar that collects on the teeth above the gums.

Pneumonia: An infection of the lungs caused by bacteria or a virus.

Poliomyelitis: A viral infection of the nervous system.

Polyp: A tumor, usually noncancerous, that protrudes from a part of the body.

Preexisting condition: An injury that occurred, a disease that was contracted, or a physical or mental condition that existed prior to the issuance of a health insurance policy. Usually, benefits will not be paid for services relating to a pre-existing condition, although some plans may make payment after an appropriate waiting period.

Preferred provider organization (PPO): An organization of doctors and hospitals that provide medical services to groups of people at discounted rates. Members of the group agree to use only the "preferred" providers.

Premenstrual syndrome (PMS): The symptoms of mental tension, irritability, depression, headaches, and bloatedness (edema, or the swelling of body tissues due to retention of fluid) that occur in women during the week before menstruation and stops at the onset of menstruation.

Presbycusis: Age-related hearing loss.

Progesterone: A female hormone produced by the ovaries during the second half of the menstrual cycle.

Prognosis: A forecast of the probable outcome of a disease; the prospects for recovery from a disease as indicated by the nature and symptoms of the case.

Prostate-specific antigen (PSA): A substance, produced exclusively by prostate cells, whose level increases in the presence of prostate cancer and rises significantly with the spread of such cancer.

Prostatitis: Inflammation of the prostate.

Psoriasis: A scaly inflammation of the skin caused by overproduction of outer skin cells.

Puberty: The stage of physical development in which sex characteristics such as breasts and pubic hair develop and reproduction becomes possible.

Regional anesthesia: Anesthesia that numbs areas of the body for up to three hours at a time.

Reye's syndrome: A childhood degenerative condition of the brain and liver that usually follows a viral disease such as influenza or chicken pox. Because doctors suspect that aspirin triggers the disease, they usually prescribe nonaspirin medication, such as acetaminophen, to control fever during infections.

Rh factor: An immune system substance present on red blood cells. Rh incompatibility between a mother and fetus may cause complications during pregnancy.

Rheumatic fever: An inflammatory disease, often a delayed reaction to bacterial infection of the upper respiratory tract.

Rider: A document that amends an insurance policy. It may increase or decrease benefits, waive the condition of coverage, or amend the original contract in other ways.

Rubella: An acute viral infection and common contagious disease of childhood. Symptoms are fever and rash. Also called *German measles.*

Schedule of benefits: The list of medical services that a particular insurance policy will cover, or the maximum amount payable for certain conditions.

Schizophrenia: A category of psychosis characterized by severely disturbed patterns of thinking that cause bizarre behavior.

Semen: A milky fluid that contains and nourishes sperm.

Sexually transmitted disease (STD): A disease that can be contracted during sex or intimate contact. STDs include AIDS, hepatitis B, chlamydial infections, gonorrhea, syphilis, genital herpes, and genital warts.

Sickle-cell anemia: A serious, long-term, incurable blood disease that attacks the red blood cells.

Side effects: Effects on the body apart from the principal action of a medicine. Side effects are usually undesirable.

Sinusitis: An inflammation of one or more of the four nasal sinus cavities. Symptoms include pain, tenderness, and a thick nasal discharge.

Slipped disc: The dislocation or herniation (bulging) of gelatinous substance through one of the cartilaginous rings that separate the spinal vertebrae.

Speculum: A duckbill-shaped instrument inserted into the vagina and locked open that allows a doctor to view the cervix and insert and withdraw instruments without touching the sides of the vagina.

Sperm: The male reproductive cell produced in the testes and present in semen. They are released during ejaculation and are capable of fertilizing a woman's egg.

Spinal tap: A sampling of cerebrospinal fluid removed from the spinal canal by means of a long needle. Used to diagnose diseases of and injuries to the brain and spinal cord, especially in suspected cases of meningitis and stroke.

Staging: The effort to determine whether cancer has spread, and what parts of the body are involved.

Stent: A small, tubelike structure that can be inserted into a vessel or passage to widen it or keep it open.

Streptococcus infection: A category of common bacterial diseases, most frequently associated with the throat.

Stroke: A sudden brain disturbance resulting from an interruption in the flow of blood to the brain.

Sudden infant death syndrome (SIDS): An unexpected infant death in which an autopsy fails to find a cause.

Systolic pressure: The measure of blood pressure when the heart is pumping blood; the upper number in the blood pressure fraction. See also *Diastolic pressure*.

Tartar: A hard, chalky substance that collects on teeth along and below the gumline.

Testosterone: A male hormone produced mainly by the testicles.

Tinnitus: Ringing in the ears.

Tonsillitis: Inflammation of the tonsils, the clusters of tissue that lie at the back of the throat and produce antibodies to fight viruses and bacteria. A common childhood condition.

Tubal ligation: A process of sterilization in which the fallopian tubes are tied to prevent egg and sperm from uniting.

Tuberculosis (TB): A long-term, grainy, tumorous infection caused by a rod-shaped bacterium and usually affecting the lungs.

Ulcer: An eroded area of normal tissue that is caused by some inflammatory, infectious, or malignant process.

Ultrasound: A procedure that bounces high-frequency sound waves off tissues and converts the echoes into images. Used to gather information about a part of the body, or on a pregnant woman to gain information about the health or development of the fetus.

Urinalysis: The physical, chemical, and microscopic analysis of urine for abnormalities.

Urinary retention: Inability to urinate.

Vaccine: A substance that contains an active or inactive germ of a specific disease. When administered, a vaccine triggers an immune system response that helps create immunity.

Varicose veins: Veins, usually at the backs and inner sides of the calves, that are swollen or enlarged and are visible through the skin as a bluish-red network of lines.

Vasectomy: An operation, generally for contraceptive purposes, in which the vas deferens (tubes that carry sperm) are sealed off.

Vertigo: The sensations of loss of balance and irregular and whirling motion of oneself or of nearby objects.

Virus: An infectious organism that's capable of growing and reproducing within a living cell. Some viruses are difficult to eradicate and may remain in the body indefinitely.

Whooping cough: An infectious disease of the mucous membranes lining the air passages that affects mainly children. Also called *pertussis*.

X-ray: A picture of the body's internal structures made with electromagnetic rays with a short wavelength.

Appendix B

Common Medical Abbreviations

octors, nurses, and other health care professionals have a long-established habit of abbreviating medical terms and everyday words, especially in charts and medical records. They have been trained to think that no one except another doctor or nurse needs to look at what's scribbled there, and they all learn the codes in the course of their training. Most patients do not know the codes, and when you look at your chart and records (which you ought to do regularly), you may understand little about your condition and your prognosis. This lack of understanding can be a major obstacle blocking your participation in your own care and that of your family.

The following list can change that. It's a collection from many sources of abbreviations frequently used in records, on forms and prescriptions, and even in everyday conversation. If something you see or hear doesn't appear on this list, ask your doctor, nurse, hospital patients' representative, or some other person to translate.

a = before

aa = of each

a.c. = before meals

ad. = to, up to

ADL = activities of daily living

ad lib. = as needed, as desired

AF = atrial fibrillation

agit = shake, stir

AM = morning

AMA = against medical advice

Api. = appendicitis

Aq. = water

ASHD = arteriosclerotic heart disease

AVAP = as soon as possible

B.E. = barium enema

b.i.d. = twice a day

Bl. time = bleeding time

B.M. = bowel movement

BMR = basal metabolic rate

BP = blood pressure

BRP = bathroom privileges

Bx = biopsy

C = centigrade

$\bar{c}$ = with

CA = cancer

CAD = coronary artery disease

cap(s) = capsule(s)

CBC = complete blood count

CBD = common bile duct

cc = cubic centimeter(s)

CC = chief complaint

CCU = coronary care unit

CHD = coronary heart disease or congenital heart disease

CHF = congestive heart failure

Chol = cholesterol

Cl. time = clotting time

cm = centimeter

CNS = central nervous system

comp = compound

cont rem = continue the medicine

COPD = chronic obstructive pulmonary disease

CPM = continue present management

CSF = cerebrospinal fluid

CV = cardiovascular

CVA = cardiovascular accident

CVP = central venous pressure

CXR = chest X-ray

d = give

D&C = dilation and curettage

D&E = dilation and evacuation

dd in d = from day to day

dec = pour off

dexter = the right

dil = dilute

disp. = dispense

div = divide

DM = diabetes mellitus

DNR = do not resuscitate

dos = dose

dur dolor = while pain lasts

D/W = dextrose in water

Dx = diagnosis

ECG; EKG = electrocardiogram

EEG = electroencephalogram

emp = as directed

ER = emergency room

ext = for external use

F = Fahrenheit

FBS = fasting blood sugar

febris = fever

FH = family history

Fx = fracture

GA = general anesthesia

garg = gargle

GB = gallbladder

GC = gonorrhea

GI = gastrointestinal

GL = glaucoma

gm = gram

gr. = grains

grad = by degrees

gravida = pregnancies

gtt = drops

GTT = glucose tolerance test

GU = genitourinary

GYN = gynecology

h = hour

Hb, Hgb = hemoglobin

HCT = hematocrit

HHD = hypertensive heart disease

HOB = head of bed

h.s. = at bedtime, before retiring

Hx = history

ICU = intensive care unit

I&D = incision and drainage

IM = intramuscular

I.M. = infectious mononucleosis

ind = daily

I&O = intake and output (measure fluids going into and out of the body)

IPPB = intermittent positive pressure breathing

IV = intravenous

IVP = intravenous pyelogram

L = left

liq = liquid

LLE = left lower extremity

LLQ = left lower quadrant

LMP = last menstrual period

LP = lumbar puncture (spinal tap)

LPN = licensed practical nurse

LUE = left upper extremity

LUQ = left upper quadrant

ⓜ = murmur

M = mix

m et n = morning and night

mg = milligram

MI = heart attack (myocardial infarction)

ml = milliliter

mor. dict. = in the manner directed

M.S. = morphine sulfate

NA = nursing assistant

neg = negative

NG = nasogastric

no. = number

noct. = at night

non rep, nr = do not repeat

non repetat = no refill

NPO = non per os (nothing by mouth)

NS = normal saline

NSR = normal heart rate

N&V = nausea and vomiting

o = none

O_2 = oxygen

oc = oral contraceptive

OD = right eye

o.d. = once a day

OL, OS = left eye

OOB = out of bed

OPD = outpatient department

OR = operating room

OT = occupational therapy

OU = both eyes

$\bar{P}$ = after

Para = number of births

Path. = pathology

pc = after meals

PE = physical examination; or pulmonary embolus

PI = present illness

PID = pelvic inflammatory disease

pil = pill

PM = evening

p.o. = per os (by mouth)

Post. = posterior

post-op = postoperative, after the operation

PR = pulse rate; or rectally

pr = per rectum (by rectum)

p.r.n. = as needed, as often as necessary

Prog. = prognosis

pt = patient

PT = physical therapy

PTA = prior to admission

Px = prognosis

q. = every

q.d. = once a day

q.h. = every hour (q.4h. = every 4 hours, q.8h. = every 8 hours, and so on)

q.h.s., qhs = every hour of sleep (bedtime)

q.i.d. = four times a day

q.n. = every night

q.o.d. = every other day

q.s. = proper amount, quantity sufficient

q.v. = as much as desired

R = right

rbc = red blood cells

RBC = red blood cell count

rep = repeat

RHD = rheumatic heart disease

RLQ = right lower quadrant

R.N. = registered nurse

ROM = range of motion

RR = respiratory rate; or recovery room

RT = radiation therapy

RTI = reproductive tract infection

rub = red

RUQ = right upper quadrant

Rx = prescription; or therapy

$\bar{s}$ = without

S&A = sugar and acetone (a urine test)

SC = subcutaneous

scop. = scopolamine

SH = social history

SICU = surgical intensive care unit

sig = write, let it be imprinted, label, directions

sig ut dict = take as directed

sing = of each

SOB = shortness of breath

sol = solution

solv = dissolve

SOP = standard operating procedure

SOS = can repeat in an emergency

ss = half

S&S = signs and symptoms

SSE = soapsuds enema

stat = right away, immediately

STD = sexually transmitted disease

STI = sexually transmitted infection

suppos = suppository

Sx = symptoms

T&A = tonsillectomy and adenoidectomy

tab = tablet

TAT = tetanus antitoxin

tere = rub

TIA = transient ischemic attack

t.i.d. = three times a day

tinc., tinct. = tincture

top = apply topically

TPR = temperature, pulse, and respiration

Tx = treatment

ung = ointment

URI = upper respiratory infection

ut dict = as directed

UTI = urinary tract infection

VD = venereal disease

VS = vital signs

wbc = white blood cells

WBC = white blood cell count

WC = wheelchair

X = times

y.o. = year old

↑ = increase

↗ = increasing

↓ = decrease

↙ = decreasing

→ = leads to

← = resulting from

= male

a = female

Index

IDG BOOKS WORLDWIDE
BOOK REGISTRATION

We want to hear from you!

Register This Book and Win!

Visit **http://my2cents.dummies.com** to register this book and tell us how you liked it!

✔ Get entered in our monthly prize giveaway.

✔ Give us feedback about this book — tell us what you like best, what you like least, or maybe what you'd like to ask the author and us to change!

✔ Let us know any other ...*For Dummies*® topics that interest you.

Your feedback helps us determine what books to publish, tells us what coverage to add as we revise our books, and lets us know whether we're meeting your needs as a ...*For Dummies* reader. You're our most valuable resource, and what you have to say is important to us!

Not on the Web yet? It's easy to get started with *Dummies 101*®: *The Internet For Windows*® *98* or *The Internet For Dummies*,® 5th Edition, at local retailers everywhere.

Or let us know what you think by sending us a letter at the following address:

...*For Dummies* Book Registration
Dummies Press
7260 Shadeland Station, Suite 100
Indianapolis, IN 46256-3945
Fax 317-596-5498

**BESTSELLING
BOOK SERIES
FROM IDG**